Ebstein's
or
R. Bun

Neonatology
Review

↑ atrial press
Resp for what
circ. Δ @ birth
= elim R→L
          shunt

Fall below ht, wt, length — viral
                          inf.

^{use}
glucose by brain
      > in asymm.
        growth
        Restrict

uteroplac / nutrit — head
      defic   spanng

              < 12 hrs
Younger gestation — quicker (Ballard)
                  GA

      Term p̄ 24

Hypochloremia
   old soy form
   insuff. intake
   ↑ Loss of Cl (GI, Renal)

Interaction c̄ parents ş infants
            is necc. for Lang. dev.

Thyroid screen 36 hr
      low T4 elev. TSH
                  ↘ have confirmatory
                    serum testing

PDA
  = L→R

Taxi — enter brain
      use cefotax

Naloxone
  0.1 mg/kg
  Q 2-3 min as needed
  close monit. 4-6 hours.

Adv. servo contre ^{skin} = more stable
                              NTE

Cold stressed infant @ risk for
            HTN — diminishe
                      bl. flow
Self infl — breathe on own
Δ ti → Flow infl.

Neonatology
Review

Dara Brodsky, MD
Neonatologist
Children's Hospital, Boston
Beth Israel Deaconess Medical Center
Brigham and Women's Hospital

Instructor of Pediatrics
Harvard Medical School
Boston, Massachusetts

Camilia Martin, MD
Associate Director of Neonatal Intensive Care Unit
Beth Israel Deaconess Medical Center

Instructor of Pediatrics
Harvard Medical School
Boston, Massachusetts

HANLEY & BELFUS, INC. / Philadelphia

Publisher: HANLEY & BELFUS, INC.
             Medical Publishers
             210 South 13th Street
             Philadelphia, PA 19107
             (215) 546-7293; 800-962-1892
             FAX (215) 790-9330
             Web site: http://www.hanleyandbelfus.com

Note to the reader: Although the information in this book has been carefully reviewed for correctness of dosage and indications, neither the authors nor the publisher can accept any legal responsibility for any errors or omissions that may be made. Neither the publisher nor the authors make any warranty, expressed or implied, with respect to the material contained herein. Before prescribing any drug, the reader must review the manufacturer's current product information (package inserts) for accepted indications, absolute dosage recommendations, and other information pertinent to the safe and effective use of the product described.

Library of Congress Control Number: 2002116190

Neonatology Review   ISBN 1-56053-491-5

Last digit is the print number: 9 8 7 6 5 4 3 2 1

Contents

Acknowledgments

We would like to acknowledge the following people for their invaluable editorial comments:

Karen Altmann, MD
Assistant Professor of Pediatrics
College of Physicians and Surgeons of Columbia University, New York, New York
Cardiology

Katrina Berlage, PharmD
Pharmacy Practice Resident
Beth Israel Deaconess Medical Center, Boston, Massachusetts
Pharmacology

Sandra K. Burchett, MD, MS
Clinical Director, Division of Infectious Diseases
Children's Hospital
Assistant Professor of Pediatrics, Harvard Medical School, Boston, Massachusetts
Infectious Diseases

Gregory J Dumas, RPh
Pharmacist, Neonatology Intensive Care Unit
Beth Israel Deaconess Medical Center, Boston, Massachusetts
Pharmacology

Deirdre Ellard, MS, RD, CNSD
Neonatal Dietitian
Brigham and Women's Hospital, Boston, Massachusetts
Nutrition

Stephen E. Gellis, MD
Program Director in Dermatology
Children's Hospital
Assistant Professor of Pediatrics, Harvard Medical School, Boston, Massachusetts
Dermatology

Catherine Gordon, MD
Assistant in Medicine, Divisions of Endocrinology and Adolescent Medicine
Children's Hospital
Assistant Professor of Pediatrics, Harvard Medical School, Boston, Massachusetts
Endocrinology

Mira B. Irons, MD
Associate Chief, Division of Genetics
Children's Hospital
Associate Professor of Pediatrics, Harvard Medical School, Boston, Massachusetts
Genetics

Kee-Hak Lim, MD
Obstetrics, Gynecology and Reproductive Biology
Beth Israel Deaconess Medical Center
Assistant Professor, Harvard Medical School, Boston, Massachusetts
Maternal-Fetal Medicine

Deborah L. Marsden, MBBS
Director, Metabolism Service
Children's Hospital
Assistant Professor of Pediatrics, Harvard Medical School, Boston, Massachusetts
Inborn Errors of Metabolism

Jordan M. Symons, MD
Division of Nephrology
Children's Hospital & Regional Medical Center
Assistant Professor of Pediatrics, University of Washington School of Medicine, Seattle, Washington
Fluids, Electrolytes, and Renal System

Mary Ellen B. Wohl, MD
Chief Emerita, Division of Respiratory Diseases
Children's Hospital
Professor of Pediatrics, Harvard Medical School, Boston, Massachusetts
Respiratory

John A.F. Zupancic, MD, ScD
Associate Director of Neonatal Intensive Care Unit
Beth Israel Deaconess Medical Center
Instructor of Pediatrics, Harvard Medical School, Boston, Massachusetts
Statistics

Preface

Welcome to the first edition of *Neonatology Review*. While preparing for the neonatology specialty boards, we were dismayed that we could not find any books synthesizing the material covered on the boards to guide us. Therefore, like our predecessors who have studied for this exam, we began the painstaking process of collecting notes, reviewing texts, and generating numerous index cards containing facts in perinatal/neonatal pathophysiology.

While studying for the boards, we never even thought of writing this book. It was only after taking the boards and looking back on our efforts that we decided to put our notes together. We hope that this book will serve not only as a study guide for those about to prepare for the perinatal-neonatal boards but also as a long-standing reference.

This book is meant to provide you with a framework for studying neonatology. You will still need to refer to the excellent comprehensive texts that already exist in neonatology. We also recommend that you supplement each subject area with more detailed readings and pictorial reviews of common findings, particularly in the areas of radiology, genetics, and dermatology. This book is not intended for direct patient care.

The chapters of the book are organized by system, and the material is similar to the content outline suggested by the American Board of Pediatrics. General references are listed at the end of each section. In addition to textbooks, we also refer to lecture notes from our residency years at Babies & Children's Hospital of New York / Columbia University (New York) and Children's Memorial Hospital/Northwestern University (Illinois) as well as our notes from lectures we attended during our fellowship training at Boston Children's Hospital/Harvard Medical School.

We wish you the best of success and hope you find this neonatology review helpful.

Dara Brodsky, MD
Camilia Martin, MD

Dedication

To my devoted parents, my three spirited brothers, my husband and best friend, Adam, and my precious little one, Zane.

DB

Many thanks to my loving family and special thanks to my supportive husband, Brad, and my gregarious daughter, Linnea.

CM

We dedicate this book to Douglas K. Richardson, MD, MBA, a compassionate clinician and talented teacher; he will be greatly missed.

CHAPTER 1

Maternal-Fetal Medicine

TOPICS COVERED IN THIS CHAPTER

I. Maternal Adaptation to Pregnancy
A. Cardiovascular changes
B. Respiratory changes
C. Renal changes
D. Hematologic changes
E. Gastrointestinal changes
F. Endocrine changes

II. Maternal Hormones During Pregnancy
A. hCG and hPL
B. Progesterone and estrogens

III. Placenta
A. Anatomy
B. Transplacental transfer
C. Placenta previa
D. Placental abruption
E. Abnormal placental adherence
F. Placental tumors
   1. Hydatidiform mole
   2. Gestational trophoblastic tumors
   3. Chorioangioma
   4. Placental metastases

IV. Umbilical Cord
A. Anatomy
B. Single umbilical artery
C. Velamentous insertion of cord

V. Maternal Disorders Affecting Fetus
A. Lupus
B. Myasthenia gravis
C. Diabetes mellitus
D. Immune thrombocytopenic purpura (ITP)
E. Advanced maternal age
F. Hypothyroidism and hyperthyroidism

VI. Hypertension in Pregnancy
A. Preeclampsia
B. Eclampsia

VII. Fetal Screening
A. Alpha-fetoprotein (AFP)
B. Triple screen
C. Ultrasonography
D. Amniocentesis (amnio)
E. Chorionic villus sampling (CVS)
F. Percutaneous umbilical blood sampling (PUBS)
G. Comparison of fetal testing techniques

VIII. Assessment of Fetal Status
A. Nonstress test (NST)
B. Contraction stress test
C. Biophysical profile (BPP)
D. Fetal heart rate (FHR)
E. Uterine activity
F. Fetal scalp sampling
G. Uterine and umbilical gases
H. Amniotic fluid

IX. Fetal Growth
A. Stages
B. General
C. Hormonal regulation of fetal growth

X. Intrauterine Growth Restriction (IUGR) and Small for Gestational Age (SGA)
A. IUGR vs SGA
B. Etiology
C. Symmetric vs asymmetric SGA/IUGR
D. Diagnosis
E. Neonatal effects
F. Management of mother
G. Prognosis

XI. Nonimmune Fetal Hydrops
A. Definition
B. Etiology
C. Diagnosis
D. Management of nonimmune fetal hydrops in utero
E. Prognosis

XII. Multiple Gestation
A. Incidence
B. Types of twins
C. Maternal and fetal risks
D. Twin-twin transfusion

XIII. Labor
A. Pathogenesis
B. Phases during labor
C. Epidural analgesia

XIV. Delivery
A. Presentations
B. Forceps delivery
C. Vacuum extraction
D. Cesarean section

TOPICS COVERED IN THIS CHAPTER (*continued*)

I. Maternal Adaptation to Pregnancy

A. CARDIOVASCULAR CHANGES

Heart rate (HR): increases 10–15 bpm

Blood volume: increases 30–50% due to an increase in both plasma volume and red blood cells (RBCs)
  Begins to increase during 1st trimester, increases rapidly during 2nd trimester, and rises more slowly during 3rd trimester
  The increase in blood volume leads to increased preload and:
    1. Protects the mother from impaired venous return when supine and erect
    2. Meets demand of extremely vascular uterus
    3. Protects the mother against large blood loss during delivery

Blood pressure (BP): decreases during 1st trimester, lowest in 2nd trimester
Widened pulse pressure (since diastolic BP decreased more than systolic BP)

Cardiac output: increases 30–50% with majority output to uterus and kidneys
  During late pregnancy, cardiac output is greater when mother is in lateral recumbent position compared with the spine position in which uterus impedes venous return

B. RESPIRATORY CHANGES

Minimal change in respiratory rate, significant increase in tidal volume, and minute ventilation with increasing gestational age (GA); decreased residual volume

C. RENAL CHANGES

Renal hypertrophy; dilated calyces and ureters

Increased glomerular filtration rate and renal blood flow by ~50%

Decreased renal bicarbonate threshold; increased protein filtration

Increased antidiuretic hormone, renin, angiotensin II, and aldosterone secretion

D. HEMATOLOGICAL CHANGES

RBCs (red blood cells): increase by ~30%
  Increased production due to increased demand for iron
  Increased mean cell volume of RBC
  Plasma volume increases greater than increase in number of RBCs, leading to *dilutional anemia*

WBCs (white blood cells): estrogen-mediated leukocytosis (greatest during labor)

Despite increased number of WBCs, decreased leukocyte function during pregnancy

Platelets: minimal change in platelet count yet platelet width and volume increases (probably due to greater proportion of younger, larger platelets following increased platelet consumption)

Hemoglobin/hematocrit: despite increased erythropoiesis, hemoglobin and hematocrit decrease slightly during pregnancy due to increased blood volume

Coagulation: increased coagulation factors and greater risk for thromboembolic disease

Fibrinogen increases 30–50% due to estrogen effect; decreased fibrinolysis

E. GASTROINTESTINAL CHANGES

Increasing size of uterus displaces stomach and intestines

Decreased gastric emptying time, altered stomach position, and decreased lower esophageal sphincter tone all increase risk of reflux

Hemorrhoids due to constipation and increased venous pressure inferior to large uterus

Impaired gallbladder contraction (may increase risk of gallstones)

F. ENDOCRINE CHANGES

Enlargement of pituitary gland by ~135% with increased prolactin production

Increased thyroxine-binding globulin, increased total T4 (yet mother remains euthyroid)

Significant increase in PTH-related hormone (PTHrP), which increases calcitriol production and leads to increased maternal intestinal absorption of Ca; thus placental transfer of maternal Ca to fetus can occur while maternal serum Ca levels remain normal

II. Maternal Hormones During Pregnancy

A. hCG AND hPL

hCG: human chorionic gonadotropin
Produced by syncytiotrophoblasts
Production begins extremely early in pregnancy, and can be detected in the blood or urine 8–9 days following ovulation
Greatest amount detected during 1st trimester
Prevents corpus luteum involution

hPL: human placental lactogen
Increases with increased gestational age
Putative functions include involvement in lipolysis and anti-insulin effect

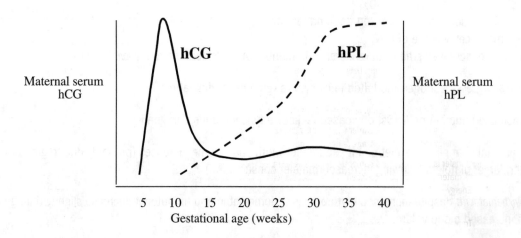

Modified from Cunningham FG, Gant NF, Leveno KJ, et al (eds): Williams Obstetrics (21st edition). New York, McGraw-Hill, 2001, p 27.

B. PROGESTERONE AND ESTROGENS

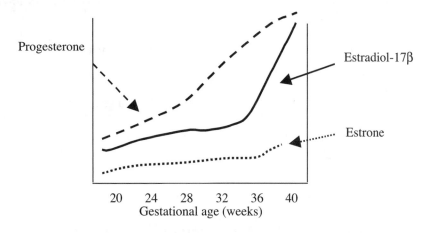

Modified from Cunningham FG, Gant NF, Leveno KJ, et al (eds): Williams Obstetrics (21st edition). New York, McGraw-Hill, 2001, p 123.

III. Placenta

A. ANATOMY

Fetal portion
   Contains numerous branching villi that are suspended in the intervillous space
   Branches of the umbilical artery enter each villus and end in a capillary plexus
   Through the walls of the villi, fetal blood can absorb appropriate components from maternal blood and return to the fetus by the umbilical vein
   Trophoblast cells are represented by cytotrophoblasts (deep layer), and syncytiotrophoblasts (superficial layer, in contact with maternal blood)

Maternal portion
   Formed by the decidua, which contain the intervillous space
   Uterine surface of placenta is divided into 10–38 lobes or cotyledons
   Maternal blood passes through the intervillous space, which is supplied by uterine arteries and drained by uterine veins

B. TRANSPLACENTAL TRANSFER

Method	Description	Examples

Simple diffusion	Passive
	No energy required for passage of compounds
	The direction of transplacental transfer is dependent on:
	   a. Concentration gradient between maternal and fetal region
	   b. Surface area of membrane
	   c. Blood flow to area
	   d. Properties of drug (e.g. lipid solubility, molecular weight, protein binding)
		O_2, CO_2
		H_2O
		Na,Cl
		Lipids
		Fat-soluble vitamins
		Most medications

Facilitated diffusion	Transfer is mediated by a carrier that moves compounds *along* the concentration gradient No energy required for passage of compounds	Glucose Cephalexin
Active transport	Transfer is mediated by a carrier that moves *against* the concentration gradient with transfer from maternal to fetal side (concentration of substance greater on fetal side) Energy required	Amino acids calcium, phosphate, magnesium, iron and iodide H_2O-soluble vitamins
Bulk flow	Transfer by hydrostatic or osmotic gradient	H_2O, dissolved electrolytes
Pinocytosis	Compounds are engulfed, packaged and transferred across cell to opposite side	Immunoglobulin G Other proteins
Breaks	Abnormalities in the placental membrane	Maternal or fetal cells

Compounds that Cross the Placenta	Compounds that Do Not Cross the Placenta
Bilirubin	Biliverdin
Aspirin, coumadin	Heparin
Dilantin, valproate	Glucagon. human growth hormone, insulin
Alcohol	Propylthiouracil (only small amounts cross)
Small amount of T_4 crosses (also converted to inactive reverse T_3 by placenta) and small amount of T_3 crosses (also converted to T_2 by placenta)	Thyroid-stimulating hormone
Thyroid-releasing hormone and iodine	Maternal IgM
Maternal immunoglobulin (Ig) G	

T_4 = thyroxine; T_3 = triiodothyronine; T_2 = diiodothyronine.

C. PLACENTA PREVIA

Definition

Abnormal implantation of placenta near or over the internal cervical os

Can be total (os completely covered by placenta), partial (os partially covered by placenta), marginal (edge of placenta is at margin of os), and low-lying (placenta implanted in lower uterine segment near os)

Type can vary depending on degree of cervical dilatation

Incidence

~1 in 200 deliveries

Common finding during 2nd trimester but decreases with increasing GA (e.g. > 90% of low placental implantations will be in normal position at term)

Increased risk if advanced maternal age, increased parity, previous cesarean section or c/s (especially if recent), maternal smoking, history of abortion

Increased risk of premature delivery, greater risk of fetal anomalies (increased by 2.5-fold, unclear reason)

Pathology

Unclear, possibly due to endometrial damage that prevents effective placentation

Clinical

Acute onset of painless vaginal bleeding (typically after late 2nd trimester) due to tearing of placenta

Initial bleeding usually ceases spontaneously and often recurs

Diagnosis

Ultrasound (transvaginal approach with greater accuracy than transabdominal)

Management

Dependent on gestational age and maternal/fetal status

If severe bleeding $\rightarrow$ deliver

If premature and no active bleeding $\rightarrow$ close observation

If mature $\rightarrow$ deliver by C/S

Closely monitor fetus if acute bleeding

Monitor for bleeding post-delivery

D. PLACENTAL ABRUPTION

Definition

Premature separation of a normally implanted placenta that can lead to concealed or apparent hemorrhage into decidua basalis

Can be total or partial

Incidence
~1 in 100 deliveries
Associated with maternal hypertension (most common association), history of prior abruption, advanced maternal age, increased parity, cigarette smoking, cocaine use, increased thrombotic maternal state, external trauma, uterine leiomyoma
Increased risk of premature delivery, stillbirth, and neonate with neurological deficits
~15-25% perinatal mortality

Clinical
Majority with external vaginal bleeding (not absolutely required since may be concealed due to retroplacental bleeding), uterine tenderness or back pain, and fetal distress
Mother may develop shock, severe anemia, consumptive coagulopathy, and/or renal failure

Diagnosis
Limited diagnosis by US

Management
Dependent on gestational age and maternal/fetal status
    If mature, well fetus and vaginal delivery not imminent → majority will do C/S
    If premature, well fetus → expectant management with frequent monitoring
    Transfusion as needed

E. ABNORMAL PLACENTAL ADHERENCE

Incidence
1 in 2500-9000
Increased risk if co-existing placenta previa (~30%), history of curettage (~25%), increased parity (~25%), gravida 6 or more, implantation in lower uterine segment, or prior uterine surgery

Types
Placenta accreta—placental villi attach to myometrium of uterine wall
Placenta increta—placental villi invade myometrium
Placenta percreta—placental villi penetrate through myometrium
May involve some or all cotyledons

Clinical
Early in pregnancy, may have elevated maternal serum alpha-fetoprotein
May lead to severe hemorrhage, uterine perforation, or possible infection
Complications at time of delivery of placenta related to implantation site, depth of myometrial invasion, and number of cotyledons involved

Management
If extensive hemorrhage, blood transfusion and prompt hysterectomy
Can consider uterine or internal iliac artery ligation or embolization

F. PLACENTAL TUMORS

1. Hydatidiform mole
Definition: = molar pregnancy
Abnormal chorionic villi with trophoblastic proliferation and villous edema that is typically contained within uterine cavity

Incidence: occurs in ~ 1 in 1000 pregnancies
Increased risk with advanced maternal age and maternal history of previous mole

Types:　1. Complete (majority 46, XX with mostly paternal origin; no fetus or amnion present; uterus large for GA; ~20% develop trophoblastic tumors; frequently with medical complications)
　　　2. Partial (majority with 69, XXX, XXY or XYY; nonviable fetus and amnion often present, uterus usually small for GA, less likely to develop trophoblastic tumors; rare to have medical complications)

Clinical: uterine bleeding (continuous or intermittent, typically mild)
　Uterus enlarges more rapidly than usual
　Absence of fetus
　May develop preeclampsia early in 2nd trimester
　Increased risk of trophoblastic tissue embolization
　Higher β-hCG than expected for GA

Management: immediately suction and evacuate mole, possible hysterectomy
　Assess for metastatic disease
　Follow closely for persistent trophoblastic proliferation or malignant changes by following β-hCG levels

2. Gestational trophoblastic disease

Types:　1. Invasive mole (excessive trophoblastic growth and extremely invasive; typically does not metastasize)
　　　2. Choriocarcinoma (very malignant trophoblastic tumor; rapidly growing mass invading uterine muscle and blood vessels; can lead to hemorrhage and/or necrosis; metastasis to lungs and vagina is common)

Clinical: typically presents with irregular bleeding
　Persistently elevated β-hCG levels

3. Chorioangioma—benign placental tumor

4. Placental metastases—rare, can be due to malignant melanoma, leukemia, lymphoma, breast and lung carcinoma or sarcoma

IV. Umbilical Cord

A. ANATOMY

Average length = 55 cm (range 30-100 cm; if < 30 cm, increased risk of poor outcome)

Extends from fetal umbilicus to the fetal side of the placenta; covered by amnion

The extracellular matrix contains Wharton jelly (to protect vessels); 2 arteries and 1 vein; spiraling most often counter-clockwise

If one umbilical artery is damaged, fetus is not compromised since there is a large arterial anastomosis near the umbilical cord insertion; in contrast, the umbilical vein is the sole supplier of oxygenated placental blood to the fetus

B. SINGLE UMBILICAL ARTERY

Incidence: one of the most common malformations
　0.5-1% all infants
　3-4x more common in twins compared with singletons
　May be associated with urogenital tract or cardiac anomalies

Management: assess for other anomalies; if other abnormalities detected on exam, do chromosomal analysis
  Controversial if renal ultrasound (US) required (some centers do US if no prenatal level II US performed; majority of centers do US only if other anomalies)

C. VELAMENTOUS INSERTION OF CORD

Occurs in 0.5–1.0% singletons, more frequently in twins, and in almost all triplets

Umbilical vessels are exposed in the membranes before they insert into the placental tissue

Vasa previa: umbilical vessels cross the internal os and are positioned ahead of fetal presenting part
  Vessels can easily tear (especially when membranes rupture), leading to significant fetal blood loss; this is more common if low-lying placenta and multiple gestation
  High fetal mortality (50–90%)

V. Maternal Disorders Affecting Fetus

A. LUPUS

Incidence
  Increased incidence of 1st trimester spontaneous abortion, intrauterine growth restriction (IUGR), and fetal death

Pathophysiology
  Associated with lupus anticoagulant antibodies and anticardiolipin antibodies (antibodies also observed in other autoimmune disorders as well as mothers without any disease)
  Both antibodies probably inhibit prostacyclin (functions as a vasodilator and inhibits platelet aggregation) production
  Can also be associated with maternal ribonucleoprotein antibodies [(anti-Ro (SSA) and anti-La (SSB) antibodies]

Diagnosis
  Measure lupus anticoagulant antibody
  Can also assess lupus anticoagulant antibody levels indirectly by prolonged clotting time
  Measure anticardiolipin antibody by assay

Neonatal Effects
  Increased risk of congenital heart block (risk is independent from the severity of maternal illness and indeed, fetal heart block may be the first sign of maternal lupus); greater risk of heart block if maternal anti-Ro (SSA) and anti-La (SSB) antibodies; fetal heart block may lead to hydrops

Management
  Heparin and low dose aspirin
  $+/-$ corticosteroids (can decrease fetal growth with prolonged use and increase risk of premature delivery)
  Monitor fetus closely for development of fetal heart block

B. MYASTHENIA GRAVIS Preg. comp. by MG is @ risk for: Malformation

Definition
  A chronic, autoimmune disease leading to progressive fatigue and weakness involving the facial, pharyngeal and respiratory muscles
  90% with antibodies (typically IgG) to acetylcholine (Ach) receptors
  The severity of maternal disease is proportional to the ability of antibodies to block Ach receptor in skeletal muscle

Pregnancy effects
  For mothers with lupus, possible exacerbation of lupus may occur
  Limited fetal effects:
    May lead to fetal arthrogryposis (low risk)

Neonatal effects (See Neurology chapter)
  10–20% of neonates will develop myasthenia signs (flat facies, weak suck, decreased cry, respiratory distress)
  Presents 12–48 hours after birth and may last as long as 15 weeks (average ~3 weeks)
  Treat with anticholinesterases

C. DIABETES MELLITUS (see Endocrinology chapter)

D. IMMUNE THROMOBCYTOPENIC PURPURA (ITP)

Etiology
  Autoimmune disorder leading to thrombocytopenia; due to unknown etiology

Diagnosis
  Low platelet number with greater proportion of large platelets
  Normal number of WBCs and RBCs; normal clotting studies

Neonatal effects
  Maternal IgG antibodies may cross to fetus and lead to fetal thrombocytopenia (this may occur even if mother had splenectomy, since maternal antibodies are still present)
  Risk of intraventricular hemorrhage (especially if vaginal delivery and premature infant)

Management
  Treat mother with corticosteroids; consider high-dose intravenous IgG if no response and severe ITP, may require splenectomy; platelet transfusions if severe ITP yet will only yield transient increase in platelet count
  C/S if fetus with thrombocytopenia (platelet count < 50,000)

E. ADVANCED MATERNAL AGE

Risks during pregnancy
  Increased miscarriage rate, chromosomal abnormalities, congenital malformations, premature delivery, pregnancy-induced hypertension, bleeding during 3rd trimester, gestational diabetes, C/S rate, and maternal mortality
  Increased risk of trisomy 13, trisomy 18, trisomy 21, Klinefelter syndrome

Frequency of trisomy 21 related to maternal age

Maternal Age	Risk of Trisomy 21 Full-Term Infant
20 years old	1 in 1667
25 years old	1 in 1250
30 years old	1 in 952
35 years old	1 in 385
40 years old	1 in 106
45 years old	1 in 30

Modified from Bianchi DW, Crombleholme TM, D'Alton ME: Fetology. New York, McGraw-Hill, 2000, p 12.

F. HYPOTHYROIDISM AND HYPERTHYROIDISM (see Endocrinology chapter)

VI. Hypertension (HTN)

A. PREECLAMPSIA

Definition
1. HTN (diastolic BP $\geq$ 90 mmHg or systolic BP $\geq$ 140 mmHg documented more than twice; severe if diastolic BP $\geq$ 110 mmHg or systolic BP $\geq$ 160 mmHg)
2. Proteinuria ($>$ 300 mg protein in 24 hours, dipstick $>$1+; severe if $>$ 5000 mg protein in 24 hours)

Incidence
6–8% of all pregnancies
Severe preeclampsia in $<$1% of pregnancies
Majority of mothers with preeclampsia during 1st pregnancy
In 14–20% of multiple gestations
In 30% of patients with major uterine anomalies
In 25% of patients with chronic hypertension
In 25–30% of patients with chronic renal disease
Recurrence rate is high (up to 65%)

Pathophysiology
Develops at time of implantation and thus is not preventable
Most recent theory: decreased trophoblastic invasion $\longrightarrow$ less dilated spiral arteries $\longrightarrow$ decreased uterine placental blood flow $\longrightarrow$ placental ischemia $\longrightarrow$ placental cytokine release $\longrightarrow$ endothelial cell dysfunction $\longrightarrow$ increased BP, fibrin deposition (leading to glomeruloendotheliosis and proteinuria), and IUGR

Clinical
Although changes occur as early as 1st trimester, not clinically symptomatic until $>$ 20 weeks gestation
Patients typically with facial and/or hand/feet edema but not a requirement for diagnosis
If severe, can have HELLP syndrome (*h*emolysis, *e*levated *l*iver enzymes, *l*ow *p*latelets) that can be associated with severe headache and/or visual disturbances

Fetal risks
IUGR and increased risk of premature delivery if severe preeclampsia
Maternal medications may affect infant (e.g. hypermagnesemia may lead to fetal hypotonia and respiratory depression)
Increased risk of low platelets and neutropenia in neonate

Outcome
Cannot predict whether preeclampsia will become severe or if it will change to eclampsia
Patients with mild preeclampsia do not have increased perinatal morbidity or mortality
However, if severe preeclampsia, there is an increased risk to mother and fetus
Glomeruloendotheliosis is reversible postpartum and typically no residual renal damage

Management
If mild $\longrightarrow$ home bed rest, daily urine tests for protein, BP 4 x/day, low sodium diet ($<$ 4 g per day), delivery should not be beyond term due to placental insufficiency
If mild or moderate$\longrightarrow$may require anti-hypertensive medications
If severe$\longrightarrow$hospitalize, bed rest, measure input and output, monitor liver function tests, creatinine and platelet count; low sodium diet, may need to deliver even if premature (if fetal lung indices immature and mother relatively stable, consider betamethasone to enhance fetal lung maturity), intravenous hydralazine if DBP $>$ 100 mmHg, magnesium sulfate to prevent seizures (monitor for toxicity: decreased respiratory effort and disappearance of knee jerks)

Postpartum period requires very close monitoring since symptoms may worsen immediately after delivery (usually lessens 48 hours after delivery)

B. ECLAMPSIA = PREECLAMPSIA + SEIZURES

Incidence
   0.1% of pregnancies

Clinical
   Seizures can occur antepartum, intrapartum or up to 7 days postpartum

Management
   Treat as in severe preeclampsia, magnesium sulfate extremely critical to prevent recurrent seizures

Prognosis
   Without treatment, maternal mortality 0.5%–17% and fetal mortality 8–37% (both are greater in underdeveloped countries)

VII. Fetal Screening

A. ALPHA-FETOPROTEIN (AFP)

Physiology
   AFP is produced by the fetal yolk sac early in gestation
   Later in gestation, AFP produced by the liver and gastrointestinal tract
   AFP passes from fetal serum to fetal urine to amniotic fluid; following, the glycoprotein is swallowed and catabolized in the gastrointestinal tract
   AFP can diffuse across the placenta into the maternal circulation
   Unknown function
   All AFP measurements require the precise GA of fetus at time of measurement since levels change dramatically with GA

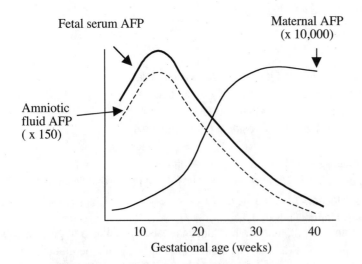

Fetal AFP: peaks at ~13 weeks gestation
Maternal serum AFP (MSAFP): Detected after 12 weeks gestation; peaks ~32 weeks gestation
Usually check level between 15 and 22 weeks gestation
Greatest sensitivity between 16 and 18 weeks gestation
Amniotic fluid AFP: Peaks at ~13 weeks gestation

Modified from Cunningham FG, Gant NF, Leveno KJ, et al (eds): Williams Obstetrics (21st edition). New York, McGraw-Hill, 2001, p 980.
Note: number in parenthesis represents scale.

Elevated Maternal AFP (≥ 2.0–2.5 MOM)	Low Maternal AFP (< 0.6 MOM)
Neurological: neural tube defects Gastrointestinal: liver necrosis, esophageal or intestinal obstruction, omphalocele, gastroschisis Renal: urinary obstruction, polycystic kidneys, renal aplasia, congenital nephrotic syndrome, cloacal exstrophy Masses: pilonidal cyst, cystic hygroma, sacrococcygeal teratoma Other: low birth weight, low maternal weight, oligohydramnios, multiple gestation, under-estimation of GA, osteogenesis imperfecta, placental chorioangioma	Genetics: trisomies Other: fetal death, increased maternal weight, overestimated GA, gestational trophoblastic disease

MOM = multiple of mean. Modified from Cunningham FG, Gant NF, Leveno KJ, et al (eds): Williams Obstetrics (21st edition). New York, McGraw-Hill, 2001, p 982.

Protocol for elevated maternal serum AFP

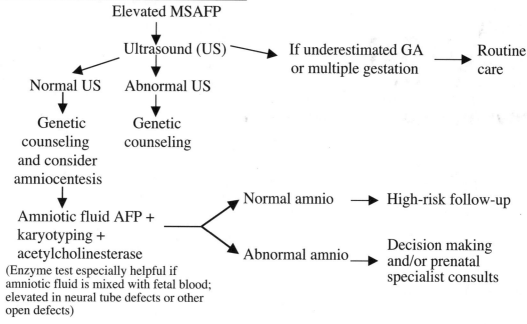

Note: high false-positive rate of MSAFP, while amniotic fluid AFP with rare false-positive rate unless mixed with fetal blood. Modified from Cunningham FG, Gant NF, Leveno KJ, et al (eds): Williams Obstetrics (21st edition). New York, McGraw-Hill, 2001, p 981.

B. TRIPLE SCREEN

Screen performed at 15–20 weeks gestation (16 weeks optimal GA) and consists of:
1. *Maternal AFP:* least sensitive of the three tests
2. *Maternal unconjugated estriol (uE$_3$):* produced by placenta from precursors provided by fetal adrenal glands and liver
3. *Maternal β-hCG:* most sensitive of the three tests for detection of trisomy 21

Trisomy 21: low AFP, high β-hCG and low uE$_3$
Triple screen will detect > 60% of trisomy 21 fetuses
There is a high false-positive that increases with advancing maternal age

A negative triple screen does *not* completely exclude fetus with trisomy 21

Inhibin A can be used as a 4th serum marker to increase detection rate of fetus with trisomy 21

Trisomy 18: low AFP, low β-hCG, low uE_3

Triple screen will detect ~60% of trisomy 18 fetuses

Trisomy 13: triple screen is NOT helpful

C. ULTRASONOGRAPHY

Detection

Pregnancy diagnosed by US by 5th week post menses

~80% of major fetal abnormalities detected by 2nd trimester US

Measurements

Crown-rump length

Best for 1st trimester assessment

Can assess GA $+/-$ 3 to 5 days (only early hCG or accurate dating of conception is better for assessing GA)

Cephalometry—biparietal diameter

Best for 2nd trimester assessment

Before 34 weeks gestation, can assess GA $+/-$ 10 days

After 34 weeks gestation, can assess GA $+/-$ 3 weeks

Measure at level of thalamus

Abdominal circumference

Measured at level of liver, using the portal vein and stomach as landmarks

Can assess GA $+/-$ 3 weeks

Important to determine fetal weight

Reliability is dependent on fetal symmetry (e.g., if asymmetric IUGR, decrease in abdominal circumference leading to an underestimation of GA; in contrast, macrosomic fetus overestimates GA)

Femur length

Measures femur diaphysis only

Can assess GA $+/-$ 3 weeks

May be affected by genetic abnormalities (e.g., trisomy 21, severe IUGR)

Vaginal ultrasound

May detect abnormal heart several weeks prior to abdominal US and can also be helpful for diagnosis of placenta previa, diagnosing the number of chorions in multiple gestations, and also helpful to visualize fetus if mother is obese

Doppler velocimetry

Assesses flow velocity in umbilical arteries during systole (S) and diastole (D)

IUGR fetuses have decreased diastolic flow velocities and thus increased S/D ratio

If imminent fetal death, may have absent (infinite S/D ratio) or reversed diastolic flow (negative S/D ratio)

Interpretation: IUGR fetuses develop medial hypertrophy of villous arterioles $\longrightarrow$ increase in fetal systemic vascular resistance (SVR)$\longrightarrow$ fetal compensation by ventricular dilation, ventricular hypertrophy or an increase in FHR

As fetal heart pushes blood into placenta through the umbilical arteries, the increased SVR may decrease diastolic flow; this diastolic flow may even become reversed when blood flows from placenta to umbilical artery

Reversed diastolic flow or negative S/D ratio is a poor prognostic indicator; thus, if abnormal S/D ratio, requires nonstress test or biophysical profile to determine degree of fetal distress

Abnormal findings on fetal ultrasound
Gastrointestinal abnormalities

Congenital diaphragmatic hernia	Abdominal organs observed in thoracic cavity
	$+/-$ polyhydramnios
Distal bowel obstruction	Dilated bowel loops typically observed during 3rd trimester
	e.g. Hirschsprung disease, anal atresia, meconium ileus
Duodenal atresia	Double-bubble observed in bowel (also in annular pancreas, malrotation, duodenal stenosis/web) due to dilated fluid-filled stomach and proximal duodenum
	Increased echogenicity of intraluminal bowel
	30% with trisomy 21
Echogenic bowel	Nonspecific
	Majority normal
	Can be associated with chromosomal abnormalities (e.g. trisomy 21), cytomegalovirus infection, cystic fibrosis (due to meconium ileus), meconium peritonitis, intestinal abnormalities and swallowed maternal blood
Gallstones	Echogenic foci within gallbladder and associated distal shadowing
	Majority resolve and minimal clinical effect
Gastroschisis	Abdominal wall defect to right of the umbilical cord insertion with herniated bowel loops that are floating freely in amniotic fluid
	May be confused with ruptured omphalocele yet gastroschisis rarely with liver involvement
Ileal/jejunal atresia	Fluid-filled intestinal loops
	Majority in proximal jejunum or distal ileum
	Possible abdominal distention, polyhydramnios (25%), and/or increased peristalsis
	Due to in utero vascular accidents
Meconium peritonitis	Peritoneal calcifications
	May also observe polyhydramnios, pseudocysts, fetal ascites, and/or bowel dilatation
Omphalocele	Midline abdominal wall defect with umbilical cord insertion into membrane covering defect; defect contains herniated intestinal loops
	Associated with Beckwith-Wiedemann syndrome, trisomy 13, trisomy 18 and cloacal exstrophy
Tracheo-esophageal fistula with esophageal atresia	Unable to visualize fluid-filled stomach
	If small fistula $\rightarrow$ may have polyhydramnios; if large fistula $\rightarrow$ may have visible stomach due to fluid passing from fistula into stomach
	Assess for VACTERL abnormalities

Limb abnormalities

Achondrogenesis	Lethal skeletal dysplasia evident by severe micromelia and lack of vertebral ossifications
Achondroplasia	Most common nonlethal skeletal dysplasia evident by rhizomelia of long bones (especially femur) observed between 21 and 27 weeks gestation
	May also have large head, frontal bossing, protuberant abdomen and trident-shaped hand
Acromelia	Short hands and feet
Mesomelia	Short forearms and legs
Micromelia	Overall shortening of limbs
Osteogenesis imperfecta type II	In utero fractures leading to long-bone deformation and limb shortening
	May observe abnormal fetal skull shape, underossification of cranial bones, and/or small thoracic cavity with broad and irregular ribs
Rhizomelia	Shortening of proximal limbs (e.g. femurs and humeri)
Thanatophoric dysplasia	Lethal skeletal dysplasia evident by severe micromelia with limited limb mobility and curved femurs
	May observe short, broad ribs, pulmonary hypoplasia and/or hypoplastic vertebral bodies

Neurological abnormalities

Anencephaly	Absence of upper portion of cranial vault
	Detected by 14–15 weeks gestation
	13–33% with other abnormalities including congenital heart disease, congenital diaphragmatic hernia, renal malformation, hypoplastic adrenal glands, and omphalocele
Choroid plexus cysts	Echolucent structures within choroid plexus with sharp margins
	Due to neuroepithelial folds filled with cerebrospinal fluid and cellular debris
	Detected by US as early as 11 weeks and usually disappear by 26 weeks gestation
	Occurs in ~0.5% of normal fetuses
	While choroid plexus cysts can be an isolated finding in small % of fetuses with trisomy 18, additional ultrasound findings are typically observed in fetuses with trisomy 18

(continued on following page)

Dandy-Walker abnormality	*Dandy-Walker malformation:* cystic dilatation of 4th ventricle, enlarged or normal-sized posterior fossa, and cerebellar vermis aplasia; often associated with obstructive hydrocephalus (typically postnatal) *Dandy-Walker variant:* direct communication between 4th ventricle and cisterna magna without enlargement of posterior fossa, mild cerebellar vermis hypoplasia, increased incidence chromosomal abnormalities (e.g., trisomy 13)
Encephalocele	Mass (can be cystic, solid or both) with skull defect 75% occipital Must differentiate from soft tissue edema or cystic hygroma by identifying bony defect High association with renal cystic disease Also associated with neural tube defects and microcephaly

Meningomyelocele	US demonstrates splaying of posterior ossification centers of spinal bones
	May have fluid-filled sac over skin
	Intracranial associations:
	  A. "Banana" sign in which there is a crescent shape around brainstem due to elongated cerebellum
	  B. "Lemon" sign in which the calvaria shape is abnormal with concave frontal bones; present between 18 and 24 weeks gestation
	  C. Microcephaly
	  D. Ventriculomegaly

Sacrococcygeal teratoma	Large posterior spinal mass that is often cystic and solid Often associated with polyhydramnios
Ventriculomegaly	Accurate diagnosis by ultrasound although clinical outcome difficult to assess by prenatal US findings Measure at same location throughout pregnancy—at level of atrium of lateral ventricles, which is at level of choroid plexus Choroid plexus often appears to be "dangling" All degrees of ventriculomegaly in utero with increased risk of morbidity and mortality

Renal abnormalities

Hydronephrosis	Note: mild dilation of renal pelvis is normal Pathologic if upper renal pelvis > 10 mm With increasing severity, leads to dilated pelvis and calices with renal parenchymal thinning Unilateral → unilateral ureteropelvic junction obstruction Bilateral → lower urinary tract obstruction (e.g. posterior urethral valves) or bilateral uteropelvic junction obstruction
Multicystic dysplastic kidney	Noncommunicating cysts in kidney that are different sizes and disorganized Size of cysts can change during gestation 40% with contralateral renal anomalies Often distorts kidney shape and associated with abnormal renal tissue
Polycystic kidney disease	Bilaterally multiple renal cysts with normal renal tissue
Posterior urethral valves	Distended bladder (with thickened wall) and hydronephrosis (typically bilateral) If severe, oligohydramnios will be present
Renal agenesis—bilateral	Kidneys and bladder not visible Severe oligohydramnios (typically observed 18–20 weeks gestation)

Other abnormalities

Cystic hygroma	Septated cystic mass or lymphangioma that is most often in neck or occiput (often with a dense midline posterior septum across width of hygroma) Increased incidence in fetus with Noonan syndrome and Turner syndrome May also be observed in deletion 13q, trisomy 13, 18 and 21

D. AMNIOCENTESIS (AMNIO)

Technique

Typically performed at 15–20 weeks gestation

Aspirate 20–30 cc amniotic fluid (contains desquamated fetal cells and amniocytes) using a 20–22 gauge spinal needle; first few ccs are discarded to decrease maternal skin cell contamination

Assessments

Chromosomal analysis within 1–2 weeks of procedure

Measure amniotic fluid AFP

Acetylcholinesterase can be measured (higher with neural tube defects)

Assess for fetal lung maturity

Measure bilirubin in Rh-sensitized patients

Assess for suspected viral or bacterial infection

E. CHORIONIC VILLUS SAMPLING (CVS)

Technique

Earliest prenatal diagnostic technique

Biopsy of chorionic villi usually at 10–13 weeks gestation (can also do later in 2nd/3rd trimester if severe oligohydramnios and unable to do amnio or circumstances in which cannot do percutaneous umbilical blood sampling)

With US guidance, transcervically or transabdominally insert catheter to edge of placenta; following, remove stylet and apply suction to syringe containing cell culture media; remove 10–50 mg chorionic villi (smaller amounts are obtained with transabdominal approach compared to transcervical technique)

Assessments

Chromosomal analysis of trophoblast cells

Difficult to assess for neural tube defects since too early

F. PERCUTANEOUS UMBILICAL BLOOD SAMPLING (PUBS)

Technique

Perform if >19 weeks gestation

With US guidance, insert 20–22 gauge spinal needle into umbilical vein at level cord inserts into placenta

After sample obtained, need to assess if fetal vs maternal cells (fetal cells with larger diameter or at later gestational ages, can use Kleihauer-Betke test to distinguish between cells)

Assessments

Chromosomal analysis if require results quickly (within 24–72 hours)

Multiple fetal blood tests including: specific hemoglobin levels, IgM or IgG levels, bacterial and viral cultures, hydrops evaluation

Transfusion of blood products

Fetal drug therapy (e.g. anti-arrhythmic drug administration)

G. COMPARISON OF FETAL TESTING TECHNIQUES

Fetal testing	Risk fetal death	Advantages	Disadvantages
Amniocentesis (typically 15–20 wks; modified early amnio is available at 11–14 wks)	Fetal loss rate ~0.5% (1 in 200) above baseline Higher fetal loss rate if early amnio	Safer than CVS Less expensive Can test for amniotic fluid AFP Low likelihood of severe fetal injury (limited to scarring or skin dimpling)	Results obtained late in gestation 1–2 week delay in diagnosis for chromosomal analysis Increased risk Rh sensitization so mother with negative blood type requires Rhogam Some increased incidence of chorioamnionitis (probably <1 in 1000) 1–2% with spotting or leakage of amniotic fluid following procedure Early amnio with increased risk of positional foot deformities and rupture of membranes; in addition, may require repeat testing
Chorionic villus sampling (10–13 wks)	Fetal loss rate ~1.0% above amnio Higher fetal loss rate if trans-cervical approach	Earliest prenatal diagnostic procedure	Increased risk infection (less likely with transabdominal approach) Increased risk of premature rupture of membranes and placental disruption Increased risk limb abnormalities and oromandibular malformations if performed < 9 weeks gestation *(continued on following page)*

Fetal testing	Risk fetal death	Advantages	Disadvantages
			Greater contamination with maternal cells compared with amnio
			Greater chromosomal mosaicism in placental tissue compared with cells of fetal origin
			Increased risk Rh sensitization so mother with negative blood type requires Rhogam
			Doesn't detect neural tube defects
PUBS (>19 wks)	Fetal loss rate ~1–2% above baseline	Rapid analysis within 48–72 hours	Increased risk of umbilical cord vessel bleeding (~50%), hematoma (~17%), fetal-maternal hemorrhage (~66%) and fetal bradycardia (~3–12%)
		Multiple studies can be done	Increased risk of preterm labor (5%)
		Can be used for therapy (e.g. in utero blood transfusion)	

Note: Percentages cited above may vary between centers.

VIII. Assessment of Fetal Status

A. NONSTRESS TEST (NST)

Technique

Assess FHR (fetal heart rate) and reactivity (beat-to-beat variability and accelerations) in response to fetal movement

No contraindications

Reactive positive result

≥ 2 accelerations within 20 minutes associated with fetal movements with an increase in 15 bpm lasting > 15 seconds

Nonreactive negative result

<2 accelerations within 20 minutes

Must r/o fetal sleep or effects from maternal sedatives

Repeat 20 minutes later

A nonreactive NST *alone* doesn't define loss of fetal well-being, so other testing is required

78% of tests that are initially nonreactive and repeated later in day are reactive

Predictability

A reactive NST is very predictive of intrauterine survival for 7 subsequent days

A nonreactive NST *may* suggest a fetus who is becoming acidotic due to decreased oxygenation

B. CONTRACTION STRESS TEST

Theory

If fetal oxygenation is marginal at rest, contractions will lead to further hypoxemia

Technique

Assess FHR × 15–20 minutes *in response to contractions*

Must have >3 palpable 40–60 second contractions within 10 minutes or a prolonged contraction lasting more than 90 seconds

If inadequate number of contractions, consider oxytocin administration or intermittent nipple stimulation

Contraindications

Preterm labor, premature rupture of membranes, classical uterine incision scar, placenta previa, multiple gestation, incompetent cervix

Results and Management

Positive stress test: late decels associated with 50% of contractions; requires prompt intervention (if term or postterm→ deliver; if premature and FHR reactivity, consider amnio to assess for lung maturity so that if mature → delivery and if immature → frequent FHR and BPP testing, administer glucocorticoids and manage expectantly)

Negative stress test: no late decels in presence of sufficient number of uterine contractions; repeat test every 7 days
Suspicious: intermittent late or variable decels; repeat testing 24 hours later
Hyperstimulatory: excessive uterine activity (contractions more frequently than every 2 minutes) with late decels
Unsatisfactory: if unable to interpret results due to extreme obesity, polyhydramnios or active fetus

Predictability
A negative contraction stress test is very predictive of intrauterine survival for 7 subsequent days
Of note, studies in fetal monkeys have found that a positive stress test *precedes* a nonreactive NST (since late decels correlate with mild fetal hypoxemia while loss of reactivity corresponds with development of metabolic acidosis)
1/2 have false-positive results
If positive stress test, increased incidence of intrauterine fetal demise, intolerance of labor, perinatal depression, IUGR, and meconium passage

C. BIOPHYSICAL PROFILE (BPP)

Technique
Composed of 5 categories with each scoring 2 or 0 (all or none):
1. NST (*some exclude this test*): ≥ 2 accelerations within 20 minutes associated with fetal movements with an increase in 15 bpm lasting > 15 seconds
2. *Fetal body movement:* at least 3 movements within 30 minute period
3. *Breathing:* ≥ 1 period of 30 seconds with continuous breathing during 30 minute period
4. *Fetal tone:* at least one extension/flexion cycle of a limb with rapid return to the flexed position observed during 30 minute period
5. *Amniotic fluid volume (AFV):* at least one pocket of fluid >1 cm in two perpendicular planes (e.g., amniotic fluid index [AFI] ≥ 5 cm—see Section VIIIH)

Results and management

Score	Interpretation	Recommended Treatment
10	Well fetus	No intervention required Repeat weekly (if diabetic or postterm, check 2× per week)
8/10 + normal AFV	Well fetus	No intervention required Repeat in 1 week unless change in circumstances
8/10 + decreased AFV	Possible chronic asphyxia	Deliver unless oligohydramnios is due to rupture of membranes

6	Possible fetal asphyxia	Deliver if abnormal AF volume
		If normal AF volume and > 36 weeks → deliver
		If normal AF volume and = 36 weeks or immature lung indices → repeat in 24 hours:
		    If repeat and ≤ 6 → deliver
		    if repeat and over 6 → as above

4	Probable fetal asphyxia	Repeat same day if normal AF If repeat is ≤ 6 → deliver
0–2	Almost certain of fetal asphyxia	Deliver

Modified from Cunningham FG, Gant NF, Leveno KJ, et al (eds): Williams Obstetrics (21st edition). New York, McGraw-Hill, 2001, p 1105.

D. FETAL HEART RATE (FHR)

Definition
Typically 110–160 beats per minute (bpm) with periodic accelerations
FHR maintained by balance between parasympathetic and sympathetic nervous system

Monitoring
Internal: electrode on scalp—monitors HR and beat-to-beat variability
Doppler: broad signal, monitors HR, cannot accurately detect beat-to-beat variability

Tachycardia
>160 bpm, due to increased sympathetic tone and /or decreased parasympathetic tone
Etiology: maternal fever, in utero infection
　　Medications (β-agonists, parasympathetic blockers)
　　Fetal tachyarrhythmia
　　Extreme prematurity, maternal thyrotoxicosis, fetal anemia
　　Hypoxia (mechanism probably due to enhanced β-adrenergic activity following hypoxemia; can have fetal
　　　tachycardia *after* hypoxic episode or *during* the gradual onset of fetal hypoxemia)
　　If presence of beat-to-beat variability with tachycardia, not ominous

Bradycardia <110 bpm
　Etiology: may be due to continuous head compression with a vagal response or well-compensated, mild hypoxemia
　　　Also may be due to hypoxemia (especially if also associated with poor variability), maternal medications (e.g., β-
　　　blockers), hypothermia, vagal response, fetal bradyarrhythmias

Fetal heart rate variability
　Variability between beats (i.e., "waviness of baseline")
　Absent if <2 bpm, decreased if <6 bpm, average if 6–15 bpm, increased if >15 bpm, and saltatory (increased
　　swings in variability) if >25 bpm
　Significance: presence of FHR variability implies an intact nervous pathway from the cerebral cortex → midbrain →
　　vagus nerve → heart
　Normal variability: low likelihood of cerebral asphyxia
　Decreased variability: In utero hypoxia can lead to decreased cerebral oxygenation → decreased cerebral input to
　　heart → decreased variability
　　　May be due to labor, fetal sleep, narcotics, magnesium sulfate, abnormal cardiac conduction, anencephaly

Decelerations (decels) of FHR
　Early decels: due to *head compression* → pressure on fetal head → changes in cerebral blood flow → vagal deceleration
　　of HR
　　　Occur at *same time as contraction*, mirror image of contraction
　　　Mild (seldom < 120 bpm), never > 20 bpm below baseline
　　　Benign, gradual onset and offset, uniform shape
　　　Deeper decelerations with increased force of contraction
　　　Typically occur when mother with cervical dilation ~4–7 cm since this corresponds to the time when the edge of the
　　　　cervix is crossing the fetus' anterior fontanel
　　　Associated with normal fetal pH, normal Apgars
　Variable decels: due to *umbilical cord compression* leading to:
　　　　1. Fetal hypertension → baroreceptor response → vagal deceleration of HR
　　　　2. Fetal hypoxemia → chemoreceptor response → vagal deceleration of HR
　　　　3. Fetal hypoxemia → myocardial depression → deceleration of HR
　　An *abrupt* decrease in FHR with abrupt resolution; usually at same time as contraction; no uniformity to shape,
　　　pattern or timing; decrease in HR typically much lower than early decel
　　　Mild decel: 1/2 pregnancies with mild decels; often associated with a brief acceleration prior to the decel
　　　Severe decel: ominous; slow return of decel to baseline FHR; can lead to hypoxia and fetal decompensation
　Late decels: due to *uteroplacental insufficiency* leading to:
　　　Smooth configuration; onset, nadir and recovery are 10–30 seconds after that of contraction
　　　　1. Fetal hypoxemia → chemoreceptor response → enhanced alpha-adrenergic activity → fetal hypertension →
　　　　　baroreceptor response → parasympathetic response → late decel (note: no acidosis)
　　　　2. Fetal hypoxemia → myocardial depression → decel (note: with acidosis)

Sinusoidal FHR

A regular smooth sine wave; frequency of 3–6 cycles per minute with an amplitude up to 30 bpm; usually without beat-to-beat variability; absence of FHR reactivity

Ominous: associated with severe chronic anemia, fetomaternal hemorrhage, asphyxia

If good reactivity before or after sinusoidal pattern = pseudosinusoidal (can be due to maternal opiates) → less likely to be ominous

E. UTERINE ACTIVITY

Tocodynamometer: records timing and duration of contractions as well as relative intensity of contraction

Intrauterine pressure catheter: more precise and can be used following rupture of membranes to quantitate contraction pressure

Associated with increased risk of chorioamnionitis and postpartum maternal infection

F. FETAL SCALP SAMPLING

Possible only if cervix > 3–4 cm dilated

Used to assess blood gas and degree of metabolic acidosis (pH > 7.25 is normal; pH = 7.20–7.25 is worrisome; pH = 7.10–7.20, consider emergent delivery; pH < 7.10 requires emergent delivery)

If concerned, recheck every 15 minutes since pH changes quickly

G. UTERINE AND UMBILICAL GASES—SEE CARDIOLOGY CHAPTER IIIA

H. AMNIOTIC FLUID (AF)

Composition

1st trimester: osmolality similar to maternal and fetal blood, minimal fetal urine output, fluid formed by active transport of Na and Cl across amniotic membrane and fetal skin with H_2O passively following

2nd trimester: fetal urine production significant ~ 12 weeks gestation and thus amniotic fluid osmolality decreases

3rd trimester: dialysis across fetal skin is blocked due to keratinization; with maturation of fetal renal function, increased intravascular sodium reabsorption leads to decreased urine and amniotic fluid osmolality

Amniotic fluid volume (AFV)

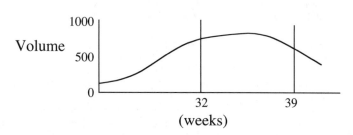

Amniotic fluid volume (AFV)

Modified from Fanaroff AA and Martin RJ (eds): Neonatal-Perinatal Medicine (6th edition). St Louis, Mosby–Year Book Inc, 1997, p 313.

Increase in AFV until ~32 weeks gestation; between 32 and 39 weeks, the mean AFV is constant (~700–800 cc); between 40 and 44 weeks, decrease in AFV to ~ 400 cc at 42 weeks

AFV determined by fetal urine output and swallowing ability of fetus

Hormonal regulation of AFV: prolactin decreases permeability of amnion to water; vasopressin increases AF osmolality; maternal dehydration will lead to decreased AFV and increased AF osmolality

Amniotic fluid index (AFI) = divides maternal uterus into four quadrants and adds the amount of AF (cm) in the largest vertical pocket in each quadrant

Normal AFI = 8–18 cm

	Oligohydramnios (oligo)	Polyhydramnios (poly)
Definition	AFI < 5 cm	AFI > 24 cm
Incidence	0.5–8.0% of pregnancies	0.1–3.0% of pregnancies
	Increased risk congenital anomalies	
Etiology	Fetal urinary tract abnormalities (e.g. ureteral and urethral obstruction, PCKD, renal agenesis)	Majority are idiopathic
	Placental insufficiency (due to decreased fetal hydration and decreased fetal urine output) associated, IUGR, severe pre-eclampsia, in utero hypoxia or postmaturity	GI anomalies (including duodenal and esophageal atresia) due to decreased amount of fluid swallowed
	Premature rupture of membranes	CNS anomalies due to decreased swallowing
	Twin-twin transfusion	Some cardiac anomalies
	Maternal medications (e.g. prostaglandin synthase inhibitors such as indomethacin due to decrease in glomerular filtration rate and angiotensin-converting enzyme inhibitors due to fetal hypotension)	Hydrops from severe fetal anemia (due to erythroblastosis fetalis, fetomaternal hemorrhage, parvovirus, twin-twin transfusion)
		Maternal diabetes
		Macrosomia
		Multiple gestation
		Genetic syndromes (e.g. trisomy 18 and 21, Turner syndrome and Beckwith-Wiedemann syndrome)
Clinical Evaluation	*Maternal assessment*—rule out rupture of membranes (often difficult to prove), assess for renal disease and HTN	*Maternal assessment*—assess for dyspnea, edema, increased weight gain, distention of uterus, rule out maternal diabetes and Rh disease
	Fetal assessment:	*Fetal assessment*—ultrasound to rule out congenital anomalies
	Evaluate fetal urinary tract—ultrasound to detect if presence of bilateral renal agenesis; assess for bilateral uteropelvic junction obstruction or PCKD	
	Evaluate fetal growth—decreased if placental insufficiency, placental abruption or placental infarction	
	Evaluate fetal lung growth—calculate lung area ratio by ultrasound (not always predictive)	
	Assess for congenital anomalies	
Management	*Fetal monitoring*	*Fetal monitoring*
	Amnioinfusion—instill fluid during labor to attempt to decrease intrapartum fetal distress; can also do if severe oligo and very premature to attempt to decrease risk of pulmonary hypoplasia (experimental); may be complicated by overdistention of uterus or amniotic fluid embolus (rare)	*In utero transfusion* if severe anemia
	Consider fetal intervention with vesicoamniotic shunt if severe oligo due to bladder obstruction	*Reductive amniocentesis*—to decrease AFV; may be complicated (~10%) by rupture of membranes, abruption or chorio-amnionitis
	Maternal hydration (especially hypotonic fluid) to increase fetal urine output	*Prostaglandin synthase inhibitors* (e.g. indomethacin)—leads to decreased fetal urine production (limited due to increased risk of complications)
	Delivery—especially if term or postterm with severe oligo; if premature, monitor closely, administer steroids and deliver if nonreassuring fetal status	
Morbidity	Increased risk of meconium passage, fetal distress, perinatal depression, and delivery by C/S	Increased risk of abnormal fetal positioning, placental abruption, premature rupture of membranes, premature delivery, and delivery by C/S
	Severe and chronic oligo may decrease fetal movements leading to contractures, Potter syndrome, thoracic compression and/or pulmonary hypoplasia (especially if severe oligo during 16-24 weeks gestation)	Increased risk of fetal distress, perinatal depression, macrosomia and admission rate to intensive care unit
		Increased risk of postpartum hemorrhage
Mortality	Increase in perinatal mortality to ~56/1000 (baseline ~2/1000)	Increase in perinatal mortality to ~4/1000
	If severe oligo, perinatal mortality increases to ~187/1000	

PCKD = polycystic kidney disease; GI = gastrointestinal; CNS = central nervous system; HTN = hypertension.

IX. Fetal Growth

A. STAGES

Stage	Time period	Physiology	Result of impairment
Hyperplastic	During embryonic and early fetal period (1st 16 weeks gestation)	Rapid increase in cell number Increased DNA	Symmetric IUGR
Hyperplastic and hypertrophic	Occurs between 16 and 32 weeks gestation	Increased cell number Increase in cellular size	Leads to asymmetric or symmetric IUGR
Hypertrophic	Occurs after 32 weeks gestation	Increase in cellular size Increased protein and RNA Period when most fetal fat and glycogen are deposited	Asymmetric IUGR

B. GENERAL

If growth expressed as % increase/day, greatest during 1st trimester; if growth expressed as grams/day, greatest with increasing gestational age

During 2nd trimester, weight gain is constant followed by an acceleration of growth during the 3rd trimester

Near term, the fetal growth rate decreases; this is probably due to limited placental function and/or uterine size

Protein increases gradually during gestation while body fat increases mostly in 3rd trimester

C. HORMONAL REGULATION OF FETAL GROWTH

Insulin: major hormone for *in utero* growth; produced by fetus

IGF (insulin-like growth factor)–I and II: mice knockouts of IGF demonstrate decreased fetal growth

Epidermal growth factor: important for ectodermal and mesodermal tissue development

Growth hormone (GH): no involvement of fetal or maternal GH; fetal tissues do not have GH receptors until late gestation

X. Intrauterine Growth Restriction (IUGR) and Small for Gestational Age (SGA)

A. IUGR VS SGA

IUGR	SGA
Rate of growth less than a fetus' predetermined genetic potential 4–8% of fetuses Pathologic	A fetus whose weight is lower than standard population (typically less than 10% of population-based weight data) May be pathologic or nonpathologic
IUGR fetuses may not necessarily be SGA since may still be within normals of population-based weight	Always smaller compared to population

B. ETIOLOGY

Maternal factors
1. Poor weight gain due to inadequate maternal nutrition will lead to decreased fetal weight gain during 3rd trimester; not important during 1st or 2nd trimester due to relatively large nutrient supply and low fetal nutrient demand
2. Smoking

3. Drugs—alcohol, amphetamines, corticosteroids, heroin, hydantoin, methadone, propanolol, warfarin
4. Hypertension—greatest if preeclampsia or chronic HTN; usually asymmetric IUGR
5. Maternal diseases—including maternal cyanotic congenital heart disease, cystic fibrosis, asthma, renal disease, sickle cell disease, lupus, inflammatory bowel disease, advanced diabetes, hyperthyroidism

Placental factors
Uteroplacental insufficiency most common
Placental factors include multiple gestation, twin-twin transfusion, placenta previa, villitis due to congenital infection, chronic placental abruption, abnormal umbilical cord insertion, multiple placental infarcts, and syncytial knots

Fetal factors
Fetal anomalies (particularly cardiovascular abnormalities and renal agenesis), genetic abnormalities, infection, multiple gestation (typically growth decreases at ~30 weeks gestation)

Unknown

Normal variant

C. SYMMETRIC VS ASYMMETRIC SGA/IUGR

Characteristic	Symmetric	Asymmetric (more common)
Head circumference (HC) relative to rest of body	HC proportional to rest of body	HC % greater than weight %
Time of onset	Early onset—prior to 3rd trimester	Late onset
Ponderal index (see diagnosis section)	Normal	Low
Growth	Decreased growth potential	Growth arrest
	Catch-up growth takes longer than 6 months	Catch-up growth by 6 months of age in majority
Risk of perinatal depression	Low risk	Increased risk
Blood flow to internal carotid artery	Normal	Increased and thus, brain growth is spared
Glycogen, fat and glucose levels	Relatively normal glycogen and fat levels	Low glycogen and fat levels
	Low risk of hypoglycemia	Increased risk of hypoglycemia
Etiology	Usually intrinsic	Usually environmental
	Due to chromosomal abnormalities, congenital infections, some inborn errors of metabolism and some maternal drugs	Due to uteroplacental insufficiency from preeclampsia, chronic hypertension, or severe diabetes

Modified from Fanaroff AA and Martin RJ (eds): Neonatal-Perinatal Medicine (6th edition). St Louis, Mosby-Year Book Inc, 1997, p 223.

D. DIAGNOSIS

History: identify patients at greater risk (e.g. multiple gestation, poor weight gain, poor prenatal care, hypertension, positive maternal antiphospholipid antibody)

Uterine fundal height: screening method that identifies ~40% of IUGR fetuses; measure between 18 and 30 weeks gestation; the # cm corresponds to GA in weeks; if difference > 2-3 cm, need to rule out IUGR

Measurements:
1. Decreased abdominal circumference compared to expected for gestational age
2. Low ponderal index (PI) if asymmetric growth

$$PI = \frac{\text{weight (grams)} \times 100}{(\text{crown-heel})^3}$$

length in cm

3. Decreased femur length

4. Decreased AFV due to decreased urine production from hypoxia and/or decreased renal blood flow
5. Decreased diastolic flow velocity in umbilical arteries with increased S/D ratio (see US section)

E. NEONATAL EFFECTS

Effect	Pathophysiology	Other
Depressed immune system	Decreased lymphocyte number and function Decreased immunoglobulin levels	May persist later in life
Hyperglycemia	Low amount of insulin Increased catecholamines	Increased sensitivity to insulin and thus, hyperglycemia is easily corrected
Hypocalcemia	Decreased vascular supply in utero	Increased risk for a difficult delivery
Hypoglycemia	Decreased glycogen stores Decreased gluconeogenesis Increased sensitivity to insulin	Particularly during first 3 days of life Optimal to initiate feeds or intravenous glucose early
Hypothermia	Decreased subcutaneous fat Large surface area to body-weight ratio	Infants will have a narrow temperature range
Perinatal depression	Uterine contractions increase hypoxic stress further	Leads to greater risk of C/S and greater risk of neonatal resuscitation
Polycythemia	Chronic hypoxia in utero leading to increased erythropoietin production	~1/2 of all SGA full-term infants have hematocrit > 60% May exacerbate hypoglycemia

Other: increased risk of meconium aspiration syndrome, gastrointestinal perforation due to focal bowel ischemia, acute renal failure, and persistent pulmonary hypertension due to prolonged in utero hypoxia

Newborn exam: decreased subcutaneous fat; rough, dry skin; skin desquamates easily due to decreased vernix production; often with increased anterior fontanel due to decreased membranous bone formation; female genitalia appear less mature due to decreased fat tissue covering the labia; often with ruddy appearance

Of note: alveolar maturation appropriate for GA in fetuses with IUGR

F. MANAGEMENT OF MOTHER

Bed rest if severe growth restriction (especially if due to uteroplacental insufficiency)

If fetus in acute distress, place mother in left lateral recumbent position to increase uterine blood flow and administer O_2 to mother

Improve maternal nutrition, manage maternal chronic illness

Serial ultrasounds to assess growth rate

Current studies to determine if low-dose aspirin will increase placental perfusion

If evidence of fetal distress, delivery fetus

G. PROGNOSIS

Prognosis dependent on etiology, duration and severity of IGUR or SGA

Increased mortality (increased ~5–20x compared to appropriate for gestational age infants)

Increased risk of perinatal complications with greater chance of admission to intensive care unit

Increased risk of neurological abnormalities (especially if persistent microcephaly)

Postnatal growth: dependent on severity of growth restriction at birth

Recent evidence suggests that adults have an increased risk of hypertension, glucose intolerance, and obesity (Barker's hypothesis)

XI. Nonimmune Fetal Hydrops (NIFH)

A. DEFINITION

Abnormal fluid accumulation in $\geq$ 2 fetal compartments (without maternal circulating antibodies against red blood cell antigens) leading to generalized skin thickening ($>$ 5 mm), fetal ascites, pleural effusion, pericardial effusion, cystic hygroma, and /or thick placenta ($>$ 6 cm)

Occurs in 1 in 1500–4000 deliveries

B. ETIOLOGY

The increase in interstitial and total fetal body water is attributed to disorders associated with congestive heart failure (most common), obstructed lymphatic flow, or decreased plasma osmotic pressure with increased capillary permeability

Hematology: twin-twin transfusion ($\sim$10%), homozygous alpha thalassemia, red blood cell enzyme deficiencies (glucose 6-phosphate dehydrogenase deficiency), severe fetomaternal hemorrhage

Cardiac ($\sim$25%): (specifically associated with increased preload or decreased cardiac outflow leading to greater stress on right ventricle): arrhythmia (supraventricular tachycardia, heart block), congenital heart disease, cardiac mass, cardiomyopathy

Vascular malformation: arteriovenous malformation, vascular accident (e.g. renal vein thrombosis), lymphatic obstruction (cystic hygroma)

Infection ($\sim$4%): coxsackie virus (leading to myocarditis), parvovirus B19 (leading to anemia), cytomegalovirus and syphilis (leading to hepatitis, portal hypertension and hepatic failure), toxoplasmosis, rubella, herpes, adenovirus

Genetic: aneuploidy ($\sim$16%), syndrome ($\sim$11%, e.g. Turner syndrome, Noonan syndrome)

Metabolic: lysosomal storage disease, glycogen storage disease type IV

Endocrine: thyrotoxicosis

Pulmonary ($\sim$8%): chylothorax, cystic adenomatoid malformation, pulmonary sequestration

Other: unknown ($\sim$16%), congenital nephrotic syndrome, congenital diaphragmatic hernia, skeletal dysplasias, placental/cord abnormalities

C. DIAGNOSIS

Mean GA at diagnosis = 24–25 weeks

Can present with maternal symptoms (increased uterine size, acute increase in weight gain, abdominal pain, respiratory compromise)

If assess all patients with polyhydramnios, HTN, maternal anemia or fetal tachycardia, will detect $\sim$ 60–80% nonimmune fetal hydrops

Ultrasound—diagnosis requires excessive fluid accumulation in $\geq$ 2 sites
  Abnormalities include ascites ($\sim$85%), scalp edema, thickened placenta, body wall edema, polyhydramnios, pleural effusion, and pericardial effusion

D. MANAGEMENT OF NONIMMUNE FETAL HYDROPS IN UTERO

Evaluation

Identify additional ultrasound findings—assess for twin gestation, anatomical abnormalities, cardiac rhythm, Doppler blood flow of umbilical, intrahepatic and intrathoracic vessels

Maternal labs—blood type, Rh, antibody screen (to differentiate from immune fetal hydrops—see Hematology section), Kleihauer-Betke, complete blood count (CBC) with differential, syphilis VDRL or RPR test, TORCH titers (*Toxoplasmosis, Rubella, Cytomegalovirus, Herpes* simplex virus), parvovirus B19 IgG and IgM titers, hemoglobin electrophoresis, glucose-6-phosphate dehydrogenase deficiency screen

Consider amniocentesis—chromosome analysis, AF culture, polymerase chain reaction (PCR) for specific infections, amniotic fluid AFP, possible metabolic studies

Consider percutaneous umbilical blood sampling (preferred invasive method if $\geq$ 18–20 weeks GA)—chromosome analysis, CBC, hemoglobin electrophoresis, specific fetal IgM levels, cultures, PCR for specific infections, liver function tests, possible metabolic studies

Postnatally—chromosome analysis, metabolic studies, CBC, blood type, hemoglobin electrophoresis, skeletal x-rays, echocardiogram, ultrasound of abdomen and chest, genetics evaluation

Multidisciplinary counseling (perinatalogist, neonatologist, geneticist, appropriate pediatric subspecialist)

If underlying cause is identified early in gestation and expected dismal prognosis, consider elective abortion

Possible fetal intervention: fetal transfusion if profound fetal anemia, maternal anti-arrhythmic if fetal arrhythmia, in utero surgery (fetal thoracentesis or surgical resection)

Regularly monitor BPP, NST, fetal growth and effusion volumes

Consider hospitalization of mother

Most recommend expectant management until 37 weeks GA or mature fetal lung indices unless nonreassuring fetal testing or other indication (e.g. severe preeclampsia); consider prenatal corticosteroids if premature

Mode of delivery controversial – majority deliver by C/S due to risk of soft tissue dystocia

Post-delivery management of neonate may include intubation, paracentesis and/or thoracentesis, placement of lines, fluid resuscitation; echocardiogram, subspecialist consultation

E. PROGNOSIS

Prognosis dependent on etiology of NIFH

Perinatal mortality = 40–90%; prognosis significantly worse if oligo, and/or structural cardiac disease

Complications include polyhydramnios (40–75%), malpresentation (25%), preeclampsia (10–20%), preterm labor (~90%), perinatal depression, pulmonary hypoplasia

XII. Multiple Gestation

A. INCIDENCE

Frequency = $80^{(n-1)}$ with n = number of fetuses

Spontaneous twins ~1 in 80 pregnancies; triplets ~1 in 8000 pregnancies

Monozygotic twins—incidence 1 in 3.5 per 1000 with uniform frequency throughout world

Dizygotic twins—incidence varies by locale, race, maternal age (increased risk with increased age until 37 years old)

B. TYPES OF TWINS

Dizygotic (2/3): fertilization of 2 eggs leading to fraternal twins; dichorionic (2 placentas)
   If implant sites are near, placentas may fuse yet vascular communications do not occur

Monozygotic (1/3): 1 fertilized egg splits during first 2 weeks of development
   Although monozygotic twins are genetically identical, there may be phenotypic differences
   Dichorionic, diamniotic: due to early division
   Monochorionic, diamniotic: due to later division (>3 days after fertilization); most common type of monozygotic twins; increased risk of twin-twin transfusion
   Monochorionic, monoamniotic: due to even later division (after amnion has formed); greater risk of cord problems; high mortality rate; acardiac twin is a rare complication (twin reversed-arterial-perfusion sequence with structurally normal donor twin yet recipient twin without a normal heart and lacking other structures)

C. MATERNAL AND FETAL RISKS

Maternal risks: hyperemesis, anemia, preeclampsia, gestational diabetes, postpartum hemorrhage, placenta previa

Fetal risks: congenital anomalies, growth restriction or discordant growth, twin-twin transfusion, fetal demise, premature delivery

Second twin: increased risk of malpresentation, in utero hypoxia, and hyaline membrane disease

D. TWIN-TWIN TRANSFUSION

Incidence
   Occurs in only 5–15% of *monochorionic, diamniotic* twins despite ~ 85% with vascular anastomoses
   Does not occur in dichorionic twins
   Interestingly, also does not occur in monochorionic, monoamniotic twins

Etiology
   Placental vascular anastomoses (typically deep) leading to acute or chronic transfer of blood from one twin to the other

Diagnosis
   Ultrasound findings: size disparity between fetuses, amniotic sacs and umbilical cords; single placenta; hydrops or congestive heart failure in recipient twin

Clinical (in extreme cases)
   Mother may present with an acute increase in abdominal girth that may lead to discomfort, respiratory distress or preterm labor
   Donor twin: anemia, hypovolemia, oligohydramnios (if severe, fetus appears "stuck" against uterine wall due to amnion adhering to fetus), decreased urine output, lower birth weight
   Recipient twin: polycythemia, hypervolemia, polyhydramnios, cardiac hypertrophy, may develop hydrops, increased birth weight
   If the difference in hematocrits is large yet the weight difference is small, suggests that transfusion occurred around time of delivery
   Both twins with poor outcome, especially if transfusion occurs before 24 weeks gestation

Management

Gestational age is most significant factor in deciding management

Serial removal of amniotic fluid if polyhydramnios to relieve some pressure differences between the two circulations (treatment of choice if > 20 weeks gestation)

Some centers create an opening in amnion between the two fetuses (amniotic septostomy) to allow fluid exchange and potentially equilibrate the pressure differences

Endoscopic laser ablation of vascular anastomoses is also possible yet with high complication rate and often difficult since anastomoses may be deep in placenta

If severe and early in utero and thus high risk of death in both twins, consider selective fetal reduction of donor twin

XIII. Labor

Maternal fever during labor May accelerate fetal brain injury

A. PATHOGENESIS

Unclear pathogenesis

Theories of labor include:

Decrease in progesterone levels (yet while levels in sheep decline prior to labor, human levels typically decline after placental delivery and despite administration of progesterone, labor still continues)

Fetus may trigger labor (supported by sheep studies in which adrenalectomy or hypophysectomy in utero delayed labor)

Uterine modifications (perhaps due to increase in myometrial oxytocin receptors, increase in gap junctions between myometrial cells, increased responsiveness or levels of one or more compounds that lead to uterine contractions)

Potential role of amnion, chorion and/or decidua

B. PHASES DURING LABOR

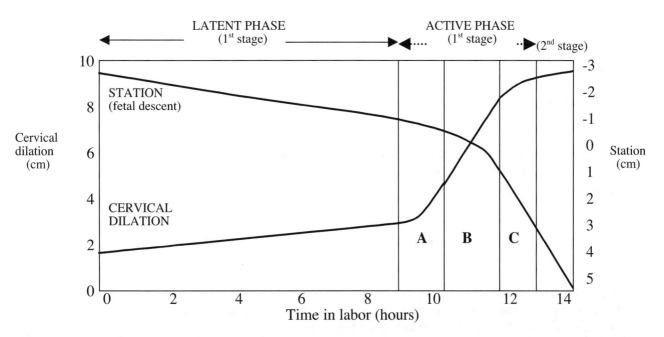

A = acceleration phase; B = phase of maximum slope; C = deceleration phase. Modified from Cunningham FG, Gant NF, Leveno KJ, et al (eds): Williams Obstetrics (21st edition). New York, McGraw-Hill, 2001, p 260.

First stage of labor = latent phase + active phase

Latent phase: begins when regular uterine contractions lead to effacement and dilatation of cervix

Prolonged if >20 hours in nullipara and >14 hours in multipara women; can be prolonged due to excessive analgesia or unfavorable cervix

Active phase: greatest rate of cervical dilatation

    Begins when cervix is ~3–4 cm dilated and ends when cervix is fully dilated (~10 cm); note that there is large variability of time and rate of cervical dilatation between women

    Descent begins during later stage of active dilatation

    Arrest of dilatation (2 hours without cervical change) and arrest of dilatation (1 hour without fetal descent) can be due to excessive sedation and/or fetal malposition

Second stage of labor

    Begins when cervical dilatation is complete

    Ends with delivery of fetus

    Arrest if > 2 hours for nullipara and > 1 hour for multipara women; if regional analgesia, 1 more hour added

Third stage of labor

    Begins after delivery of fetus

    Ends with delivery of placenta

C. EPIDURAL ANALGESIA *Regional anesthetic is @ ↑ risk for bradycardia*

Procedure: injection of local anesthetic into epidural space to block 10th thoracic to 5th sacral dermatome if vaginal delivery and 8th thoracic to 1st sacral dermatome for C/S

Complications: include low-grade maternal fever, spinal block if *subarachnoid* injection, hypotension (due to sympathetic blockade), urinary retention, headache, seizures, meningitis, cardiorespiratory arrest, vestibulocochlear dysfunction; may lead to long-term headaches, neck ache, or hand/feet tingling

Contraindications: maternal hemorrhage (severe), infection, or neurological disease

XIV. Delivery

A. PRESENTATIONS

Breech presentation

    ~3–4% of singleton deliveries

    When fetal buttocks enter pelvis first

    Frank breech: lower extremities are flexed at hips and extended at knees

    Complete breech: one or both knees are flexed

    Incomplete or footling breech: one or both hips are not flexed, and one or both feet or knees are lowermost in canal

    Increased risk with increased parity, multiple gestation, abnormal AFV, hydrocephalus, anencephaly, previous breech delivery, uterine anomalies, pelvic tumor, or fetal anomalies

    Complications include increased perinatal morbidity and mortality, IUGR, prolapsed cord, and C/S

Face presentation

    1 in 600 to 1 in 2000 deliveries

    When head hyperextended with occiput contacting fetal back and chin is presenting feature

    May be due to enlarged neck, cord around neck, anencephaly

    If effective labor and pelvis not contracted, vaginal delivery usually successful

Brow presentation

    Rarest presentation

    When region of head between orbital ridge, and anterior fontanel is presenting feature

    Due to same reasons as face presentation

Typically converts to a face or occiput presentation
If no fetal distress, labor can progress without intervention

Transverse lie
~ 1 in 320 deliveries
When long axis of fetus is perpendicular to that of mother (typically shoulder is over pelvic inlet)
Due to excessive abdominal wall relaxation from high parity; also can be associated with premature fetus, placenta previa, abnormal uterus, increased AFV or contracted pelvis
Increased maternal and neonatal risks
If active labor → deliver by C/S
If prior to labor or in early labor and membranes intact → can attempt external version

Compound presentation
1 in 700 to 1 in 1000 deliveries
When extremity is presenting feature
Occurs in premature deliveries since fetal head does not completely occlude pelvic inlet
Increased risk of prolapsed cord

Shoulder dystocia
0.6–1.4% of deliveries
Typically > 60 seconds between delivery of head and body
Increased risk if obese mother, multiparity, maternal diabetes or macrosomic fetus
May lead to postpartum hemorrhage (due to uterine atony or vaginal/cervical lacerations)
Increased perinatal morbidity (including brachial plexus injury, clavicular fracture, humeral fracture) and mortality
Difficult to predict or prevent
Manage with initial gentle attempt at traction followed by episiotomy, suprapubic pressure and various obstetric maneuvers (e.g. McRoberts: flex thighs above abdomen and simultaneously apply suprapubic pressure)

B. FORCEPS DELIVERY

Incidence
Varies between centers

Indications
Functions to provide traction and/or rotation under any circumstance that threatens mother or fetus, and would be relieved by delivery of fetus
Consider usage if significant cardiac, pulmonary or neurological disease in mother, intrapartum infection, exhaustion, prolonged 2nd stage of labor

Prerequisites
Engagement of head
Vertex or face presentation with anterior chin
Complete cervical dilatation, rupture of membranes
Must know exact position of head
Cannot have disproportion between head and pelvic inlet

Complications
Increased risk of vaginal laceration and episiotomy (especially if fetus at high station and if > 45 degree rotation required); increased maternal need for blood transfusion
Increased risk of perinatal depression
Increased risk of neonate with cephalohematoma, facial injury, retinal hemorrhage, intracranial hemorrhage

C. VACUUM EXTRACTION

Incidence
  Varies between centers

Indications and prerequisites
  Similar to forceps delivery
  However, in contrast to forceps, vacuum avoids insertion of blades within vagina and does not require precise
    placement over fetal head, and less intracranial pressure is applied

Complications
  Scalp laceration, facial bruising, subgaleal hematoma, cephalohematoma, intracranial hemorrhage, clavicular fracture,
    shoulder dystocia, facial injury, retinal hemorrhage

Contraindications
  Face or nonvertex presentation, extreme prematurity, fetal coagulopathy, macrosomia, s/p fetal scalp sampling

D. CESAREAN DELIVERY

Incidence
  ~20%
  1 in 10 with history of prior C/S

Indications
  Prior C/S due to increased risk of uterine rupture to 4–9% (especially if classical incision)
  Labor dystocia
  Fetal distress
  Breech presentation

Incisions
  Vertical incision: infraumbilical midline vertical incision with length corresponding to estimated fetal size; can rapidly
    extend incision around umbilicus
  Transverse incision: lower transverse slightly curved incision at pubic hairline and extended beyond lateral rectus muscles;
    difficult to extend incision
  Classical incision: vertical (can also be transverse) incision into body of uterus above lower uterine segment and reaching
    into uterine fundus

Complications
  Dependent on reason C/S is performed
  Include hysterectomy, operative injury to pelvic structures, blood loss, wound infection

Vaginal birth after C/S (VBAC)
  Recommended if 1 or 2 prior low-transverse C/S, adequately sized pelvis, no history of previous uterine rupture, no
    other uterine scars, and must have staff available for emergent C/S

E. FETAL DISTRESS

Diagnosis
  Persistent late decels, persistent severe variable decels (especially if slow return to baseline FHR) or prolonged decels
    and poor HR variability
  Note: presence of meconium alone does not always correlate with fetal hypoxemia/acidosis

Management
  Consider discontinuing oxytocin since this medication increases uterine tone

Change maternal position—avoid supine position (inferior vena cava compressed by enlarged uterus); left lateral decubitus position is preferred position

Monitor maternal BP closely and correct hypotension with intravenous fluids

Administer O_2 to mother

Close fetal monitoring; consider sampling of fetal scalp pH

May need to deliver emergently by C/S if persistent and/or severe

F. APGAR SCORES

Clinical sign	Apgar Score = 0	Apgar Score = 1	Apgar Score = 2
Respirations	None	Gasping, poor, irregular	Strong cry
Heart rate	No heart rate	<100 beats/min	>100 beats/min
Color	Cyanotic	Acrocyanosis	Pink
Muscle tone	Floppy	Some flexion of extremities	Active
Reflex irritability	None	Grimace	Cough, sneeze or cry

Modified from Apgar V: A proposal for a new method of evaluation of the newborn infant. *Anesth Analg* 1953; 32:260.

G. NEONATAL RESUSCITATION

1. Protocol

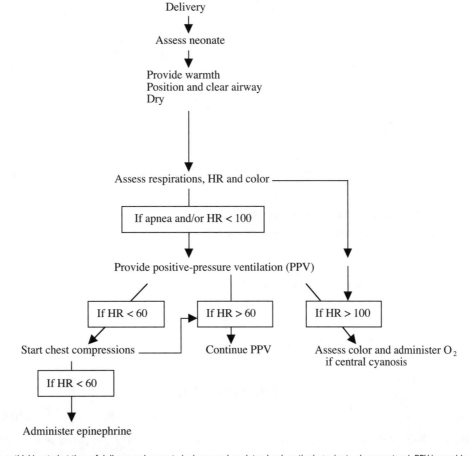

If meconium (mild, moderate or thick) noted at time of delivery and neonate is depressed, endotracheal suctioning prior to above protocol; PPV is provided at 40-60 breaths per minute (if simultaneous chest compressions, PPV at 30 breaths per minute); chest compressions to a depth of ~1/3 of anterior-posterior diameter of chest and rate of 90 compressions per minute; Modified from Kattwinkel J (ed): Textbook of Neonatal Resuscitation (4th ed). American Academy of Pediatrics and American Heart Association, 2000, pp 1-9 (please refer to most recent version for any changes to protocol).

2. Medications

Medication	Dosage/Route	Other
Epinephrine (1:10,000)	0.1–0.3 cc/kg intravenous (IV) or endotracheal (ET)	Administer rapidly Follow with 0.5–1.0 cc normal saline

Volume
  Normal saline
  O-negative blood
  Ringer's lactate
	10 cc/kg IV	Administer over 5–10 minutes
		If time allows, cross-match blood with mother's

Sodium bicarbonate (0.5 mEq/cc or 4.2% solution)	2 mEq/kg IV	Administer slowly (not faster than 1 mEq/kg/min)
Naloxone (1.0 mg/cc)	0.1 mg/kg (IV, ET, intramuscular, or subcutaneous)	Administer rapidly IV or ET method preferred Do not administer if mother suspected of narcotic addiction or receiving methadone

3. Ventilation bags

Flow-Inflating Bag (Anesthesia Bag)	Self-Inflating Bag

Fills only when O_2 from a compressed source flows into it
Collapsed when not in use
Has an adjustable flow-control valve with pressure manometer to regulate pressure
Advantages:
  100% O_2 administered at all times
  Easy to assess when there is a complete seal on patient's face
  Lung stiffness can be "felt" when squeezing bag
  Can deliver free-flow 100% O_2
Disadvantages:
  Requires a tight seal to maintain inflation
  Requires a gas source to inflate
  Typically without a safety pop-off valve
	Fills spontaneously after it is squeezed
	Remains inflated at all times
	Has a pressure-release valve (or pop-off valve) to limit amount pressure
	Advantages:
	  Always refills after being squeezed (even without compressed gas source)
	  Pressure-release valve decreases risk of overinflation
	
	Disadvantages:
	  Inflates even without tight seal
	  Requires a reservoir to deliver close to 100% O_2 (without a reservoir, only ~40% O_2 can be delivered)
	  Cannot reliably deliver free-flow 100% O_2

4. Indications for endotracheal intubation in the delivery room

Presence of meconium-stained amniotic fluid in a depressed neonate

Ineffective bag-mask ventilation

Prolonged positive-pressure ventilation

Chest compressions (to maximize efficiency of ventilation)

Epinephrine administration

Extreme prematurity

Surfactant administration

Congenital diaphragmatic hernia

XV. Prematurity

A. INCIDENCE

In US, 6–10% of all births; disproportionately greater % morbidity and mortality compared with full-term infants

Can be categorized by birth weight:

LBW (low birth weight) = infant < 2500 g at birth
VLBW (very low birth weight) = infant < 1500 g at birth
ELBW (extremely low birth weight) = infant < 1000 g at birth
"Micropremie" if infant < 750 g at birth

While premature survival rate has increased, risk of cerebral palsy has remained constant

B. RISK FACTORS

Demographic and behavioral factors	Decreased risk in Caucasians Low maternal age (< 17 years old) or advanced maternal age (> 35 years old) Maternal smoking or cocaine use
Maternal factors	Previous preterm delivery is the most significant risk factor with recurrence risk between 17 and 40% History of second-trimester abortions (unclear if first-trimester abortions related) Uterine malformations (3–16% of all preterm deliveries) History of maternal DES exposure (15–28% increased risk) Myomas Poor maternal nutrition Inadequate prenatal care Maternal illness (e.g. preeclampsia, autoimmune disease, diabetes)
Pregnancy complications	Chorioamnionitis (highest correlation with preterm labor-30%) Cervical incompetence Vaginal bleeding due to placental abruption or placenta previa Multiple gestation (~30–50% will deliver prematurely) Asymptomatic bacteriuria
Fetal factors	Fetal anomalies Oligohydramnios or polyhydramnios

C. POSSIBLE PREDICTORS OF PREMATURITY

Pathogenesis of prematurity unclear

Possible biological indicators of premature labor:
  Elevated fetal fibronectin levels (thus far, one of the best indicators)
  Decreased progesterone (yet no proven correlation)
  Elevated corticotropin releasing hormone—made by placenta 2nd or 3rd trimester
  Increased serum collagenase and cervical granulocyte elastase activity
  Elevated prolactin

D. TOCOLYTIC MEDICATIONS

Medication	Action	Complications
Terbutaline (PO, IV, SQ)	β2 agonist Binds to β2 receptors on myometrium of uterus, which activates adenyl cyclase → ATP converted to cAMP → decreases intracellular Ca → decreases uterine contractility	Maternal—tachycardia, glucose intolerance, pulmonary edema; also can lead to hypokalemia, hypotension, cardiac insufficiency, arrhythmias or myocardial ischemia
Magnesium sulfate (IV)	Decreases uterine contractility by decreasing Ach release from neuromuscular junction and by acting as a Ca antagonist	Maternal—fluid overload, pulmonary edema, decreased deep tendon reflexes, respiratory depression, cardiac arrest Neonatal—decreased RR, decreased peristalsis, hypotension, hypotonia

(continued on following page)

Medication	Action	Complications
Indomethacin (PO or PR)	Prostaglandin synthase inhibitor	Increased risk with prolonged usage Maternal—gastrointestinal bleeding, transient cholestasis, pulmonary edema, renal insufficiency Fetal—oligo (due to decreased fetal urine output), premature closure or constriction of PDA Neonatal—renal insufficiency, PHTN, ileal perforation, NEC
Calcium-channel blocking agent—2nd line (nifedipine—PO or sublingual)	Decreases uterine contractility by inhibiting transmembrane Ca influx	Maternal—hypotension, possible uteroplacental insufficiency Fetal—complications from uteroplacental insufficiency

PO = oral; IV = intravenous; SQ = subcutaneous; cAMP = cyclic adenosine monophosphate; Ach = acetylcholine; PR = rectal; PDA = patent ductus arteriosus, PHTN = pulmonary HTN; NEC = necrotizing enterocolitis.

XVI. Complications During Pregnancy

A. CERVICAL INCOMPETENCE

Definition: painless dilation of cervix beginning between 12th and 20th week gestation

Risk factors: in utero DES exposure, uterine abnormalities, trauma, 2nd trimester abortion

Diagnosis: typically made after history of 1 or more 2nd trimester losses
   If risk factors → cervical exams weekly and vaginal ultrasound to assess for cervical changes

Management:
   Cerclage—placed early 2nd trimester (ideal if placed 12–14 weeks gestation rather than waiting for cervical changes to be present)
      Cannot place if premature ROM, infection, congenital anomalies, active vaginal bleeding or active labor
      Remove at 36–37 weeks gestation

B. SPONTANEOUS ABORTION

Definition: termination of pregnancy prior to 20 weeks gestation without any medical intervention

Incidence: occurs in ~12% of women < 20 years of age and ~26% of women > 40 years of age
   >80% in 1st 12 weeks gestation with majority due to chromosomal abnormalities
   Increased risk with advanced maternal and paternal age
   Increased incidence if conception 3 months after a term birth

Etiology

Maternal factors	Chronic infection (e.g. HIV, tuberculosis) Maternal illness (e.g. insulin-dependent diabetes, lupus) Drug usage (e.g. tobacco, alcohol) Environmental toxins (see Section XVIIC) Autoimmune factors (particularly antiphospholipid antibodies) Thrombophilias (e.g. factor V Leiden mutation, possibly associated with antithrombin III deficiency, protein C and S deficiency) Uterine abnormalities
Placental factors	Placental abnormalities
Fetal factors	Abnormal zygote development Chromosomal abnormalities

(continued on following page)

C. PREMATURE RUPTURE OF MEMBRANES (PROM)

Diagnosis
AF is observed pooling in posterior fornix or clear fluid is passing from cervical canal
If diagnosis is uncertain—test pH of vaginal fluid with *nitrazine* as indicator
If pH = 6.5 suggests ruptured membranes (normal vaginal fluid pH = 4.5–5.5 and amniotic fluid pH = 7.0–7.5)
False-positive tests with blood, semen or bacterial vaginosis
False-negative test if inadequate amount of vaginal fluid
Ferning of vaginal fluid suggests amniotic fluid

D. CHORIOAMNIONITIS (CHORIO)

Definition: clinical signs of amniotic infection with fever, elevated WBC, foul-smelling amniotic fluid, maternal or fetal tachycardia, uterine tenderness

Incidence
1% of pregnancies
Only ~10% of neonates born to mothers with chorio will develop neonatal sepsis

Pathogenesis

Excess overgrowth of organisms within vagina and cervical canal
↓
Organism infects decidua, chorion and finally amnion and amniotic cavity
↓
Fetus aspirates or swallows infected amniotic fluid or becomes infected by direct contact
↓
Generalized sepsis

Management: broad-spectrum antibiotics and deliver fetus

E. UTERINE RUPTURE

Incidence: varies significantly between centers

Risks: previous C/S scar (usually classical), previous uterine trauma (prior curettage, myomectomy), overdistended uterus (multiple gestation, macrosomic fetus, polyhydramnios), breech extraction, difficult forceps delivery, internal version

Types: Complete—uterine rupture extends through myometrium with contact with peritoneal cavity
Incomplete—uterine rupture that does not extend through myometrium

Clinical: mother can present with abdominal pain, vaginal bleeding, cessation of uterine contractions, shock, diaphragmatic or suprapubic pain

Management: repair or hysterectomy

F. POSTTERM PREGNANCY (> 42 WEEKS GESTATIONAL AGE)

Incidence: ~10% of all pregnancies
Can be associated with anencephaly or placental sulfatase deficiency

Etiology: unknown; probably of fetal origin

Outcomes
1. Fetus will have decreased growth due to placental insufficiency (majority) leading to small, dysmature infant (wasting skin and nails, small umbilical cord) with greater risk of fetal distress during labor and meconium aspiration syndrome
2. Fetus may continue to grow in utero and be macrosomic at birth leading to greater risk of birth trauma
Increased mortality rate

Management:
Monitor fetus after 41 weeks gestation (e.g. biweekly NST, BPP with assessment of AFV and/or contraction stress test)
If any signs of fetal distress → deliver
If cervix favorable at 42 weeks → may induce with oxytocin and/or ROM
If cervix not favorable and > 42 weeks gestational age → controversial
  · Some physicians would continue biweekly monitoring
  · Some physicians recommend prostaglandin E_2 intracervical gel to induce cervical changes; however, studies show that this is not necessarily more effective than a placebo
  · Some physicians recommend induction or C/S

XVII. Human Teratogens

A. FDA CATEGORIES OF DRUGS AND MEDICATIONS

Category	Definition	Example(s)
A	Well-controlled human studies show no fetal risks	Prenatal vitamins
B	Animal studies show no fetal risks yet no human studies OR Adverse fetal effects in animal studies but *not* in well-controlled human studies	Penicillins
C	No adequate animal or human studies OR Adverse fetal effects in animal studies but no human studies available	Acyclovir β-blockers Calcium antagonists
D	Evidence of fetal risk but benefits outweigh risks	Carbamazepine Phenytoin
X	Fetal risks clearly outweigh benefits	Isoretinoin

Modified from Cunningham FG, Gant NF, Leveno KJ, et al (eds): Williams Obstetrics (21st edition). New York, McGraw-Hill, 2001, p 1009.

B. TERATOGENIC EFFECTS OF DRUGS AND MEDICATIONS

Drug	Teratogenic Effect
Angiotensin-converting enzyme inhibitors (e.g. captopril, enalapril)	Greater risk if exposure during 2nd and 3rd trimester Increased risk prenatally of oligohydramnios Increased risk postnatally of hypotension, oliguria May lead to hypoplasia of skull, fetal compression syndrome with limb deformations and pulmonary hypoplasia, renal tubular dysgenesis
Alcohol	Most common teratogenic exposure to fetus; leads to fetal alcohol syndrome The earlier the period of exposure in utero, greater likelihood of classic clinical features Greater effect with exposure of large amounts infrequently compared with smaller chronic intake Facial: *long, smooth philtrum, thin upper lip, short palpebral fissures*, ptosis, strabismus, epicanthal folds, maxillary hypoplasia, short nose, flat nasal bridge Cardiac: *ventricular septal defect*, atrial septal defect, tetralogy of Fallot Neurological: mental deficiency (average IQ=63), *microcephaly*, heterotopias, hyperactivity during childhood, fine motor dysfunction with poor hand-eye coordination Other: *intrauterine growth restriction*, short stature, abnormal palmar creases, limited joint mobility, small distal phalanges, small 5th fingernails, renal abnormalities
Caffeine	No evidence that caffeine is a teratogen in humans Some animal studies found that large amounts of caffeine potentiate mutagenic effects of radiation and some chemicals Controversial if increased risk of spontaneous abortions
Carbamazepine	Craniofacial defects, fingernail hypoplasia, growth restriction Neural tube defects (especially meningomyelocele), developmental delay Decreased vitamin K placental transfer and thus increased risk of hemorrhagic disease of the newborn
Cigarette smoking	Effects related to number of cigarettes per day (majority effects associated with >10 cigarettes/day) Nicotine increases catecholamines leading to vasoconstriction in uterine circulation and decreased uteroplacental blood flow Carbon monoxide inhibits oxygen delivery to tissue by binding to hemoglobin; effect is greater in utero since fetal hemoglobin has a greater affinity for carbon monoxide Placenta demonstrates decidual necrosis, microinfarcts, fibrinoid changes and atrophic villi Prenatally: spontaneous abortion, preterm delivery, *intrauterine growth restriction or SGA* (100–320 g reduction in expected birth weight, symmetric IUGR), placental abruption, placenta previa Postnatally (may be due to secondhand smoke exposure): increased risk of smaller head circumference, decreased cognitive performance, lung disease later in life (e.g. asthma, bronchitis, pneumonia), sudden infant death syndrome
Cocaine	Increased risk of stillbirth, *placental abruption*, skull abnormalities, cutis aplasia, porencephaly, ileal atresia, cardiac anomalies, visceral infarctions, urinary tract abnormalities
Cyclophosphamide	Fetal abnormalities if exposure during early pregnancy Missing and/or hypoplastic digits of hands and feet, cleft palate, single coronary artery, imperforate anus, fetal growth restriction, microcephaly
Diethylstilbestrol (DES)	Between 1940 and 1971 approximately 2–10 million pregnant women took DES Fetuses that are exposed are at risk later in life of: vaginal adenocarcinoma, abnormal female reproductive organ development (e.g. uterine and cervical abnormalities) and abnormal male reproductive organ development (e.g. epididymal cysts, microphallus, cryptorchidism, testicular hypoplasia)
Hydantoin (Phenytoin)	Facial: cleft lip/palate, short nose, depressed nasal bridge, mild hypertelorism Extremities: *digit and nail hypoplasia* Other: *intrauterine growth restriction*, failure to thrive, mild mental deficiency, wide anterior fontanel, short neck, rib anomalies, umbilical and inguinal hernias, hirsutism, hypospadius, may have cardiac defects (pulmonary or aortic valvar stenosis, ventricular septal defect) Decreased vitamin K placental transfer and thus increased risk of hemorrhagic disease of the newborn
Isotretinoin (Retinoic acid)	Spontaneous abortion and stillbirths are common Abnormalities described only with 1st trimester exposure *Cardiac*—transposition of the great arteries, truncus arteriosus, tetralogy of Fallot, ventricular septal defect, double outlet right ventricle, hypoplastic or interrupted aortic arch, retroesophageal subclavian artery Facial—*microtia* or anotia with or without stenosis of external ear canal, anterolateral displacement of hair whorl, hypertelorism, may have down-slanting palpebral fissures and/or epicanthal folds, depressed nasal bridge, facies may appear triangular due to hypoplastic maxilla and mandible, facial nerve paralysis (typically ipsilateral to malformed ear), narrow sloping forehead Neurology—*hydrocephalus*, cerebellar hypoplasia, microcephaly, mental deficiency Other—thymic and/or parathyroid abnormalities, limb reduction
Lithium	Ebstein anomaly Case reports of fetal goiter, hypotonia, arrhythmias, seizures, diabetes insipidus, premature birth
Methotrexate	6–8 weeks after conception is a critical period for exposure Facial—*cranial dysplasia, broad nasal bridge, low-set ears*, wide fontanels, synostosis of lamboid or coronal sutures, shallow supraorbital ridges, micrognathia, epicanthal folds

(continued on following page)

	Neurology—microcephaly
	Other—intrauterine growth restriction, short stature, talipes equinovarus, syndactyly
Phenobarbital	Cleft lip and palate
	Cardiac abnormalities
	Increased risk of withdrawal
	Decreased vitamin K placental transfer and thus increased risk of hemorrhagic disease of the newborn
Salicylates	Possible risk of thrombocytopenia and bleeding
	Possible intrauterine closure of PDA, pulmonary hypertension
Tetracycline	Yellow-brown discoloration of deciduous teeth
	Can be deposited in fetal long bones
Thalidomide	Epidemic of thalidomide-induced deformities occurred between 1959 and 1962 when it was commonly used as a sedative
	Teratogenic effect occurs between day 27 and 33 after conception
	Extremities: *phocomelia*, radius, ulna and humerus may be hypoplastic or absent, may have rudimentary or malformed hand, may have polydactyly and/or syndactyly, lower limbs may have malformations (usually not as severe as upper limbs)
	Facial: midline facial hemangioma, depressed nasal bridge, *microtia*
	Other: may also have intestinal atresia, congenital heart disease
Valproic acid	Facial—narrow bifrontal diameter, high forehead, epicanthal folds, telecanthus, broad nasal bridge, short nose, anteverted nostrils, midface hypoplasia, long philtrum, small mouth, may have cleft lip
	Cardiac—coarctation of aorta, hypoplastic left heart, aortic valve stenosis, interrupted aortic arch, secundum atrial septal defect, pulmonary atresia with intact ventricular septum
	Extremities—long, thin fingers and toes, hyperconvex fingernails
	Neurology—*neural tube defects* (in 1% of affected fetuses exposed in 1st trimester, especially meningomyelocele), may have mental deficiency
	Other—hypospadius
Warfarin (Coumadin)	Fetal effects if exposure between 6 and 12 weeks gestation with risk of syndrome ~25%
	If exposure following 12th week, decreased risk of fetal effects
	If mother receiving drug during delivery, increased risk of hemorrhage
	Facial—*nasal hypoplasia*, depressed nasal bridge, often with deep groove between nasal alae and nasal tip
	Neurology—severe mental deficiency, seizures, may have microcephaly and/or hydrocephalus
	Orthopedic—*stippled bone epiphyses*
	Other—low birth weight, mild nail hypoplasia, may have upper airway obstruction
	Note: while warfarin does cross the placenta, heparin does not cross the placenta and thus does not lead to any teratogenic effects

Note: italics represents most common features.

C. ENVIRONMENTAL TOXINS

1. **Lead:** increased risk spontaneous abortion, premature delivery, neurological abnormalities

2. **Radiation:** irradiation < 5 rad with minimal fetal effect; threshold probably > 15–20 rad and may lead to microcephaly (most common), growth restriction, and mental deficiency
   Other possible adverse effects include abnormal genitalia, microphthalmia, cataracts

3. **Other**
   Arsenic: increased risk spontaneous abortion, low birth weight
   Carbon monoxide: low birth weight, fetal death
   Ethylene oxide, inorganic mercury, benzene and formaldehyde: all increase risk of spontaneous abortion

XVIII. Fetal Disorders Amenable to In Utero Surgery

Majority are still experimental

Fetal surgeries only offered at specific centers

Chylothorax: thoracic shunt is placed to prevent pulmonary hypoplasia; also possible for pulmonary sequestration, congenital cystic adenomatoid malformation and tumors of the chest; variable success

Congenital cystic adenomatoid malformation and pulmonary sequestration: if these lesions rapidly enlarge in utero with early hydropic changes, consider cyst drainage or in utero surgical resection

Congenital diaphragmatic hernia: in utero surgery to allow for adequate lung development and prevent pulmonary hypoplasia
  Possible procedures include surgical correction (yet increased risk of premature rupture of membranes and preterm labor) and technique to "plug" the trachea (**P**lug the **L**ung **U**ntil it **G**rows)
  Since surgery during neonatal period recently with improved outcomes and in utero procedures have not been consistently successfully, prenatal intervention not commonly done

Neural tube defects: current experimental procedures include in utero surgical resection and coverage of defect to prevent exposure to amniotic fluid (exposure may result in permanent neurological damage)

Obstructive uropathies: urinary shunt with fetal urine shunted into uterine cavity to decrease the risk of pulmonary hypoplasia and other effects

Sacrococcygeal teratoma: complete excision has been unsuccessful in majority of cases; palliation by debulking to prevent hydrops with good results

References

Bianchi DW, Crombleholme TM and D'Alton ME: Fetology. New York, McGraw-Hill, 2000.

Boyle RJ: Effects of certain prenatal drugs on the fetus and newborn. *Ped Rev* 2002; 23(1):17–24

Creasy RK and Resnik R (eds): Maternal-Fetal Medicine (4th edition). Philadelphia, WB Saunders, 1999.

Cunningham FG, Gant NF, Leveno KJ, et al (eds): Williams Obstetrics (21st edition). New York, McGraw-Hill, 2001.

Fanaroff AA and Martin RJ (eds): Neonatal-Perinatal Medicine (6th edition). St Louis, Mosby–Year Book Inc, 1997.

Granger JP, Alexander BT, Bennett WA and Khalil RA. Pathophysiology of pregnancy-induced hypertension. *Am J Hypertension* 2001;14:178S–185S.

Hay WW, Thureen PJ and Anderson MS. Intrauterine growth restriction. *NeoReviews* 2001; 2(6): e129–138.

Jones KL: Smith's Recognizable Patterns of Human Malformations (5th edition). Philadelphia, WB Saunders, 1997.

Jorde LB, Carey JC, Bamshad MJ and White RL: Medical Genetics (2nd ed). St. Louis, Mosby, Inc., 2000.

Kattwinkel J (ed): Textbook of Neonatal Resuscitation (4th ed). American Academy of Pediatrics and American Heart Association, 2000.

Thureen PJ, Anderson MS and Hay WW. The small-for-gestational age infant. *NeoReviews* 2001; 2(6): e139–149.

Alcohol 3-12°p̄ deliv.
- onset 0-1 days
  lasts 1-2 days
  mild NAS
  Teratogenic *
  Br.fd. OK

Nicotine
  ↑risk GBS colon.
  SIDS 2x↑
  OK br fd
  LBW — neuroexcitable
  ↓FBM - ↓lung growth

Methadone
  Long ½ life (24-36°)
  * stored in body fat
  Br.fd OK
  Later onset withdraw *
    (3-7day c̄ peak 10-21d)
  Lasts 2-6wk
  More severe than heroin
  ↓Jaundice

Cocaine
  Ø Br fd
  ↑NAS, PPHN, IVH
  CNS IMH
  SIDS 3-7x↑

Heroin
  - Quick w/draw symp 24-48°
  - duration 2-4wk
  - Ø Teratogenic
  - Accele FLM (↓RDS)
  - Fetal w/draw mimic mat. w/draw
    └ don't detox
  - ↓jaundice

CHAPTER 2

Respiratory System

TOPICS COVERED IN THIS CHAPTER

BPD

I. Morphologic Development of the Lung

The structural development of the lung determines the effectiveness of gas exchange

Lung and airway formation
  Respiratory tract derived from *endoderm*
  The lung forms from a ventral bud of the esophagus, i.e., arises from foregut
  Branching dependent on the underlying mesodermal mesenchyme
  Branching of airways complete by 12–14 weeks gestation

Vascular supply
  Pulmonary vasculature formed from branches off the 6th aortic arch
  The bronchial arterial system from the aorta supplies the conducting airways, visceral pleura, connective tissue, and
    pulmonary arteries

Alveolarization
  Increase in bronchioles and alveoli occur in the alveolar phase
  Alveoli develop in late gestation and continue their development until 2-6 years of age
  Alveolarization delayed by:
    1) Antenatal steroids (despite the benefit of increased fetal lung surface area)
    2) Supplemental oxygen
    3) Nutritional deficiencies
    4) Mechanical ventilation

Lung development

Phase	Embryonic	Pseudoglandular	Canalicular	Terminal Sac	Alveolar
Gestation (weeks)	~0–5	~5–16	~16–25	~25–36	~36+
Structures	Trachea Bronchi	Nonrespiratory bronchioles		Alveolar ducts	
	Conducting Airways		Terminal Respiratory Units		

Modified from Hansen TN, Cooper TR and Weisman LE (eds): Neonatal Respiratory Diseases (2nd edition). Newtown, Pennsylvania, Handbooks in Health Care Co, 1998, p 2.

(Note: mnemonic for phases—"**E**ach **P**ulmonary part **C**omes **T**hrough **A**ge")

Abnormal development
  During the embryonic phase, common malformations include: tracheal stenosis and tracheo-esophageal fistula
  During the pseudoglandular phase, common malformations include: bronchogenic cysts, congenital diaphragmatic
    hernia, branching anomalies of the lung, cystic adenomatoid malformation

A. TYPE I AND II PNEUMOCYTES = PULMONARY CELLS THAT LINE ALVEOLAR SPACES

Type I pneumocyte	Type II pneumocyte
Shaped like a fried-egg; tight junctions	Cuboidal shape
Spread thinly and flatly across the alveolar surface (covers ~ 90% of the surface)	Comprises ~10% of alveolar surface
Fewer number of cells in alveolar lining	Greater number of cells in alveolar lining
Important role in gas exchange	Important role in surfactant metabolism and secretion
No gene material for surfactant	
Derived from type II cells	Progenitor to type I cells

II. Fetal Respiration

Fetal lung fluid (FLF) plays a critical role in lung development

Postnatally, FLF *clearance* is important for normal postnatal adaptation

During fetal respirations, the larynx opens, allowing for minimal but steady flow of FLF out of the trachea; this fluid can then be swallowed or mixed with amniotic fluid; when the larynx is closed, the lung can maintain a distended pressure, which is vital for lung growth

FLF maintains airway volume that is similar to the functional residual capacity (FRC) at birth (20–30 cc/kg)

Near-term FLF production rate is low (4–5 cc/kg/hr)

A. FETAL LUNG FLUID COMPOSITION

Chloride is *actively* transported across pulmonary epithelial cells into air spaces, creating an osmotic gradient that induces the flow of liquid into the fetal lung

The pulmonary epithelial cells actively transport bicarbonate out of the lung

FLF is low in bicarbonate and protein, yet high in chloride, Na and K

FLF production can be inhibited by epinephrine (naturally increased with stress of delivery) and β-adrenergic agonists

B. FETAL LUNG FLUID CLEARANCE

Prenatal
FLF decreases by 35% during the days prior to birth (sheep model); prenatal clearance occurs by:
1. Decreased formation and secretion of FLF
2. Chloride secretion markedly decreases and eventually stops; simultaneously, epithelial cells pump sodium from the alveolar spaces into the interstitium and FLF follows
3. Increased lymphatic oncotic pressure and low fetal alveolar protein leading to movement of fluid from alveoli to pulmonary lymphatics

Active labor
During active labor, ~30% FLF is further cleared from the alveoli and airways

Postnatal
~35% remains to be cleared postnatally, accomplished by:
1. Lung distention leading to an increase in transpulmonary pressures, which drives fluid into the interstitium

2. Increased lymphatic oncotic pressure and low fetal alveolar protein leading to movement of fluid from alveoli to pulmonary lymphatics

III. Surfactant ↓ risk of pneumo

A. COMPOSITION

Mostly lipid (majority is DPPC or *di*palmitoyl *phos*phatidylcholine—most physiologically active component)

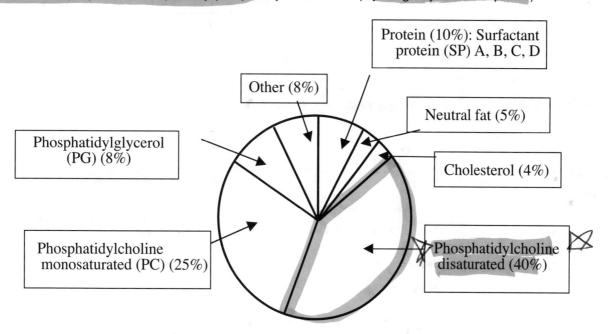

Protein (10%): Surfactant protein (SP) A, B, C, D

Other (8%)

Neutral fat (5%)

Phosphatidylglycerol (PG) (8%)

Cholesterol (4%)

Phosphatidylcholine monosaturated (PC) (25%)

Phosphatidylcholine disaturated (40%)

Modified from Hansen TN, Cooper TR and Weisman LE (eds): Neonatal Respiratory Diseases (2nd edition). Pennsylvania, Handbooks in Health Care Co, 1998, p 42.

B. SURFACTANT PROTEINS

	Origin	Characteristics	Role(s)
SP-A	Type II mostly, also nonciliated bronchiolar cells = Clara cells Chromosome 10 Expressed early in third trimester	28, 32 kDa Most abundant Induced by steroids (in vitro) Hydrophilic Collectin member	Tubular myelin formation (with SP-B and calcium) Surface adsorption of phospholipids Enhances phospholipid uptake and inhibits phospholipid secretion Host defense: significant role of opsonization, also involved in agglutination, reduction of viral infectivity, and modulation of inflammation SP-A null mice: increased lung inflammation, ineffective pulmonary clearance of organisms, no tubular myelin formation
SP-B	Type II and Clara cells Chromosome 2 Expressed at end of first trimester	8 kDa—final active form Hydrophobic Induced by steroids (in vitro)	Tubular myelin formation (with SP-A and calcium) Surface adsorption of phospholipids FT infants with SP-B deficiency: death from severe respiratory failure with alveolar proteinosis; require lung transplantation for survival
SP-C	Type II cells Chromosome 8 Expressed at end of first trimester	4 kDa—final active form Hydrophobic Induced by steroids (in vitro)	Surface adsorption of phospholipids SP-C null mice: minimal effect on postnatal respiratory function or survival
SP-D	Type II cells Also present in many nonpulmonary cells Chromosome 10 Expressed last—after early third trimester	43 kDa preprotein Hydrophilic Structurally similar to SP-A Collectin member	Host defense: significant role of agglutination and reduction of viral infectivity, also involved in opsonization and modulation of inflammation SP-D null mice: altered surfactant homeostasis (mice with increased alveolar surfactant pool), susceptible to viral pathogens

Modified from McCormack FX and Whitsett JA. "The pulmonary collectins, SP-A and SP-D, orchestrate innate immunity in the lung." *J Clin Invest* 2002; 109(6):707–712 and from lecture by Karen McAlmon, MD "Neonatal Core Conference: Pulmonary Surfactant" Children's Hospital, Boston, MA 1996.

C. SURFACTANT PRODUCTION AND SECRETION

Type II pneumocytes obtain the precursors of surfactant (glucose, glycerol, fatty acids, choline and lipids) by uptake from the circulation; fatty acids can also by synthesized in the microsomes and mitochondria; PC, PG and phosphatidylinositol (PI) are produced in the microsomes and transported to the lamellar bodies

Surfactant proteins are made in the endoplasmic reticulum of type II pneumocytes, glycosylated in the Golgi bodies and stored in lamellar bodies

Lamellar contents are then released into alveoli, form tubular myelin, and line interface

Surfactant components are recycled by endocytosis, reincorporated into lamellar bodies, and then resecreted (thus decreasing the need for *de novo* synthesis) *Lamellar count >50,000 assoc. lung maturity*

~95% secreted surfactant is recycled; surfactant turnover = 10 hrs

Influences of surfactant production

Lung maturation	Pregnancy-related conditions	Effector substances
Accelerated	Chronic maternal hypertension Maternal cardiovascular disease Placental infarction Intrauterine growth restriction Pregnancy-induced hypertension Prolonged rupture of membranes Incompetent cervix Hemoglobinopathies	Corticosteroids Thyroid hormones Thyroid stimulating and releasing hormone Cyclic adenosine monophosphate Methylxanthines Beta-agonists Prolactin Estrogens Epidermal growth factor Transforming growth factor-alpha
Delayed	Diabetes Rh isoimmunization with hydrops fetalis 2nd born twin Male sex Cesarean section Prematurity History of RDS in sibling Perinatal asphyxia	Insulin Transforming growth factor-beta Androgens

RDS = respiratory distress syndrome; Modified from Fanaroff AA and Martin RJ (eds): Neonatal-Perinatal Medicine (6th edition). St Louis, Mosby-Year Book Inc, 1997, p 1008.

Influences of surfactant secretion and flow of fetal fluid
Purines, prostaglandin, β-agonists and lung distention increase surfactant secretion prostaglandin, β-agonists and fetal breathing increase flow of fetal lung fluid

D. SURFACTANT CHANGES DURING DEVELOPMENT

	Immature lung	Mature lung
Type II cells		
Glycogen lakes	Large number	None
Lamellar bodies —*surf proteins stored*	Few	Many
Surfactant composition		
Saturated phosphatidylcholine (PC)/total PC	0.6	0.7
Phosphatidylglycerol	Absent or low	10%
Phosphatidylinositol	10%	2%
SP-A	Low	5%
Surfacant function	Decreased	Normal

Modified from Fanaroff AA and Martin RJ (eds): Neonatal-Perinatal Medicine (6th edition). St Louis, Mosby-Year Book Inc, 1997, p 997.

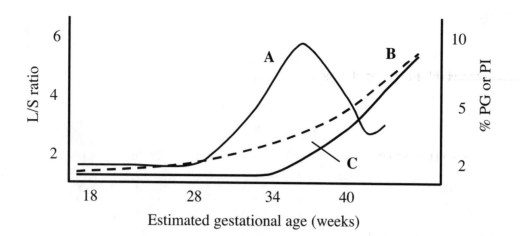

L/S = lecithin/ sphingomyelin; PG=phosphatidylglycerol; PI= phosphatidylinositol; Modified from Fanaroff AA and Martin RJ (eds): Neonatal-Perinatal Medicine (6th edition). St Louis, Mosby-Year Book Inc, 1997, p 1001.

L/S > 2 = Lung mature
L: Reflect Lung maturity
S: ↓ p̄ 32wk, Ø Related to maturity
LS = 2 @ ~35wk

Curve A **% phosphatidylinositol** (PI) within amniotic fluid
PI present in FLF before PG and falls during lung maturation

Curve B **L/S ratio = lecithin/sphingomyelin**
Sphingomyelin is a membrane lipid within amniotic fluid that decreases after 32 weeks gestation yet is *not* related to lung maturity
Lecithin content increases with increase in gestational age (GA) and *does* reflect lung maturity
Since sphingomyelin measurement standardizes for amniotic fluid volume changes that occur during gestation, the L/S ratio reflects lung maturity
If L/S > 2 ⟶ lung maturity; L/S = 2 typically at 35 weeks

Curve C **% phosphatidylglycerol** (PG), increases after 34–35 weeks * Lung maturity of IDM
More accurately reflects lung maturity; not present in infants with respiratory distress syndrome (RDS); infant with resolving RDS will have increasing PG levels in lung
Since PG is not present in meconium or blood there is low risk of contamination
Interestingly, although presence of PG demonstrates lung maturity, it is not necessary for normal surfactant function

* Blood & Meconium ↑ immature L/S Ratio and depress a mature L/S Ratio

E. FETAL LUNG MATURITY TESTING

Amniotic fluid L/S ratio	Risk of RDS (%)
> 2.0	< 0.5
< 1.0	100
PG present	< 0.5
> 2.0, no PG	> 80
> 2.0, + PG	0
2–3; and diabetes or Rh isoimmunization	13

Modified from Hansen TN, Cooper TR and Weisman LE (eds): Neonatal Respiratory Diseases (2nd edition). Newtown, Pennsylvania, Handbooks in Health Care Co, 1998, p 46.

Foam stability or shake test: if mix amniotic fluid with ethanol and foam is present ⟶ mature lung; due to presence of phosphatidylglycerol
Test has a high false-negative rate

F. ARTIFICIAL SURFACTANT TYPES

Natural	Survanta	Minced bovine lung DPPC Contains SP-B and C No SP-A Available in US for administration
	4ml/kg	
	Infasurf	Bovine lung lavage DPPC Contains SP-B, C (more SP-B than Survanta and Curosurf) No SP-A Available in US for administration
	3ml/kg Q12	
	Curosurf	Minced porcine lungs DPPC Contains SP-B and SP-C No SP-A Available in Europe for administration
	2.5/kg then 1.25/kg Q12	
Synthetic	Exosurf	Mixture of synthetic lipids DPPC Hexadecanol and tyloxapol also added to accelerate surfactant surface adsorption Protein-free (no SP) Available in US for administration

G. ROLE OF SURFACTANT: LAPLACE'S LAW

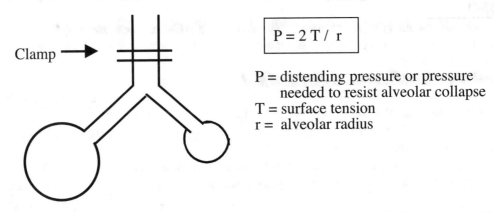

Clamp →

$$P = 2T / r$$

P = distending pressure or pressure needed to resist alveolar collapse
T = surface tension
r = alveolar radius

Role of surfactant in maintaining alveolar distention is explained by Laplace's Law: Laplace's law states that the pressure required to keep alveoli distended is directly proportional to the surface tension and indirectly proportional to the alveolar radius

The above diagram represents a large and a small alveolus—if the clamp is released, air will be displaced from the smaller alveolus (with greater pressure) to the larger alveolus; this process will continue until the smaller alveolus collapses; this is similar to infants with surfactant deficiency who have overdistention of large alveoli and collapse of smaller alveoli

Surfactant provides a stabilizing effect by decreasing alveolar surface tension and thus decreases the pressure needed to keep alveoli open
- As an alveolus becomes smaller, surfactant becomes more concentrated, decreasing the surface tension further and preventing air from leaving
- In contrast, as the alveolus becomes larger, surfactant spreads more thinly, increasing the surface tension further and increasing lung recoil pressures
- As lung inflates, surface tension increases and as lung deflates, lung surface tension decreases

IV. Extrauterine Pulmonary Transition

Decrease in pulmonary vascular resistance accomplished by: ↓PVR
1. Lung inflation—with lung expansion, there is activation of stretch receptors leading to reflex pulmonary vasodilation
2. Gas exchange—establishing adequate oxygenation and ventilation
3. Vasoactive mediators (i.e., nitric oxide production)

V. Control of Breathing

A. MECHANICAL

Inspiration

During inspiration, inspiratory muscles of the chest wall and diaphragm contract; this leads to expansion of the thorax and more negative pleural pressure (P)

This change in pleural P leads to a decrease in alveolar P

The negative pressure gradient between the airway opening and the alveolus results in inspiratory gas flow from the airways to the alveoli

Expiration

During expiration, the respiratory muscles relax

The lung recoil pressure results in a positive alveolar pressure

The positive pressure difference between the alveolus and airway opening results in gas leaving the lung

B. RESPIRATORY REFLEXES

Hering-Breuer: during inflation, airway stretch receptors limit the duration of inspiration, which may lead to apnea; important during neonatal quiet sleep

Paradoxical reflex of Head: augmented inspiratory effort following a rapid increase in lung inflation; greater in REM (rapid eye movement) sleep

C. CONTROL OF RESPIRATION

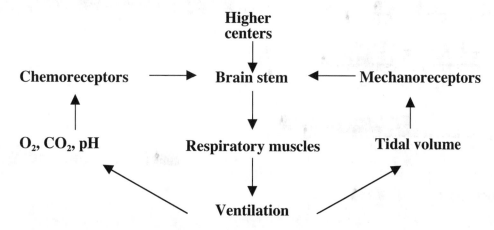

Modified from Fanaroff AA and Martin RJ (eds): Neonatal-Perinatal Medicine (6th edition). St Louis, Mosby-Year Book Inc, 1997, p 1055.

Response to carbon dioxide (CO_2) changes

CO_2 changes are dependent on *chemoreceptors* on ventrolateral surface of the medulla

These receptors sense the hydrogen ion concentration in the extracellular fluid; an increase in $paCO_2$ (partial pressure of CO_2 in arterial blood) leads to increased hydrogen ion concentration and increased respiratory rate

Metabolic acidosis and alkalosis have a strong influence on respiratory drive, independent of $paCO_2$
Sensitivity to CO_2 levels increases with advancing GA
Higher O_2 levels increase the sensitivity to CO_2 levels
Mechanoreceptors are also important for control of respiration; these are stretch receptors in airway smooth muscle that respond to changes in tidal volume

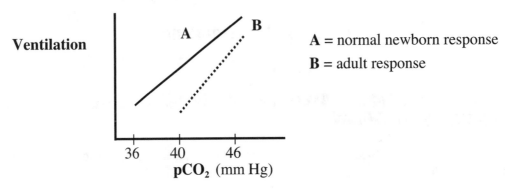

Ventilation

A = normal newborn response
B = adult response

pCO_2 (mm Hg)

Modified from Greenough A, Milner AD and Roberton NRC (eds): Neonatal Respiratory Disorders. Arnold, London and Oxford University Press Inc, New York, 1996, p 33.

Response to oxygen (O_2) changes
The response to O_2 changes is mediated by peripheral chemoreceptors in carotid bodies and in aortic bodies
In the *full-term* infant—response to hypoxia includes hyperpnea and an initial increase in ventilation, followed by a decrease in ventilation
Response to hyperoxia (2+ days in 100%) results in decreased respirations followed by an increase in ventilation; this is probably secondary to alveolar collapse sensed through mechanoreceptors and modest increases in $paCO_2$
In the *preterm* infant—decreased O_2 does not result in initial hyperpnea, but rather respiratory depression (poor peripheral chemoreceptors)

D. APNEA: A Disorder of Respiratory Control

Definition	Absence of air flow for ≥ 20 seconds (note: this is in contrast to periodic breathing, which is defined as 3 respiratory pauses with more than 3 seconds in between for up to 20 seconds–this is normal, unless associated with bradycardia or cyanosis)
	Three types:
	Central: no airflow, no respiratory effort
	Obstructive: no airflow despite respiratory effort
	Mixed: often begins as central and later becomes obstructive
	More common in REM sleep compared with quiet sleep
Etiology	Prematurity, infection, metabolic abnormalities
	Maternal medications (e.g., narcotics, magnesium, β-blocker)
	Hypoxemia, anemia, hypo or hyperthermia, arrhythmia
	Infant medications (e.g., prostaglandin), gastroesophageal reflux
	Upper airway malformation leading to increased secretions or anatomical blockage (e.g., tracheo-esophageal fistula, Pierre-Robin sequence)
	Central nervous system disorder (e.g., intracranial hemorrhage, congenital anomaly)
Diagnosis	Pneumogram (combine with EEG, pH probe)
	Impedance monitor: monitors change in chest dimension, detects only central apnea since obstructive apnea still moves chest wall
	Thermistor: registers air current, detects both obstructive and central apnea
	Note: if premature, testing not usually required unless atypical of apnea of prematurity
Prevention	Maintain normal hematocrit, electrolytes and paO_2
	Avoid neck flexion and abdominal distention
Management	Methylxanthines (see therapeutics section in this chapter)
	Consider continuous positive airway pressure
	Possible intubation if severe
	If possible, treat underlying etiology (e.g., antibiotics, adjust electrolyte supplementation, anti-reflux medications, anti-seizure medications)

E. CLINICAL SYMPTOMS OF RESPIRATORY DISEASE

Nasal flaring: a compensatory endeavor to decrease nasal airway resistance

Retractions: neonates with excessive chest wall compliance and/or noncor
will have a greater negative intrapleural pressure during inspiration, an
The presence of retractions often demonstrates worsening lung compliance
blood gas abnormalities
The severity of retractions correlates with degree of negative intrapleural pressure

Grunting: occurs when vocal cords are partially closed at the end of expiration
Generates a positive end expiratory pressure that stents open small airways, increasing ventilat
the ventilation/perfusion ratio
Improves functional residual capacity (FRC) and improves compliance

VI. Ventilation and Perfusion of the Lung

A. PERFUSION ZONES OF THE UPRIGHT ADULT LUNG

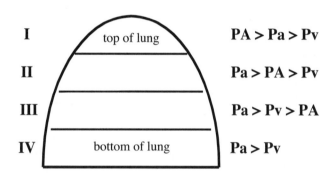

I	top of lung	PA > Pa > Pv
II		Pa > PA > Pv
III		Pa > Pv > PA
IV	bottom of lung	Pa > Pv

Modified from Goldsmith JP and Karotkin EH (eds): Assisted Ventilation of the Neonate (3rd edition). Philadelphia, WB Saunders Co, 1996, p 55.

PA = alveolar pressure (P); Pa = pulmonary arterial P; Pv = pulmonary venous P

Zone I—uppermost part of lung, almost no blood flow due to collapse of capillaries in the walls of alveoli

Zone II—some pulmonary blood flow because Pa > PA

Zone III—flow is dependent on pressure difference between arterial and venous system

Zone IV—decreased blood flow because of increased interstitial pressure leading to compression of blood vessels

B. PERFUSION ZONES OF THE NEONATAL LUNG

Entire neonatal lung functions as Zone III; Pa > Pv > PA

If air trapping or alveolar distention, the lung may functionally shift to Zone I or Zone II leading to decreased pulmonary blood flow

If increased extravascular fluid (e.g., patent ductus arteriosus (PDA), fluid overload, leaky capillaries), the lung functionally shifts to Zone IV with increased pulmonary vascular resistance (PVR) and decreased blood flow

C. DISTRIBUTION

Alveolus

pO_2 (mm Hg)
pCO_2
pN_2
pH_2O
Total (a

	FiO_2 = RA	FiO_2 = 100%
	100	671
	42	42
	570	0
	47	47
m P)	760	760

The partial pressure (p) of all gases in each alveolus must equal atmospheric (atm) pressure

If 100% FiO_2 is administered for several hours, all of the N_2 will be washed out

Since the pCO_2 is relatively constant (determined by venous pCO_2) and pH_2O is similarly stable (dependent on body temperature), the alveolar pO_2 must increase to maintain atmospheric P=760

If the airway is blocked, the alveolus will collapse because oxygen will enter the capillary from the alveolus

D. SCHEMATIC EFFECTS OF LOCAL VENTILATION/PERFUSION ($\dot{V}/\dot{Q}$) MISMATCH ON OVERALL GAS EXCHANGE

V/Q = 0	V/Q < 1	V/Q = 1	V/Q > 1	V/Q = infinity
No alveolar ventilation (no gas exchange between atm and blood)	Under ventilation of alveoli	Normal alveolar ventilation	Normal alveolar ventilation, increased dead space or *wasted ventilation*	Normal alveolar ventilation, **dead space**
Normal perfusion = intrapulmonary **shunt**	Normal perfusion	Normal perfusion	Decreased perfusion	*No perfusion*
pAO_2 ↓↓↓↓	pAO_2 ↓↓ to ↓↓↓	pAO_2 = paO_2	pAO_2 ↑	pAO_2 ↑
pa O_2 ↓↓↓↓	paO_2 ↓↓ to ↓↓↓ (decrease is dependent on the degree of mismatch)	paO_2 = pAO_2	paO_2 normal	paO_2 normal
A-a gradient O_2 ↑	A-a gradient O_2 ↑	A-a gradient O_2 normal	A-a gradient O_2 ↓	A-a gradient O_2 ↓↓
$paCO_2$ no change	$paCO_2$ ↓ to ↑↑↑	$paCO_2$ no change	$paCO_2$ ↓ to ↓↓	$paCO_2$ ↓↓

Alv=alveolus; awy=airway; mv=mixed venous blood; cap= capillary; atm=atmosphere; A = alveolar; a=arterial; A-a=alveolar/arterial gradient; this chart was created with the assistance of Mary Ellen B. Wohl, MD (Professor, Harvard Medical School; Chief Emerita, Division of Respiratory Diseases, Children's Hospital, Boston).

Shunt equation: (areas with low ventilation/perfusion ratio); often termed venous admixture

$$\frac{Qs}{Q\ total} = \%\ shunt = \frac{\text{Content pulm cap } O_2 - \text{Content pulm art } O_2}{\text{Content pulm cap } O_2 - \text{Content pulm mixed venous } O_2}$$

Qs = shunted blood; Q total = total blood flow; pulm = pulmonary; cap = end capillary; art=arterial

A number of indices (such as the oxygenation index—see XVI D of this chapter) are short-cut versions of the shunt equation since much of neonatal lung disease is manifested by large degrees of venous admixture or shunt

Dead space (Bohr equation): (areas with high ventilation/perfusion ratio)

Anatomic dead space = lung areas (i.e., conducting airways) that are not involved in gas exchange

Can measure alveolar CO_2 by determining end tidal CO_2

$$\text{Anatomic dead space} = \frac{(\text{end tidal } CO_2 - \text{expired } CO_2)}{(\text{end tidal } CO_2)} \times \text{TV (tidal volume)}$$

Alveolar dead space = alveoli that are not involved in gas exchange with vasculature (i.e. $\dot{V}/\dot{Q} > 1$)

Physiologic dead space = anatomic dead space + alveolar dead space

$$\text{Physiologic dead space} = \frac{paCO_2 - \text{expired } CO_2}{paCO_2} \times \text{TV}$$

$paCO_2$ = arterial CO_2

VII. Respiratory Mechanics: Resistance (R)

A. TOTAL RESPIRATORY SYSTEM RESISTANCE

$$R = \frac{\text{change in pressure (cm } H_2O)}{\text{change in flow (L/sec)}}$$

Total respiratory system R = chest wall R (~25%) + airway R (~55%) + lung tissue R (~20%)

Total respiratory R values are 40–55 cm H_2O/L/sec

Resistance
Airway 55%
Chest 25%
Lung Tissue 20%

B. CHEST WALL RESISTANCE (~25% of total R in neonatal lung)

The chest wall R is measured by oscillatory and occlusion techniques

It is unlikely to increase with lung disease

The neonate has a higher chest wall resistance compared with older child or adult

C. AIRWAY RESISTANCE (~55% of total R in neonatal lung)

In neonate, ~50% of the airway R is due to nasal resistance

During inspiration, airways dilate, decreasing airway R

During expiration, airways have less tethering, increasing airway R

Gas flow can move by:

1. Laminar flow (small airways)

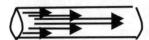 Gas travels in *straight* lines, faster-moving molecules are in the center

R increases with increased length of airway and increased viscosity of gas
R decreases with increasing radius
Laminar flow is unaffected by density of gas
Poiseuille's law for laminar flow

$$\text{Since } R = \frac{\text{change in pressure (cm H}_2\text{0)}}{\text{change in flow (L/sec)}} \text{ and R also} = \frac{\text{(length} \times \text{viscosity)}}{\text{(radius)}^4}$$

$$\rightarrow \text{flow} = \frac{\text{change in pressure} \times \pi \times \text{(radius)}^4}{8 \text{ (length} \times \text{viscosity)}}$$

2. Turbulent flow (large airways and at branching of airways, = convective acceleration)

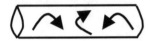 gas travels in *chaotic* movements

R increases with increased length of airway (as in laminar flow)
R decreases with increasing radius (as in laminar flow)
However, now R increases with density of gas (unlike laminar flow)

$$R \propto \frac{\text{(length} \times \text{density)}}{\text{(radius)}^5}$$

D. LUNG TISSUE RESISTANCE (~20% of total R in neonatal lung)

Due to friction between tissues of lung and chest wall

Higher in neonates due to increased tissue density (increased pulmonary interstitial fluid, especially in first few days of life)

VIII. Respiratory Mechanics: Volume (V)

A. LUNG CAPACITIES AND VOLUMES OF NORMAL NEONATE

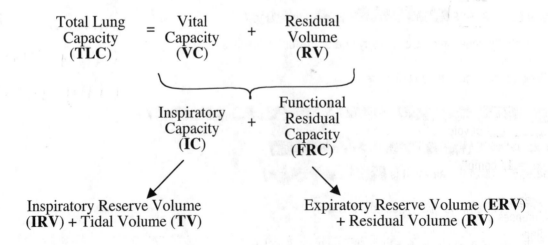

Insp. capacity
IC approximately = FRC

Tidal vol.
Dead space is approximately 1/3 TV (2 cc/kg)

TV approximately 5–7 cc/kg

Total Lung Capacity
TLC approximately 50–60 cc/kg

FRC approximately 20–30 cc/kg; FRC is actively maintained in the newborn
   In older children and adults, FRC is the volume at which the collapsing pressure of the lung is equal to the distending
      pressure of the chest
   Since premature and full-term infants breathe above resting FRC, they maintain FRC by active laryngeal braking leading
      to interruption of expiration

B. LUNG CAPACITIES AND VOLUMES OF NEONATE WITH HYALINE MEMBRANE DISEASE (HMD)

All above (TLC, VC, RV, IC, FRC, IRV, TV, ERV) are decreased in neonate with HMD

The volume in HMD lung is lower at end exhalation

Dead space is greater in neonate with HMD

IX. Respiratory Mechanics: Volume-Pressure

A. STATIC VOLUME-PRESSURE CURVES

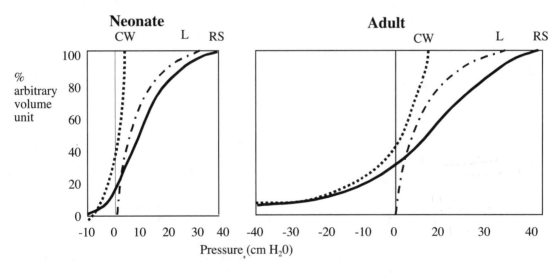

CW = chest wall; L = lung; RS = respiratory system. Modified from Fishman AP (ed): Handbook of Physiology Section 3: The Respiratory System. Bethesda, American Physiology Society, 1986, p 181.

Compliance (slope of volume-pressure curve) = change in volume/change in pressure

Elastance = 1/ compliance

Volume-pressure curve of the chest wall (CW)
   The differences between the volume-pressure chest wall curves of the neonate and adult are due to increased ratio of
      cartilage to bone, thinner cartilage, and softer bones (due to incomplete mineralization)

Neonate has greater chest wall compliance compared with adults
Premature infants have an even STEEPER chest wall curve due to greater chest wall compliance
Adults have a less compliant chest wall and thus volume-pressure curve is less steep

Volume-pressure curve of the lung (L)
Premature infants without lung disease have a more compliant lung compared with full-term infants, after correcting for volume
Premature infants with HMD have stiffer lungs leading to a FLATTER volume-pressure curve (i.e. less compliant lung)
Older children and young adults have stiffer lungs than infants

B. CREATION OF STATIC VOLUME-PRESSURE CURVES

To create static volume-pressure curves, volume is increased and related to the distending pressures using formulas below; pressures are measured at different inflation volumes

Static Pressures Across:	Distending Pressure = P inside − P outside	Simplified Distending Pressure
Lung (transpulmonary)	Alveolar P − pleural P	Airway P − pleural P
Chest wall	Pleural P − atmospheric P	Pleural P
Total respiratory system	Alveolar P − atmospheric P	Airway P

Modified from Hansen TN, Cooper TR and Weisman LE (eds): Neonatal Respiratory Diseases (2nd edition). Pennsylvania, Handbooks in Health Care Co, 1998, p 64.

Alveolar pressure: can't measure directly, so measure by occluding airway until absent gas flow and then measure airway P with transducer via face mask or endotracheal tube

Pleural pressure: measure using a P transducer from an intraesophageal balloon

Transthoracic pressure: across chest wall = pleural pressure − atmospheric pressure, assume atmospheric P = 0

Transpulmonary pressure: across lung = alveolar pressure − pleural pressure, assume alveolar P = airway P (note that during rapid inflation, transpulmonary P increases)

C. DYNAMIC LUNG VOLUME-PRESSURE CURVE

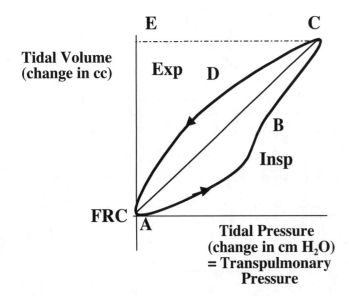

In contrast to static curves, the dynamic lung volume-pressure curves:
- Can be measured during *spontaneous* breathing
- Measure overall lung compliance at the volume the child is breathing
- Measure the work done to overcome different types of resistance
- Have two points with absent flow (A and C)

The dynamic compliance can be calculated from the slope of AC = compliance = $\dfrac{\text{change in V}}{\text{change in P}}$

Exp = expiration; Insp = inspiration; Modified from Goldsmith JP and Karotkin EH (eds): Assisted Ventilation of the Neonate (3rd edition). Philadelphia, WB Saunders Co, 1996, p 33.

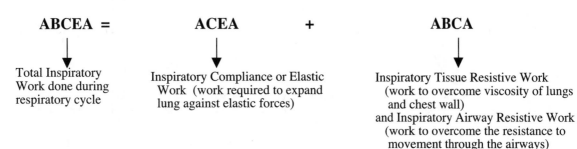

WORK of breathing = area under curve = Pressure (or force) × Volume (or displacement)

POWER = Work (kg cm) × Frequency (per min)

ABCEA =   ACEA   +   ABCA

↓   ↓   ↓

Total Inspiratory   Inspiratory Compliance or Elastic   Inspiratory Tissue Resistive Work
Work done during   Work (work required to expand   (work to overcome viscosity of lungs
respiratory cycle   lung against elastic forces)   and chest wall)
                                                                        and Inspiratory Airway Resistive Work
                                                                        (work to overcome the resistance to
                                                                        movement through the airways)

ACDA = Expiratory Resistive Work

ADCEA = Expiratory Elastic Work to stretch inspiratory muscles

In a normal lung, expiration is passive due to elastic recoil of lung; thus the majority of work occurs during inspiration

However, during rapid deep breathing or when airway resistance and/or tissue resistance increases, expiratory work is required

During normal breathing, most of the work is needed to expand the lungs (ACEA)

During rapid deep breathing, air flow is increased and a greater amount of work is needed to overcome airway resistance

D. DYNAMIC LUNG VOLUME-PRESSURE CURVES IN DIFFERENT DISEASE STATES

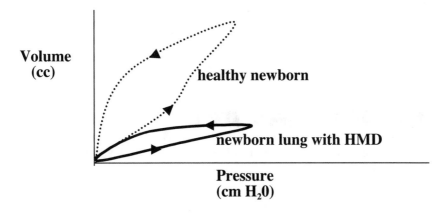

Modified from Goldsmith JP and Karotkin EH (eds): Assisted Ventilation of the Neonate (3rd edition). Philadelphia, WB Saunders Co, 1996, p 32.

HMD—very little difference (i.e., decreased hysteresis) between inspiratory and expiratory P/V loops due to stiff lungs
  Decreased compliance represented by decreased slope
  A greater change in pressure is required for a given change in volume

CLD (chronic lung disease)—similar curve to newborn lung with HMD but at *higher lung volumes*
  Decreased compliance represented by decreased slope
  A greater change in pressure is required for a given change in volume

E. TIDAL FLOW/VOLUME LOOPS IN DIFFERENT DISEASE STATES

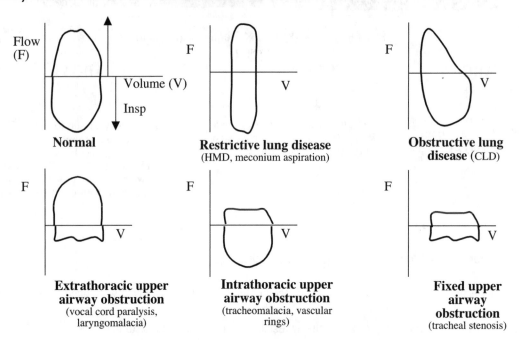

Normal

Restrictive lung disease
(HMD, meconium aspiration)

Obstructive lung disease (CLD)

Extrathoracic upper airway obstruction
(vocal cord paralysis, laryngomalacia)

Intrathoracic upper airway obstruction
(tracheomalacia, vascular rings)

Fixed upper airway obstruction
(tracheal stenosis)

X. Respiratory Mechanics: Time Constant

Time constant = resistance × compliance

$$\text{Time} = \frac{P\ (cm\ H_2O)}{flow} \times \frac{V\ (cc)}{P\ (cm\ H_2O)}$$

$$\text{Time} = \frac{P\ (cm\ H_2O)}{V/time} \times \frac{V\ (cc)}{P\ (cm\ H_2O)}$$

$$\text{Time} = \frac{time}{V} \times V$$

The time constant is an index of how rapidly the lung can empty

The lower the resistance or the lower the compliance (i.e., the stiffer the lung), the faster the lung empties and the shorter the time constant

normal = 0.12–0.15 sec

Inspiratory time must be 3–5 × time constant
  One time constant = time for alveoli to discharge 63% of its volume through the airways
  Two time constants = 84% of volume leaves
  Three time constants = 95% of volume leaves

Time constant changes with different disease states:
  1. HMD: during initial phase of HMD, require a longer I time since lung will empty rapidly but require more time to fill; however, during the recovery phase, a short expiratory time may fail to provide adequate emptying time and thus may need to increase E time (which will decrease I time)
  2. CLD: decrease ventilator rate, which allows one to lengthen the I time and E time

XI. Respiratory Mechanics: Neonate vs Adult

Increased in neonates compared with adults	Decreased in neonates compared with adults	Similar in neonates and adults
Respiratory rate (RR)	Tidal volume	Dead space
Residual volume	Total lung capacity	Functional residual capacity
Minute ventilation (TV × RR)	Inspiratory capacity	
Alveolar ventilation [(TV − dead space) × RR]	Vital capacity	
Oxygen consumption		

XII. Respiratory Mechanics: Neonatal Disease

	Lung Compliance (cc/cmH₂O)	Resistance (cc/cmH₂0/sec)	Time Constant (sec)	FRC (cc/kg)	V̇/Q̇ Matching	Work
Normal full term	4–6	20–40	0.25	20–30	–	–
HMD	↓↓	–	↓↓	↓	↓/↓↓	↑
Meconium aspiration	↓/–	↑/↑↑	↑	↑/↑↑	↓↓	↑
CLD	↑/↓	↑↑	↑	↑↑	↓↓/↓	↑↑
Air leak	↓↓	–/↑	–/↑	↑↑	↓/↓↓	↑↑
VLBW infant with apnea	↓	–	↓↓	–/↓	↓/–	–/↑

FRC = functional residual capacity; V/Q = ventilation/perfusion; HMD = hyaline membrane disease; VLBW = very low birth weight ; – = minimal change; ↑ increase; ↓ decrease; / = or; Printed with permission from Cloherty JC and Stark AR (eds): Manual of Neonatal Care (4th edition). Philadelphia, Lippincott-Raven Publishers, 1998, p 344.

XIII. Oxygen (O₂) Physiology

A. OXYGEN ALVEOLAR/ARTERIAL (A-a) GRADIENT

A's c worsening oxygenation

$$A\text{-a gradient of } O_2 = [FiO_2(p_B - pH_2O)] - (paCO_2/RQ) - (paO_2)$$

P_B = barometric pressure; $pH_2O = 47$; RQ = respiratory quotient, which is the ratio of excreted CO_2 to the O_2 taken up by the lungs and is typically = 0.8; FiO_2 in decimal form (i.e. use 0.7 if 70% FiO_2); note that the A-a gradient = (ideal alveolar oxygen equation) − (paO_2)

The A-a gradient increases with higher levels of inspired oxygen; the A-a gradient in room air is 10–15 and ~80–100 if FiO_2 is 100% in normal individuals

The A-a gradient in room air increases with increasing ventilation/perfusion mismatch

The A-a gradient in 100% FiO_2 increases with shunting

If the A-a gradient in 100% FiO_2 is >600 for 8–12 hours, extracorporeal membrane oxygenation (ECMO) needed

B. EFFECT OF ALTITUDE ON paO₂

As altitude increases, barometric pressure decreases and the partial P of O_2 decreases; thus, need to increase FiO_2 to maintain equal paO_2

$$(p_{B\#1} - pH_2O) \times FiO_{2\#1} = (p_{B\#2} - pH_2O) \times FiO_{2\#2}$$

i.e., if a neonate with RDS is requiring 100% O_2 in Denver where the p_B is 687, what percent O_2 is needed to result in the same paO_2 in Boston (at sea level)?

Since $pH_2O = 47$ in both locales and p_b at sea level = 760 then, $(687−47) \times 1.0 = (760−47) \times ?; ? = 89\%$ oxygen

C. OXYHEMOGLOBIN DISSOCIATION CURVE

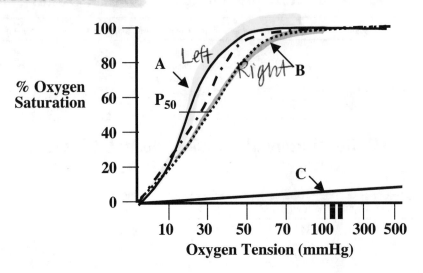

Modified from Fanaroff AA and Martin RJ (eds): Neonatal-Perinatal Medicine (6th edition). St Louis, Mosby–Year Book Inc, 1997, p 1011.

A = curve to LEFT (or *L* for LOW suggesting low acid, low $paCO_2$, low 2,3-DPG, low temperature)
Lower P_{50} (defined as the paO_2 at which hemoglobin (Hb) is 50% saturated)
Decreased release of oxygen from Hb (poor O_2 delivery)
Occurs with:
   Alkalosis/ high pH
   Lower $paCO_2$
   Increased fetal Hb
   Decreased temperature
   Decreased 2,3-diphosphoglycerate (DPG)
   HbCO (carboxyhemoglobin)

B = curve to RIGHT (or RIGHT as in *R* for release with *I* (increased) 2,3-DP*G*, increased *H*ydrogen and increased
   *T*emperature
Higher P_{50}
Increased release of oxygen (improved O_2 delivery)
Occurs with:
   Acidosis/low pH
   Higher $paCO_2$
   Increased adult Hb
   Increased temperature
   Increased 2,3-DPG
   α-Thalassemia (associated with decreased fetal Hb)

C = linear curve
Oxygen dissolved in plasma $=0.003$ cc O_2/dL torr $\times$ paO_2 (torr)

D. OXYGEN DELIVERY (cc/kg/min)

To alveoli → = (alveolar minute ventilation) $\times$ (FiO_2)
           = (tidal volume − dead space) (frequency)(FiO_2)
To tissues → = (O_2 carrying capacity)(cardiac output)(10)
           = (O_2 bound to Hb + dissolved O_2) (cardiac output) (10)

E. OXYGEN CARRYING CAPACITY

$$\text{O}_2 \text{ content of blood} = \text{O}_2 \text{ bound to Hb} + \text{dissolved O}_2$$

$$[(1.34 \text{ cc O}_2/\text{gHb}) \times \text{Hb (g/dL)} \times \text{O}_2 \text{ sat}] + [(.003 \text{ cc O}_2/\text{dl torr}) \times \text{paO}_2]$$

sat = saturation—use decimal; paO$_2$ in torrs

A small change in pO$_2$ will give a large increase in oxygen content on the steep part of the curve (40–60 torr)

There is a profound effect in O$_2$ content with changes in Hb concentration

There is very little change in O$_2$ content following a change in dissolved O$_2$

Fetal Hb has a higher affinity for oxygen than the adult, so 1.37 cc O$_2$/gHb is often used instead of 1.34

F. OXYGEN CONSUMPTION = FICK PRINCIPLE = $\dot{\text{V}}\text{O}_2$

The Fick principle states that the oxygen consumption is the difference between the O$_2$ delivered to the tissues (blood flow $\times$ oxygen content in the arterial blood) and the O$_2$ returning from the tissues (blood flow $\times$ oxygen content in the venous blood)

$$\dot{\text{V}}\text{O}_2 = \text{CO (dL/min)} \times (\text{CaO}_2 - \text{CvO}_2)$$

CO = cardiac output; CaO$_2$ = oxygen content of blood in arterial system; CvO$_2$ = oxygen content of mixed venous blood

Since oxygen content in either arterial or venous system = (1.34) (Hb concentration) O$_2$sat + .003 $\times$ paO$_2$, and .003 $\times$ paO$_2$ is minimal:

$$\dot{\text{V}}\text{O}_2 = \text{CO} \times (1.34 \text{ cc/g Hb}) \text{ (Hb concentration) (arterial sat} - \text{venous sat)}$$

note: use dL/min for CO; Hb concentration in g/dL; use decimal for saturation, i.e., arterial sat = 90% then use 0.9

If O$_2$ delivery to issues is decreased (e.g., lung disease, decreased O$_2$ carrying capacity, decreased tissue perfusion), tissues will attempt to maintain tissue O$_2$ levels by:
1. *Increasing O$_2$ extraction*—leading to decreased venous pO$_2$ and an increased difference between arterial and venous O$_2$ content
   Tissue extraction ability is limited since a tissue/blood O$_2$ gradient is necessary for diffusion to occur
2. *Recruiting more capillaries*—leading to enhanced O$_2$ delivery
   However, if the amount of O$_2$ delivered reaches a critical level, cells can become anoxic and change from *aerobic* metabolism (produces 38 moles of adenosine triphosphate (ATP) per mole of glucose) to *anaerobic* metabolism (produces 2 moles of ATP per mole of glucose and 2 moles of lactic acid per mole of glucose) to meet cellular energy requirements

Increased oxygen consumption:
1. Increased caloric intake
2. Decreased body temperature
3. Neonate >> adult (6–8 vs 3.2 cc/kg/min)
4. Term > premature infant
5. Appropriate for gestational age infant > small for gestational age infant

G. OXYGEN TRANSFER

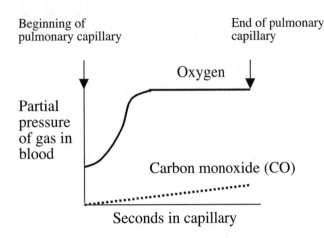

Beginning of pulmonary capillary

End of pulmonary capillary

Oxygen

Partial pressure of gas in blood

Carbon monoxide (CO)

Seconds in capillary

This graph demonstrates that the partial pressure of *oxygen* along the pulmonary capillary is *alinear and limited by perfusion*.
In contrast, the linear slope of the *CO* curve depends solely on the time in the capillary and thus, transfer is *diffusion-limited*.

Modified from West JB: Respiratory Physiology (6th edition). Philadelphia, Lippincott, Williams & Wilkins, 2000, p 23.

XIV. Carbon Dioxide Physiology

A. CARBON DIOXIDE TRANSPORT

While O_2 transport evolved to maximize O_2 carrying capacity, CO_2 transport evolved to maximize CO_2 transfer from the body (with high concentrations) to the atmosphere (with low concentrations)

$$\text{Total } CO_2 = \text{dissolved } CO_2 \ (7\%) + \text{bicarbonate or } HCO_3^- \ (70\%) + HbCO_2 \ (23\%)$$

Since CO_2 is $20 \times$ more soluble in blood compared to O_2 and the CO_2 dissociation curve is almost linear, CO_2 can be transported in large amounts in the blood

CO_2 can be extracted from blood with only a small change in blood CO_2 levels

B. BOHR EFFECT

Changes in $paCO_2$ can shift the oxyhemoglobin dissociation curve leading to increased oxygenation of blood in the lungs and also increased release of O_2 from blood to the tissues

Alveolar CO_2 increases as blood passes through the lungs; thus $paCO_2$ decreases and the oxyhemoglobin curve shifts to the left, leading to increased amount of O_2 bound and increased O_2 transport to tissues

After traveling to the tissues, CO_2 now enters the blood from the tissues, leading to increased $paCO_2$ levels and the oxyhemoglobin curve is shifted to the right; this allows for improved O_2 delivery

C. HALDANE EFFECT

This effect is the reverse of the Bohr effect

The Haldane effect is more important in assisting CO_2 transport than the Bohr effect in promoting O_2 transport

The binding of O_2 to Hb in alveolar capillaries increases CO_2 unloading from the capillary blood into the alveoli

In tissue capillaries, O_2 is removed from Hb and thus, increases CO_2 binding to Hb

CO_2 dissociation curve shifts upwards when O_2 decreases

CO_2 dissociation curve to right when O_2 saturation increases

D. HENDERSON-HASSELBALCH EQUATION

$$\text{Hydrogen concentration} = \frac{(24 \times pCO_2)}{\text{bicarbonate concentration}}$$

An increase in bicarbonate concentration leads to an increase in pH

An increase in pCO_2 leads to a decrease in pH

Since one can change pCO_2 by changing RR, the respiratory system can alter the pH

The kidney can alter the bicarbonate concentration and thus, change the pH

XV. Abnormal Hb Binding States

A. CARBOXYHEMOGLOBINEMIA (shift to Left on Oxghgb. curve)

Etiology
Excess carbon monoxide (CO) from tobacco smoke, fires, motor vehicle exhaust

Physiology
CO and O_2 bind to Hb at the same heme site
CO binds to Hb much better than O_2 so even very low levels of CO will compete with O_2 for Hb binding and impair O_2-carrying capacity of red blood cells
In addition to decreasing the amount of O_2 bound to Hb, CO increases the affinity of Hb for the remaining bound O_2 (shifts oxyhemoglobin curve to left) and decreases O_2 delivery to the tissues
Since HbCO absorbs light similar to O_2 bound to Hb, HbCO will falsely elevate O_2 saturation

Fetal effects
CO does cross placenta and bind to fetal Hb; the fetus is at risk even if there is a low amount of CO since fetal Hb already leads to poor O_2 delivery

Management
If CO poisoning, treat with 100% O_2 since high levels of O_2 can displace CO from Hb; can also add some CO_2 to increase respiratory drive

B. METHEMOGLOBINEMIA

Etiology
Excess nitrates, nitrite, maternal prilocaine, aniline dyes, hemoglobin M disease (heme iron more stable in ferric state)

Physiology
Everyone accumulates metHb daily yet normally red blood cells (with intact cytochrome b5 reductase system) will reduce it
In methemoglobinemia, the iron of Hb changes from ferrous (reduced) to ferric (oxidized) state, decreasing O_2 carrying capacity

Normal paO_2 yet decreased O_2 sat (less O_2 bound to Hb)
Calculated O_2 sat is normal in contrast to the measured O_2 sat

Diagnosis
Arterial blood appears brown following exposure to O_2

Management
Can treat with methylene blue (after treatment, urine appears blue/green)

XVI. Mechanical Ventilation Parameters

A. MEAN AIRWAY PRESSURE (MAP)

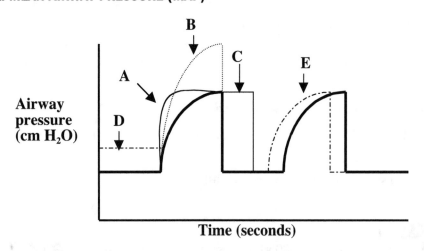

Curve **A** increased flow
Curve **B** increased PIP
Curve **C** increased I time and
    decreased E time
Curve **D** increased PEEP
Curve **E** increased rate

PIP=peak inspiratory pressure; PEEP=
positive end expiratory pressure; I time =
inspiratory time; E time = expiratory time

Modified from Goldsmith JP and Karotkin EH (eds): Assisted Ventilation of the Neonate (3rd edition). Philadelphia, WB Saunders Co, 1996, p 60.

$$MAP = \frac{\text{area under curve}}{\text{time}}$$

Oxygenation is most dependent on MAP

The most effective way to increase MAP: $\uparrow$ PEEP $>$ $\uparrow$ PIP $>$ $\uparrow$ I time: E time

If increase PEEP, this occurs at the expense of ventilation with a decrease in TV

$$MAP = K\,(PIP\text{-}PEEP) \times I\,time\,(I\,time + E\,time) + PEEP$$

K = a constant

B. BENEFITS AND RISKS OF ADJUSTING VENTILATOR PARAMETERS

Parameter	Benefits	Risks
Increase PEEP	Maintains high FRC and prevents alveolar collapse Increases MAP (improves oxygenation) Splints obstructed airways	Increased risk of air leak Decreases TV if no change in PIP Can obstruct venous return CO_2 retention (associated with decreased TV) Shifts to stiffer compliance curve (i.e. less compliant)

(continued on following page)

Parameter	Benefits	Risks
Increase PIP	Increases MAP (improves oxygenation) Prevents atelectasis	Can obstruct venous return Increased risk of barotrauma leading to air leak and/or CLD
Increase rate	Increases MAP (improves oxygenation) Decreases PIP requirement	Inadvertent PEEP (i.e., inadequate emptying time leading to air trapping) May lead to inadequate TV
Increase I time	Increases MAP (improves oxygenation)	Can obstruct venous return May lead to inadequate emptying time Leads to slower rates and increased PIP requirement with increased risk of barotrauma
Increase flow	Increases MAP (improves oxygenation)	Increased risk of barotrauma, increased resistance

PEEP = positive end expiratory pressure; PIP = peak inspiratory pressure; Modified from Cloherty JC and Stark AR (eds): Manual of Neonatal Care, 4th edition. Philadelphia, Lippincott–Raven Publishers, 1998, pp 340 and 342.

C. ACUTE RESPIRATORY DETERIORATION IN THE VENTILATED NEONATE

Possible etiologies
Endotracheal tube malposition (right mainstem or extubated)
Mucous plugging and/or excessive secretions
Air leak
Pleural effusion
Pulmonary edema

D. OXYGEN INDEX (OI)

$$OI = \frac{(MAP \times FiO_2)}{postductal\ paO_2} \times 100$$

Note: FiO_2 in decimal form

As severity of lung disease worsens, OI will increase (> 25 consistent with very severe lung disease)

E. PARAMETERS TO DECREASE PCO$_2$

1. *Increase rate:* however, this can lead to inadvertent PEEP (stacked breaths) which would decrease TV and increase CO_2

2. *Increase PIP:* however, this can increase barotrauma

3. *Decrease PEEP:* to decrease dead space and increase tidal volume
   However, this will also decrease MAP

4. *Increase flow:* however, this can increase barotrauma

5. *Increasing E time:* however, this will shorten I time and decrease MAP

XVII. Mode of Ventilation

CPAP: ↑FRC
*may interfere c̄ venous return
↓ frequ. of obstructive or mixed apnea ↓CO
*does ∅ improve ventilation

A. CONTINUOUS POSITIVE AIRWAY PRESSURE (CPAP)

Indications
Mild HMD, apnea, transitional mode following intubation

Function
Maintains positive pressure in airways during spontaneous breathing
Improves oxygenation of alveoli that are partially or complete open (i.e., CPAP is ineffective for collapsed alveoli)

Increases functional residual capacity
Decreases total airway resistance
Decreases lung compliance
Decreases work of breathing
Improves gas exchange by preventing atelectasis during expiration

Complications
Abdominal distention due to increased air flow into esophagus
Nasal obstruction from increased secretions
Nasal septum erosion

B. MODES OF CONVENTIONAL VENTILATION (CV)

Mode of Ventilation	Traits	Infant with Good Compliance	Infant with Poor Compliance
Volume-cycled	Set volume needed		
	Pressure generated to attain volume required	Pressure generated: ↑	Pressure generated: ↑↑
	Pressure generated is indirectly related to lung compliance	Volume generated: ↑↑↑	Volume generated: ↑↑↑
Pressure-cycled	Set pressure needed		
	Volume generated to attain pressure required	Pressure generated: ↑↑	Pressure generated: ↑↑
	Volume generated is proportional to compliance	Volume generated: ↑↑↑	Volume generated: ↑↑
Time-cycled	Set time and flow		
	Pressure unlimited	Pressure generated: ↑	Pressure generated: ↑↑
	Pressure generated is indirectly related to lung compliance		
	Volume generated is proportional to compliance	Volume generated: ↑↑↑	Volume generated: ↑↑

Modified from Goldsmith JP and Karotkin EH (eds): Assisted Ventilation of the Neonate (3rd edition). Philadelphia, WB Saunders Co, 1996, p 17.

C. HIGH FREQUENCY VENTILATION (HFV) ✳ *Homogeneous lung disease*

Mechanism
HFV delivers high MAP using small TVs (often less than anatomical dead space, attempting to limit barotrauma) and rapid rates
Mechanisms not well understood with gas transport occurring by:
Bulk convection (bulk axial flow of gas)
Pendelluft (gas moves between neighboring alveoli due to different time constants)
Asymmetric velocity (altering velocities of gas during inspiration and expiration)
Taylor dispersion (parabolic movement of inspired gas with the highest velocity in the middle; provides an increased area for diffusion to occur)
Molecular diffusion (diffusion gradient leads to transport of gases across alveoli)

Indications
Homogeneous lung disease (in contrast to heterogeneous disease that responds better to lower frequency), air leak, hypercarbia, persistent hypoxemia not responsive to CV

Clinical
High volume and high MAP (2-5 cm greater than CV) strategy to recruit alveoli;
Low volume and low MAP (~= CV) strategy to prevent extension of air leaks

Complications of HFV

Decreased cardiac output (often secondary to increased MAP and lung overexpansion, which may lead to secondary hypoxemia)

Air trapping (consider if low paO_2 despite well-inflated lungs—need to consider decreasing MAP to improve paO_2)

Tracheal injury, mucous impaction, unclear if increased risk intraventricular hemorrhage

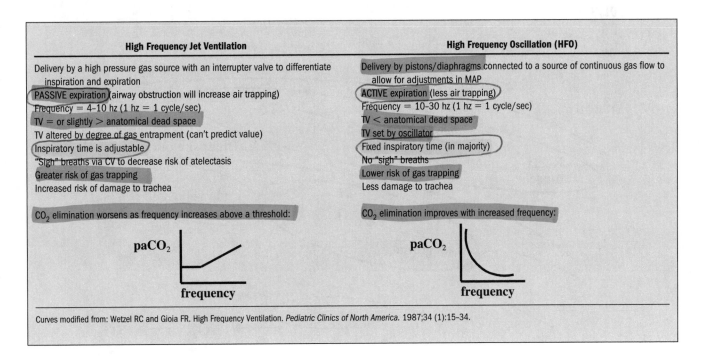

High Frequency Jet Ventilation	High Frequency Oscillation (HFO)
Delivery by a high pressure gas source with an interrupter valve to differentiate inspiration and expiration	Delivery by pistons/diaphragms connected to a source of continuous gas flow to allow for adjustments in MAP
PASSIVE expiration (airway obstruction will increase air trapping)	ACTIVE expiration (less air trapping)
Frequency = 4–10 hz (1 hz = 1 cycle/sec)	Frequency = 10–30 hz (1 hz = 1 cycle/sec)
TV = or slightly > anatomical dead space	TV < anatomical dead space
TV altered by degree of gas entrapment (can't predict value)	TV set by oscillator
Inspiratory time is adjustable	Fixed inspiratory time (in majority)
"Sigh" breaths via CV to decrease risk of atelectasis	No "sigh" breaths
Greater risk of gas trapping	Lower risk of gas trapping
Increased risk of damage to trachea	Less damage to trachea
CO_2 elimination worsens as frequency increases above a threshold:	CO_2 elimination improves with increased frequency:

Curves modified from: Wetzel RC and Gioia FR. High Frequency Ventilation. *Pediatric Clinics of North America.* 1987;34 (1):15–34.

XVIII. Extracorporeal Membrane Oxygenation (ECMO)

A. CRITERIA (note: may vary slightly between centers)

1. Failing maximal ventilatory support with FiO_2 = 100%, typically PIP > 35 cm and paO_2 < 40 mm Hg

2. A-a O_2 gradient > 600 while on ventilatory support receiving 100% O_2 for 8–12 hours (correlated with 80% predicted mortality without ECMO)

3. Oxygenation index > 40 (correlated with 80% predicted mortality without ECMO)

4. Acute deterioration with paO_2 < 30–40 mm Hg

B. CONTRAINDICATIONS

1. Premature infant (GA < 34 weeks) due to increased risk of intraventricular hemorrhage

2. Severe intraventricular hemorrhage

3. Irreversible lung disease (e.g., CLD)

4. Irreversible severe neurological abnormalities

5. Congenital anomalies incompatible with a good long-term outcome

XIX. Nitric Oxide (NO)

A. DEFINITION

An endogenous endothelium-derived gaseous molecule that relaxes vascular tone

B. METABOLISM

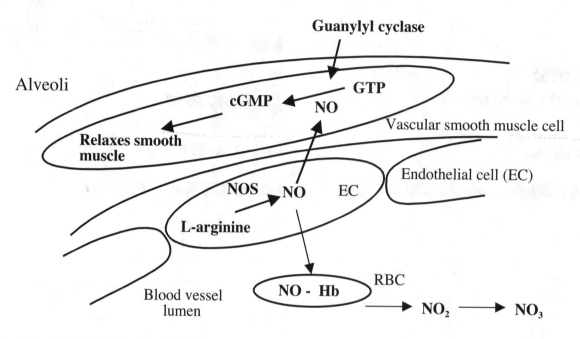

Modified from Fratacci MD, Frostell CG, Chen TY, et al: Inhaled nitric oxide. A selective pulmonary vasodilator of heparin-protamine vasoconstriction in sheep. *Anesthesiology.* 1991;75(6): 990–999.

Endogenous NO is formed from L-arginine by nitric oxide synthase (NOS) in endothelial cells lining the blood vessel walls

Some NO then diffuses into the adjacent vascular smooth muscle cell and activates guanylyl cyclase

This leads to increased cyclic guanosine monophosphate (cGMP) with vascular smooth muscle relaxation and decreased vascular tone

The remaining NO diffuses into the intravascular space, quickly binds with Hb, and becomes oxidized to NO_2 and NO_3 (leading to inactivation)

Exogenous NO has the same effect as endogenous NO; when given in the inhaled form, NO reaches the alveoli and then diffuses into adjacent vascular smooth muscle and endothelial cells

C. EFFECT OF INHALED NO ✻ contraindicated c̄ cong. ♡ c̄ dependant R→L shunt

Exogenous NO decreases pulmonary vascular resistance (PVR) (similarly, endogenous NO has been shown to be important in decreasing PVR at time of birth with levels of cGMP increasing within minutes after onset of breathing)

Inhaled NO selectively dilates pulmonary blood vessels that are ventilated, thereby improving ventilation/perfusion matching and providing effective pulmonary vasodilation (in contrast to intravenously administered vasodilators that dilate the entire pulmonary vascular bed, even those areas that are not well ventilated)

In contrast to intravenous pulmonary vasodilators, inhaled NO does not cause peripheral vasodilation since the gaseous molecule binds rapidly to Hb when it reaches the vasculature

By decreasing intrapulmonary shunting, increasing arterial O_2, and decreasing ventilation/perfusion mismatching, NO enables ventilation to occur at lower mean airway pressures, improving tissue oxygenation and decreasing FiO_2 requirement

D. INDICATIONS

Pulmonary hypertension associated with lung disease, sepsis and congenital heart disease

E. SIDE EFFECTS

1. Methemoglobinemia (especially with prolonged exposure at high doses >20 parts per million or ppm)

2. Increased oxidants (nitrogen dioxide and peroxynitrite) that can lead to pulmonary injury (especially with dose > 20 ppm)

3. Uncertain long-term effects (especially in premature infants who are more susceptible to oxidant injury because of decreased endogenous antioxidant defense system)

4. Uncertain if NO affects bleeding time or platelet function in neonates

F. CLINICAL USE

Approved by FDA—December 1999 (infants $\geq$ 34 weeks gestation)

Clinical studies have shown that NO enhances oxygenation and decreases ECMO requirement (especially if combined with HFO) in a majority of neonates with PHTN

Dosage typically between 2 and 20 ppm

Even small amounts of inhaled NO are very effective

After inhaled NO is discontinued, infant can have rebound pulmonary vasoconstriction (partly due to suppression of endogenous NO production)

Need to follow MetHb levels and possibly nitrogen dioxide levels

Contraindicated if congenital heart disease with dependent right-to-left shunting or high baseline MetHb levels

XX. Pulmonary Diseases

A. RESPIRATORY DISTRESS SYNDROME (RDS) OR HMD ↓ compliance (stiff lungs)

		diffuse atelectasis
Pathophysiology	Surfactant deficiency Uncomplicated course characterized by peak severity at 1–3 days Onset of recovery at ~72 hrs (usually coinciding with diuresis)	V/Q mismatching
Risk factors	Low gestational age Male predominance Maternal diabetes Perinatal depression	* c̄ surf Replacement: ↑comp-risk pneumo, TC lengthens

(continued on following page)

Clinical	Respiratory distress (grunting, flaring, retractions, tachypnea)
	Cyanosis
Pulmonary function	Decreased lung compliance
	Unstable alveoli (smaller alveoli will collapse during exhalation—Laplace's law)
	Decreased FRC
	Shunting of blood through atelectatic areas leading to hypoxia
Pathologic	Hyaline membranes located at junction of dilated respiratory bronchioles and dilated alveolar ducts
	Hyaline membranes contain cellular debris from injured epithelium and fibrinous matrix components
	Minimally aerated lungs, diffuse alveolar atelectasis
Prevention	Antenatal corticosteroid administration (at least 24–48 hours prior to delivery)
	Tocolytic agents to arrest premature labor
Management	Artificial surfactant replacement *Avoid peep ↑6 = interfere c̄ CO
	Respiratory support and monitoring
	Oxygen supplementation
	Fluid and metabolic management

B. TRANSIENT TACHYPNEA OF THE NEWBORN (TTN)

Pathophysiology	Delayed clearance of fetal lung fluid
	Usually resolves by 48 to 72 hours
Risk factors	Delivery by cesarean section
	Maternal diabetes
	Perinatal depression
	Maternal sedation
	Precipitous delivery
Clinical	Tachypnea
	Respiratory distress typically mild, +/− cyanosis
Management	Respiratory support and monitoring
	Oxygen supplementation
	Some may require CPAP

C. PNEUMONIA persistant focal opacifications on xray are uncommon in neonatal pneum: consider CCAM, pneum sequestration

Pathophysiology	Transplacental
	Aspiration of contaminated amniotic fluid (and/or meconium)
	Hematogenous
	Inhalation
Pathogens	⊗ Early: Group B streptococci (GBS), *Escherichia coli, Klebsiella, Listeria* , H.flu
	Late: above plus *Staphylococcus aureus, Pseudomonas,* fungal, chlamydia
	Other: ureaplasma viral (cytomegalovirus, herpes, respiratory syncytial virus, enterovirus, rubella), syphilis
	BPD
Risk factors	Prolonged rupture of membranes > 24 hrs and other sepsis risk factors
	Gasping due to fetal asphyxia (leads to increased risk of aspiration)
Clinical	Respiratory distress, possible cyanosis *Tracheal aspirates
	Poor feeding, lethargy c̄ in 8hrs of birth
	Fever (especially if herpes or enterovirus) showing bacteria &WBC
	Diagnosis by CXR (typically abnormal 24–72 hours after symptoms) on Wright's stain = highly
	CXR findings can appear very similar to RDS (especially if GBS) predictive of pneumonia
Management	Respiratory support and monitoring
	Gram stain and culture of blood and tracheal secretions
	Antibiotics Broad spectrum (PCN, aminoglycoside OR cephalosporin)
	Overall good prognosis

ASSO w/BPD(CLD)

* ureaplasma - if chronically ventilated
       *sensitive to erythromycin
       └ Requires special cx. condition

D. AIR LEAK

1. Pneumothorax

Physiology	Air between parietal pleura lining the chest wall and the visceral pleura covering the lung
Risk factors	Aspiration of blood, meconium, amniotic fluid Lung diseases including meconium aspiration syndrome, RDS (especially if pulmonary interstitial emphysema), pulmonary hypoplasia, congenital diaphragmatic hernia, pneumonia High ventilatory pressures Intubated infant with improving compliance Ventilated infant with expiratory efforts opposing ventilated breaths Spontaneous pneumothorax can occur in 1–2% of healthy FT infants, often asymptomatic
Clinical	Respiratory distress, cyanosis, apnea, and bradycardia Affected side with decreased breath sounds and increased anterior posterior (AP) diameter Displaced point of maximal impulse If under tension, acute decrease in BP, heart rate, and respiratory rate Increased risk of intraventricular hemorrhage due to decreased venous return if tension pneumothorax or sudden improvement in cerebral perfusion following chest tube placement Increased risk of syndrome of inappropriate anti-diuretic hormone Transilluminate: place probe bilateral axilla region and below diaphragm; falsely negative if large infant (increased skin thickness) or small air leak; falsely positive if subcutaneous edema, pneumomediastinum, lobar emphysema
Management	Ventilator: decrease PEEP, decrease PIP, decrease I time, increase rate Conservative management if no underlying lung disease, not ventilated, minimal respiratory distress, and no continuous leak Observe closely for signs of deterioration, follow CXRs, minimize crying (typically, extrapulmonary air will resolve in 24–48 hours) Consider 100% oxygen to obtain nitrogen washout if smaller leaks Needle aspiration Chest tube if continuous air leak, ventilated, and/or underlying pulmonary disease

2. Pneumomediastinum air leakage into mediastinum

Occurs in healthy infants, infants with RDS or pneumonia, s/p delivery room resuscitation due to direct trauma to posterior pharynx and/or airways, mechanical ventilation

Majority asymptomatic since air is seldom under tension

If symptomatic, may have tachypnea, muffled heart sounds, cyanosis

✳ Resolves spontaneously ✳

3. Pneumopericardium air leakage into pericardial sac

Symptoms dependent upon level of tension and include cyanosis, muffled heart sounds, hypotension (due to inferior vena cava compression and decreased cardiac venous return leading to decreased stroke volume)

Pericardial needle aspiration if symptoms severe

High mortality rate

4. Pulmonary interstitial emphysema (PIE) air leakage into interstitial space

PIE = position on side affected

Majority of infants are premature and ventilated with severe RDS

Interstitial air leads to decreased lung compliance, ventilation/perfusion mismatch, increased dead space

Manage by decreasing MAP; consider HFV; if unilateral involvement, can position infant on side of affected lung; consider selective bronchial intubation in rare, severe cases

E. CHRONIC LUNG DISEASE (CLD)

provide more cal c̄
✳ more lipid & carb b/c ↓resp.quotient which dimin. CO_2 production

Pathophysiology	Pulmonary immaturity
	   Imbalance of proteases/anti-proteases
	   Imbalance of oxidants/anti-oxidants
	Inflammation
	Oxygen toxicity
	Mechanical ventilation leading to barotrauma and/or volutrauma
	Above leading to areas of atelectasis, overdistention and fibrosis
	Associated with ureaplasma pneumonia

✳ can cause RV hypertrophy & cor pulmonale

(continued on following page)

Pulmonary function	*Lower lung compliance*
	Increased airway resistance
	Increased work of breathing
	Impaired gas exchange
	Greater volumes, overdistention
	Small tidal volumes, increased RR
	Ventilation/perfusion mismatch and increased work of breathing leading to CO_2 retention
	Can lead to right ventricular hypertrophy and cor pulmonale
Management	Vitamin A for first 12 weeks of life to attempt prevention
	Supportive care and adequate nutrition
	Fluid restriction $+/-$ diuretics
	Bronchodilators
	Corticosteroids (extremely controversial due to studies demonstrating long-term neurological effects and disrupted alveolarization)

Northway radiographic staging of bronchopulmonary dysplasia (BPD) 1967

I. Indistinguishable from acute RDS—poor inflation, generalized granular pattern, air bronchograms

II. Opacification of lung fields 4–10 days of age

III. Small diffuse *cystic* changes

IV. Gross distortion of lung architecture, typically beyond 1 month of age

  Large cystic areas

  Interstitial fibrosis

  Atelectasis

  Hyperinflation

Note: since surfactant therapy, the clinical and radiographic features that previously defined BPD in 1967, have changed and today, stage IV is less common

Wilson-Mikity syndrome

A rare neonatal lung disease with decreasing incidence, unknown pathophysiology

Clinical

  Typically, infant initially with minimal lung disease followed by progressively worsening lung disease over 1–4 weeks of life with slow recovery

  Radiographically indistinguishable from CLD

F. MECONIUM ASPIRATION SYNDROME

Pathophysiology	Mechanical obstruction
	Chemical inflammation
	Surfactant inactivation
	Associated with air leaks
Risk factors	Full-term or postmature
	Fetal distress
	In utero hypoxia
	Meconium-stained amniotic fluid
Clinical	Severe respiratory distress beginning shortly after birth
Pulmonary function	Decreased lung compliance
	Decreased alveolar ventilation and perfusion of poorly ventilated areas leading to hypoxemia
	Increased pulmonary vascular resistance (due to local pulmonary vasoconstriction, general pulmonary vasoconstriction following induction of vasoactive mediators, maldevelopment of pulmonary vasculature if exposed to chronic hypoxia)
Prevention	If meconium-stained amniotic fluid, suction nasopharynx at the perineum and direct tracheal suctioning if newborn is not vigorous
Management	Respiratory ventilator support and monitoring—ideal to maintain adequate expiratory time to prevent air trapping
	Manage pulmonary hypertension, monitor for signs of pneumothorax
	Surfactant administration due to surfactant inactivation by meconium and decreased surfactant production following alveolar injury
	Antibiotics since (1) meconium increases bacterial growth; (2) often cannot distinguish from pneumonia; and (3) sepsis may be precipitant for aspiration

G. PULMONARY HYPERTENSION (PHTN)

(handwritten note: Single or narrowly split S_2)
(handwritten note: R→L shunting)

Incidence	1–2 per 1000 births
Etiology	*Maladaptation:* normal structure of pulmonary vascular bed but PVR remains elevated e.g., hypoxia (can be associated with growth-restricted infants), asphyxia, hypothermia, hyperviscosity (polycythemia), pneumonia (meconium aspiration, amniotic fluid aspiration, bacterial), sepsis
	Maldevelopment: abnormal structure of pulmonary vascular beds leading to vascular smooth muscle hypertrophy e.g., intrauterine hypoxia, perinatal asphyxia, meconium aspiration, fetal ductus arteriosus closure, congenital heart disease (e.g., obstructive total anomalous pulmonary venous return), pulmonary hypoplasia, diaphragmatic hernia, alveolar capillary dysplasia
Pathophysiology	Increased PVR leads to right-to-left shunting at the atrial or ductal level
	The resultant decrease in pulmonary blood flow leads to hypoxemia
Clinical	Usually full-term or post-term
	Infant typically presents within the first 24 hours of life with severe cyanosis, respiratory distress
	Severe hypoxemia (less effect on CO_2 retention), labile oxygenation
	Single or narrowly split, loud S2
	If there is no atrial shunting and patent ductus arteriosus then, preductal O_2 sat > postductal O_2 sat (= differential cyanosis)
CXR	Decreased pulmonary vascular markings, normal, or increased heart size
EKG	May have ST changes due to subendocardial ischemia
Management	Obtain ECHO to rule out congenital heart disease; ECHO findings consistent with PHTN include pulmonary pressures similar to systemic pressures, tricuspid regurgitation, bowing of ventricular septum into LV, right-to-left shunting across PDA
	Treat with antibiotics since may be associated with sepsis
	Treat any underlying lung disease
	Administer 100% oxygen to increase pulmonary vasodilation
	Sedation, maximize oxygen carrying capacity with PRBC, maintain cardiac output (inotropic support if needed) with SBP slightly elevated to increase left-to-right shunting, ventilatory support (PEEP—yet may decrease cardiac output; hyperventilation with alkalinization; consider HFV)
	Inhaled nitric oxide
	In past, used nitroprusside (need to monitor cyanide levels) and tolazoline as pulmonary vasodilators yet these drugs also lead to systemic vasodilation
	ECMO if above therapies fail

PVR=pulmonary vascular resistance; ECHO= echocardiogram; LV= left ventricle; PRBC=packed red blood cells; SBP=systolic blood pressure

H. PULMONARY HEMORRHAGE

Pathophysiology	Due to an acute increase in capillary hydrostatic pressure (secondary to a left-to-right shunt from PDA or vasoconstriction following perinatal depression)
	This increased pressure leads to capillary vessel breakage and large amount of fluid leakage
Risk factors	PDA, sepsis, left ventricular failure, ?? surfactant administration
Clinical	Bloody tracheal secretions
	Respiratory distress, cyanosis
	Cardiovascular instability
Pulmonary function	Acute decrease in lung compliance
	Severe hypoxemia
Management	Increase PEEP to enhance alveolar distention and impede pulmonary blood flow
	Assess clotting factors and administer blood products as needed
	Treat PDA
	Consider echocardiogram to assess left ventricular function

I. TRACHEO-ESOPHAGEAL FISTULA (see Gastroenterology chapter)

XXI. Airway Obstruction

A. STRIDOR

Symptom that occurs as a result of turbulent air flow through a narrowed airway

Neonates are at increased risk of stridor due to small upper airways and incomplete development of supporting upper airway cartilages, leading to easy collapse

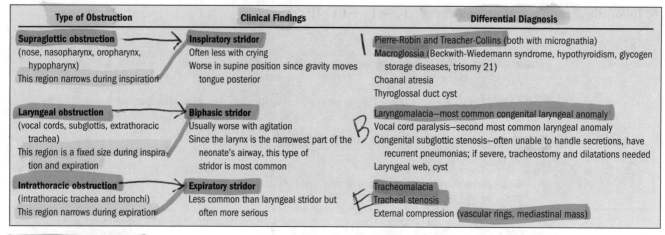

Type of Obstruction	Clinical Findings	Differential Diagnosis
Supraglottic obstruction (nose, nasopharynx, oropharynx, hypopharynx) This region narrows during inspiration	**Inspiratory stridor** Often less with crying Worse in supine position since gravity moves tongue posterior	Pierre-Robin and Treacher-Collins (both with micrognathia) Macroglossia (Beckwith-Wiedemann syndrome, hypothyroidism, glycogen storage diseases, trisomy 21) Choanal atresia Thyroglossal duct cyst
Laryngeal obstruction (vocal cords, subglottis, extrathoracic trachea) This region is a fixed size during inspiration and expiration	**Biphasic stridor** Usually worse with agitation Since the larynx is the narrowest part of the neonate's airway, this type of stridor is most common	Laryngomalacia—most common congenital laryngeal anomaly Vocal cord paralysis—second most common laryngeal anomaly Congenital subglottic stenosis—often unable to handle secretions, have recurrent pneumonias; if severe, tracheostomy and dilatations needed Laryngeal web, cyst
Intrathoracic obstruction (intrathoracic trachea and bronchi) This region narrows during expiration	**Expiratory stridor** Less common than laryngeal stridor but often more serious	Tracheomalacia Tracheal stenosis External compression (vascular rings, mediastinal mass)

B. VASCULAR RINGS

=aortic arch anomalies

Types
1. *True or complete vascular ring:* complete circle around trachea and esophagus, presents with feeding and respiratory symptoms
   A. Double aortic arch (40%)—most common, due to prevailing right and left 4th brachial arches
   B. Right aortic arch with ligamentum arteriosum/PDA (30%)—due to persistence of right 4th brachial arch
2. *Incomplete vascular ring:* incomplete circle around trachea and esophagus
   A. Anomalous innominate artery (10%)—innominate artery branches further left from aortic arch or branches more posterior
   Mild respiratory symptoms (often with stridor, cough)
   B. Aberrant right subclavian artery (20%)—right subclavian artery arises from descending aorta; mild feeding symptoms
   C. Aberrant left pulmonary artery (PA)(rare)—left PA arises from right PA to reach the lung, crosses right bronchus, behind trachea and in front of the esophagus; both respiratory and feeding difficulties

Clinical
Respiratory distress ($+/-$ stridor) and feeding difficulties with severity dependent on completeness of ring; may have swallowing difficulties; frequent pneumonias due to aspiration; atelectasis; normal physical exam and EKG

Management
Barium swallow is diagnostic except for anomalous innominate artery
Confirm with angioplasty
Diagnosis can also be made with echocardiogram
Surgery may be necessary if more severe symptoms

C. CHOANAL ATRESIA Inspiratory Stridor

Pathophysiology
Occlusion may be secondary to thin membranous covering or dense cartilaginous occlusion

Clinical
Unilateral (2/3) (right side > left side 2:1) > bilateral (1/3); females > males (2:1)
If severe and bilateral, may present in the delivery room
If bilateral choanal atresia, infant with respiratory distress and cyanosis during rest (improves with crying due to air entry through mouth)

Unilateral choanal atresia typically doesn't cause symptoms unless other nares obstructed with suction catheter or feeding tube

1/2 with congenital abnormalities (e.g., CHARGE syndrome: coloboma, *heart* disease, choanal *atresia*, mental deficiency/ *retardation*, genital hypoplasia and ear anomalies)

Diagnosis
Unable to pass nasogastric tube through nasal passage
CT or MRI helpful for more definitive diagnosis

Management
Oral airway for temporary improvement
Surgical repair (can delay if not severe)

D. VOCAL CORD PARALYSIS *insp. or Biphasic stridor, 2nd most common laryngeal anom.*

Risks
Increased risk if birth trauma, neurological abnormalities (e.g., asphyxia, Arnold-Chiari malformation, hydrocephalus) or prolonged intubation

Clinical
Unilateral > bilateral (increased risk of neurological abnormalities)
Greater on left since left recurrent laryngeal nerve with longer and winding course and thus more susceptible to trauma; if there is enlargement of great vessels, can lead to traction
Weak, hoarse, feeble cry (may be aphonic if bilateral paralysis)
Inspiratory stridor (often louder when agitated and may be positional since gravity can help move paralyzed cord away from midline); can have biphasic stridor

Management
Fiberoptic assessment
Observe if mild and/or unilateral paralysis (typical resolution by 1 year of age)
Bilateral paralysis often requires tracheostomy

E. TRACHEOMALACIA AND LARYNGOMALACIA

most common cong. laryngeal anom.

	Tracheomalacia — *collapse during E*	Laryngomalacia *collapse during I*
Pathophysiology	Cartilaginous rings supporting the trachea are soft and tend to collapse during expiration	Collapse of epiglottis and/or arytenoid cartilages and/or larynx leading to prolapse into glottis during *inspiration*
	Can be associated with chronic ventilation	Unknown etiology
Clinical	Although most common cause of intrinsic congenital tracheal narrowing, it is rare	Most common cause of congenital stridor
	Expiratory stridor	Coarse, inspiratory stridor that is worse with agitation and improved in prone position
		Can have expiratory component to stridor
		Typically benign, self-limited, male > female (2:1)
		Presents with stridor between birth and first month of life
		Majority without respiratory distress or feeding difficulties
Diagnosis	Bronchoscopy (anterior and posterior tracheal walls approximate during expiration)	Laryngoscopy
Management	Consider CPAP	Conservative
	If severe, may need tracheostomy	
Outcome	Majority with spontaneous resolution by 6–12 months of age	Spontaneous resolution by about 2 years of age
		Rare to require tracheotomy

XXII. Pleural Effusions

A. HYDROTHORAX

Characteristic	Transudate	Exudate
pH	> 7.40	< 7.40
WBC (per mm^3)	< 1000	> 1000
Protein concentration	< 3 g/dL	> 3 g/dL
Glucose concentration	Same as serum	Less than serum
Specific gravity	< 1.016	> 1.016
LDH (IU)	< 200	> 200
Pleural fluid LDH : serum LDH	< 0.6	> 0.6
Etiology	Congestive heart failure	Infections (increased polymorphonuclear cells)
	Hypoproteinemia (nephrotic syndrome)	
	Nonimmune hydrops fetalis	
	Iatrogenic (catheters, ventricular-peritoneal shunts)	

B. CHYLOTHORAX

Pathophysiology

Secondary to intrauterine obstruction of thoracic duct (isolated or with other lymphatic abnormalities); can also be acquired post-traumatic delivery or post-operatively

Thoracic duct obstruction leads to fistula between thoracic duct and pleural space

More common in fetuses with chromosomal anomalies and/or major malformations

May lead to pulmonary hypoplasia if large and develops early in gestation

Clinical

Right lung > left lung > bilateral

In utero—may spontaneously resolve (5–10%); risk of polyhydramnios, preterm labor, and hydrops

Respiratory distress with decreased breath sounds over side of effusion

Postnatally, may resolve by ~1 month of age

If prolonged thoracentesis required with large amount of drainage, may lead to lymphopenia

Management

In utero—fetal thoracentesis if large, bilateral and mediastinal shift; some consider thoracentesis immediately prior to delivery yet risk of rapid recurrence leading to hypovolemia at birth and thus others prefer to wait until after delivery

Manage respiratory distress

Definitive diagnosis and acute therapy by thoracentesis—clear fluid if not being fed, milky if feeding; fluid with large amount of lymphocytes (~90%)

Chromosomes, echocardiogram   *Portagen, Progestimil*

Recommended to feed with formula rich in medium-chain triglycerides to bypass lymphatic system and thus direct absorption into bloodstream

Ligation of thoracic duct in severe cases

XXIII. Congenital Malformations of the Lung

A. CONGENITAL LOBAR EMPHYSEMA

Incidence

Most common neonatal cystic lung malformation

Left upper lobe (~45%) > right middle lobe (~30%) > right upper lobe (~20%)

Increased risk of congenital heart disease

Pathophysiology

Postnatal overdistention of one or more lobes of lung due to air trapping

Probably due to cartilaginous deficiency within large airways

Clinical

Initially with mild respiratory distress (usually by first week of life) which may require CPAP; can have mediastinal shift to contralateral side

Management

Symptoms may resolve without treatment; if symptoms persist and/or severe, may need lobectomy

B. CONGENITAL CYSTIC ADENOMATOID MALFORMATION (CCAM)

Pathophysiology

Numerous cysts composed of lung tissue that *does* communicate with tracheobronchial tree via a small tortuous passage

Typically, involves only one lobe of lung (~80-95%)

In contrast to (bronchopulmonary sequestration) majority with blood supply from pulmonary circulation

see pg. 80

Clinical

Increased incidence of polyhydramnios, hydrops, prematurity and pulmonary hypoplasia

If significant size, typically presents with respiratory distress that begins after delivery and increases in severity as cysts fill with air; a mediastinal shift with compression of opposite lung occurs as cysts increase in size

Majority symptomatic by 1 year of age

Increased risk of developing hamartomas (focal dysplasia) and/or infection

Types and Outcome

Type I (50-70%): single or multiple large cysts (2-10 cm)

   One lobe of lung filled with air or fluid, usually communicating with bronchi

   ~10% with associated anomalies

   1/3 present after 1 year of age with cough and/or difficulty breathing

   Excellent prognosis: 90% survival

Type II (20-40%): multiple medium-sized cysts (0.5-2 cm)

   Clinical symptoms during infancy

   1/2 with associated anomalies (including renal agenesis, congenital heart disease, jejunal atresia, congenital diaphragmatic hernia, hydrocephalus, skeletal anomalies)

   Prognosis poor due to anomalies: 60% survival

Type III (10%): large bulky lesion containing numerous small cysts (< 0.2 cm)

   High risk of mediastinal shift

   Clinical symptoms in utero or during infancy

   Poor prognosis: 60% survival

Differential diagnosis

Includes congenital diaphragmatic hernia, bronchogenic cyst, enteric cyst, and neuroblastoma

Management

Chromosomes, echocardiogram, in utero—monitor closely for hydrops and possible fetal surgery if large

Manage respiratory distress (possible ventilation, ECMO if severe)

Consider selective intubation of contralateral bronchus if unilateral CCAM

Complete resection usually recommended in all types due to risk of complications

C. BRONCHOGENIC CYST

Pathophysiology
Cystic mass that can be air-filled if it communicates with the airways or solid if there is no airway connection
Central (often single) or peripheral (often multiple and may communicate with airway)
Majority are posterior to trachea but can be intraparenchymal
Some may communicate with gastrointestinal tract

Clinical
Symptoms dependent on location and size; majority are asymptomatic
If multiple cysts, respiratory distress often shortly after birth
If airway connection, may have rapid cystic enlargement leading to tension and sudden onset of respiratory distress
May also have stridor (due to airway obstruction), hemoptysis, or development of malignant malformation
May develop infection and present with fever, cough, secretions

Differential diagnosis
Includes lymphangioma, pericardial cyst, congenital diaphragmatic hernia, enteric duplication cyst, and CCAM

Management
Surgical excision (even if asymptomatic due to risk of complications)

D. CONGENITAL LYMPHANGIECTASIA

Incidence
Rare, increased in males (2:1), increased in patients with Noonan syndrome and trisomy 21

Pathophysiology
Dilatation of the lymphatic vessels of the lung due to abnormal development or lymphatic obstruction

Clinical
Respiratory distress soon after birth
Increased risk of pleural effusions
Diagnosis often requires biopsy, which further increases risk of pleural effusions

Prognosis
If severe, poor prognosis

E. BRONCHOPULMONARY SEQUESTRATION

Pathophysiology
Nonfunctioning lung tissue that receives vascular supply from anomalous systemic vessels
Intralobar (75%): abnormal tissue within normal lung; typically located in the lower lobes (L > R); majority do not communicate with bronchial tree
Slightly greater in males (1.5:1)
~10% risk of anomalies
Extralobar (25%): less common; abnormal tissue outside the visceral pleura (can be intrathoracic or sub diaphragmatic)
Greater in males (3:1)
Increased risk of other congenital anomalies (~60%) including congenital diaphragmatic hernia, tracheoesophageal fistula, congenital heart disease
Majority located on left side between lower lobe and diaphragm

Clinical

Often asymptomatic

In utero, can lead to polyhydramnios (due to esophageal obstruction or decreased swallowing), pleural effusions, mediastinal shift, hydrops (due to obstruction of inferior vena cava and decreased cardiac output), and/or pulmonary hypoplasia

Can present during infancy with respiratory distress (if pulmonary hypoplasia, will be severe and may require ECMO)

Can present during childhood with a history of recurrent pneumonias

Differential diagnosis

Includes type III CCAM, mediastinal teratoma and congenital diaphragmatic hernia

Management

Chromosomes, echocardiogram due to possible association with congenital heart disease

Manage respiratory distress

Lobectomy for intralobar sequestration due to potential complications; some centers manage extralobar lesions nonoperatively since minimal risk of infection

Prognosis

Regression in utero (~75%) even if mediastinal shift

Postnatally, prognosis dependent on degree of pulmonary hypoplasia

F. PULMONARY HYPOPLASIA

Pathophysiology

Abnormal development of the lungs leading to decreased number of alveoli, airways and vascular bed

Can result from extrathoracic, intrathoracic or thoracic compression in utero

Also due to functional compression from neuromuscular disease leading to decreased fetal respiratory activity

Greater severity if prolonged oligohydramnios

Clinical

Severe respiratory distress and cyanosis

Often with associated pulmonary hypertension

Associated with Potter's syndrome (see Renal chapter)

Management

Utilize minimal pressures to maintain adequate oxygenation

Outcome

Variable, dependent on etiology; majority with poor survival

XXIV. Radiographic Findings in Respiratory Diseases

RDS	Low lung volumes
	Alveolar atelectasis—diffuse reticulogranular pattern or ground-glass appearance
	Air bronchograms well-visualized due to contrast against diffuse atelectasis
Transient tachypnea of the newborn	Hyperinflation, perihilar linear densities (fluid in the interstitium)
	Fluid in pleural fissure
	Pleural effusions may be present
Pneumonia	Unilateral or bilateral streaky densities
	Opacifications
	Granular with air bronchograms (GBS pneumonia and RDS are often indistinguishable)

(continued on following page)

Pneumothorax	Hyperlucent area without pulmonary parenchymal markings
	Lateral decubitus film with suspected side of pneumothorax UP will demonstrate leak more clearly than AP view
Pneumo-mediastinum	"Spinnaker sail" sign due to elevated, well-visualized thymus
	Hyperlucency in the superior retrosternal space
Pneumopericardium	Hyperlucency around entire heart
CLD	Heterogeneous lung disease with cystic changes, areas of atelectasis, and possibly pulmonary interstitial emphysema
Pulmonary interstitial emphysema	Air bubbles that follow the perivascular sheaths, often more prominent near the hilum
	Small cysts may coalesce into larger cysts
Meconium aspiration syndrome	Diffuse, patchy, intraparenchymal densities
	Areas of overdistention (due to air trapping from airway obstruction)
Pulmonary hemorrhage	Distinctive opacification (s)
Pleural effusions	Obscured diaphragmatic border
	Lateral decubitus film with suspected side of pleural effusion DOWN will demonstrate layering of fluid
Congenital lobar emphysema	Hyperinflated lobes, multiple large cysts, may lead to compression of opposite lung
	In contrast to pneumothoraces, this lesion demonstrates lung markings to the periphery
Congenital cystic adenomatoid malformation	Multiple cysts that increase in size as air enters
	Compression of surrounding lung tissue
Congenital lymphangiectasia	Hyperinflated lungs
	Diffuse granular densities representing dilated lymphatic vessels
	Increased risk of pleural effusions
Pulmonary sequestration	Unilateral lung mass often triangular or oval
	Can have a cystic component
Pulmonary hypoplasia	Small, hyperlucent lungs

XXV. Therapeutic Agents in Respiratory Diseases

A. DIURETICS

Drug	Mode of action	Site of action	Side effects
Acetazolamide (Diamox)	Carbonic anhydrase inhibitor Inhibits $NaHCO_3$ reabsorption	Proximal tubule	Mild hyperchloremic metabolic acidosis Hypokalemia Other uses: can decrease progression of hydrocephalus by decreasing CSF production; anticonvulsant if refractory seizures; glaucoma
Furosemide (Lasix) Bumetanide (Bumex, 40 × more potent)	Blocks active chloride transport	Ascending loop of Henle	Increased urine losses of K, Na, Cl, Ca and Mg leading to serum deficiencies of these electrolytes Hypercalciuria and nephrocalcinosis Contraction hypochloremic metabolic alkalosis ↑ renin, hyperuricemia Ototoxicity Relief of symptoms sometimes precedes diuresis secondary to pulmonary venous dilation
Spironolactone (Aldactone)	Competitive antagonist of aldosterone	Collecting system	Decreased urinary losses of K and thus, *K- sparing* Increased urine losses of Na, Cl, Ca and Mg Contraindicated if hyperkalemia or anuria
Chlorothiazide (Diuril)	Inhibits NaCl reabsorption	Distal loop of Henle	Increased urinary losses of Na, K, Mg, Cl, HCO_3 and phosphate Decreased renal excretion of Ca Mild hypochloremic alkalosis Inhibits pancreatic release of insulin leading to hyperglycemia Displaces bilirubin from albumin—use cautiously if hyper-bilirubinemia Hyperuricemia

B. METHYLXANTHINES (e.g., theophylline—oral; aminophylline—intravenous; caffeine—oral and intravenous)

Mechanism
Probably acts by increasing cyclic AMP production as well as by changing intracellular calcium levels

Metabolism

Liver-P_{450} cytochrome system
Aminophylline and theophylline are partly metabolized to caffeine—this breakdown is decreased with increasing age
Metabolism inhibited by cimetidine, erythromycin and ketoconazole (i.e., higher levels)
Metabolism induced by phenobarbital (i.e., lower levels)

Comparisons

Caffeine has a greater therapeutic index with less toxicity compared to aminophylline or theophylline

Effects

Respiratory—relaxes pulmonary airway smooth muscle; decreases frequency of apnea by acting centrally; increases diaphragmatic contractility
Neurological—increased sensitivity of medullary respiratory center to CO_2, increases central nervous system activity, hyperreflexia, jitteriness, seizures if toxic levels
Cardiovascular—increases heart rate, increased cardiac output due to increased catecholamine sensitivity, arrhythmias, some decrease in peripheral vascular resistance; hypotension if rapid infusion
Muscular—stimulates skeletal muscle, increases diaphragmatic contractility
Renal—diuresis, increased urinary Ca excretion
Gastrointestinal—increases gastric acid secretion
Metabolic—hyperglycemia

We would like to thank Dr. Mary Ellen Wohl for her tremendous effort during the editing process. She has made an enormous and invaluable contribution to this chapter.

REFERENCES

Ashcraft KW (ed): Pediatric Surgery (3rd edition). Philadelphia, WB Saunders Co, 2000.

Bianchi DW, Crombleholme TM and D'Alton ME: Fetology. New York, McGraw-Hill, 2000.

Britton JR: The transition to extrauterine life and disorders of transition. *Clinics of Perinatology.* 1998; 25 (2): 271-94.

Fanaroff AA and Martin RJ (eds): Neonatal-Perinatal Medicine (6th edition). St Louis, Mosby-Year Book Inc, 1997.

Fishman AP (ed): Handbook of Physiology, Section 3: The Respiratory System. Bethesda, MD, American Physiology Society, 1986.

Goldsmith JP and Karotkin EH (eds): Assisted Ventilation of the Neonate (3rd edition). Philadelphia, WB Saunders Co, 1996.

Guyton AC, Hall JE and Schmitt W (eds): Human Physiology and Mechanisms of Disease (6th edition). Philadelphia, WB Saunders Co, 1997.

Hlastala MP and Berger AJ (eds): Physiology of Respiration (2nd edition). New York, Oxford University Press, 2001.

Hansen TN, Cooper TR and Weisman LE (eds): Neonatal Respiratory Disease (2nd edition). Pennsylvania, Handbooks in Health Care Co, 1998.

Leff AR and Schumacker PT: Respiratory Physiology—Basics and Applications. Philadelphia, WB Saunders Co, 1993.

Park MK: Pediatric Cardiology for Practitioners (3rd edition). St Louis, Mosby, 1996.

Polin RA and Fox WW (eds): Fetal and Neonatal Physiology (2nd edition). Philadelphia, WB Saunders Co, 1998.

Simon, NP. Evaluation and management of stridor in the newborn. *Clinical Pediatrics.* 1991; 30(4): 211-216.

Teusch HW and Ballard RA (eds): Avery's Diseases of the Newborn (7th edition). Philadelphia, WB Saunders Co, 1998.

West JB: Pulmonary Physiology and Pathophysiology: An Integrated, Case-Based Approach. Philadelphia, Lippincott, Williams & Wilkins, 2001.

West JB: Respiratory Physiology (6th edition). Philadelphia, Lippincott, Williams & Wilkins, 2000.

CHAPTER 3

Cardiology

TOPICS COVERED IN THIS CHAPTER

I. **Morphologic Development of the Heart**

II. **Cardiovascular Physiology – Prenatal, Transitional and Postnatal**
   A. Fetal circulation
   B. Hemodynamic changes at birth
   C. Cardiac output
   D. Stroke volume and stroke work
   E. Frank-Starling curve
   F. Ventricular function curves utilizing Frank-Starling law
   G. Qp/Qs
   H. Resistance

III. **Incidence of Congenital Heart Disease**

IV. **Congenital Heart Disease**
   A. Cyanotic heart disease
      1. Transposition of the great arteries (TGA)
      2. Tetralogy of fallot (TOF)
      3. Pulmonary atresia
      4. Truncus arteriosus
      5. Tricuspid atresia
      6. Ebstein's anomaly
      7. Single ventricle
      8. Total anomalous pulmonary venous return (TAPVR)
      9. Double outlet right ventricle
   B. Left-to-right shunts
      1. Ventricular septal defect (VSD)
      2. Atrial septal defect (ASD), ostium secundum type
      3. Patent ductus arteriosus (PDA)
      4. Complete atrioventricular canal (endocardial cushion defect)
      5. Partial anomalous pulmonary venous return
   C. Left and right-sided obstructive lesions
      1. Coarctation of the aorta
      2. Pulmonic stenosis and aortic stenosis
   D. Valvular heart disease
   E. Other diseases
      1. Hypoplastic left heart syndrome
      2. Cardiomyopathy
      3. Eisenmenger's complex
      4. Cor pulmonale
      5. Pericardial effusion

   6. Anomalous left coronary artery
   7. Cardiac tumors
   8. Asplenia and polysplenia
   9. Cor triatriatum

V. **Clinical Manifestations of Congenital Heart Disease**
   A. Central cyanosis
      1. Definition
      2. Differential diagnosis of cyanosis
      3. Hyperoxia test
   B. Physical exam
      1. Heart sounds
      2. Pulse pressure
      3. Murmurs
      4. Blood pressure
   C. Congestive heart failure

VI. **Radiographic Findings in Cardiac Disease**

VII. **EKG and Arrhythmias**
   A. EKG rhythm
   B. EKG axis
   C. Arrhythmias
      1. Premature beats
      2. Tachycardia
      3. Atrioventricular conduction abnormalities
      4. Other arrhythmias
      5. Electrical management of arrhythmias
   D. Supraventricular tachycardia
   E. Electrolyte abnormalities

VIII. **Echocardiography (echo)**
   A. M-mode
   B. 2-dimensional imaging
   C. Doppler echo
   D. Fetal echo

IX. **Pressure Tracings**

X. **Therapeutic Agents in Cardiac Disease**
   A. Sympathetic receptors
   B. Inotropic agents
   C. Diuretics
   D. Indomethacin
   E. Prostaglandin
   F. Endocarditis prophylaxis

XI. **Surgical Repair of Cardiac Defects**

XII. **Associations with Congenital Heart Disease**

XII. Associations with Congenital Heart Disease
(continued)
  A. Syndromes associated with heart disease
  B. Infectious diseases associated with congenital heart disease

C. Maternal medications associated with congenital heart disease
D. Maternal diseases associated with congenital heart disease

I. Morphologic Development of the Heart

Development
Cardiovascular system is the *first system* to function in utero
Heart arises from *mesoderm*
Initially two endocardial tubes are formed from angiogenic cell clusters; the tubes then fuse together; following
  subdivision of the tube into primordial heart chambers, the tube bends and forms a bulboventricular loop; septa grow
  between the atria, ventricle and bulbis cordis (leading to 2 atria, 2 ventricles and 2 great vessels)
Heart formation complete by 7–8 weeks gestation
Designation of structures:
  1st letter refers to atrial situs relative to the viscera → S = solitus, I = inversus, or A = ambiguous
  2nd letter refers to ventricular situs → D-loop = morphologically right ventricle on the right side, L-loop with mirror
    image, or X = unknown
  3rd letter refers to the great arteries → S = solitus with aorta to right and posterior of pulmonary artery or I =
    inversus or mirror image of S
  Normal = {S, D, S}
  D-transposition of great vessels (TGV) = {S, D,D} and L-TGV = {S, L, L}
  Situs inversus totalis = {I, L, I}

Abnormal development
  Embryogenesis: most cardiac abnormalities develop by 8 weeks gestation
  Morphogenesis: some cardiac abnormalities may be acquired in utero or progress during pregnancy due to decreased
    forward blood flow

II. Cardiovascular Physiology—Prenatal and Transitional

A. FETAL CIRCULATION

In utero blood flow

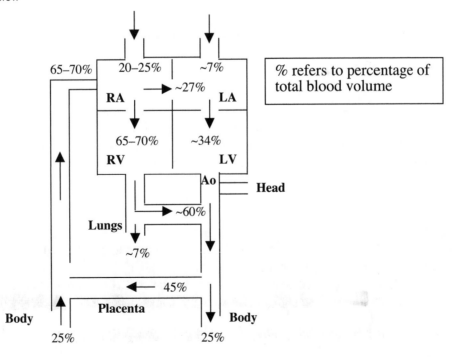

RA = =right atrium; LA=left atrium; RV=right ventricle; LV=left ventricle; Ao=aorta. Modified from Fyler DC (ed): Nadas' Pediatric Cardiology. Philadelphia, Hanley & Belfus, 1991, p 58.

Blood from the upper body drains into the superior vena cava (SVC), and most then goes to the right ventricle (RV); blood then flows through the pulmonary arteries and the patent ductus arteriosus (PDA) to the descending aorta

Blood from the lower body and the placenta (well-oxygenated) drains into the inferior vena cava (IVC); $\sim$1/3 of the IVC blood travels through the foramen ovale and leads to a greater O_2 saturation of blood in the cerebral and coronary vasculature (supplied by the left ventricle—LV)

The RV is the dominant ventricle supplying more cardiac output (CO) compared with the LV

The RV supplies the descending aorta (placenta and lower body), and the LV supplies the ascending aorta (upper body)

Placenta receives the greatest percentage of fetal cardiac output (45%) and is the organ with the lowest vascular resistance

The lungs receive only a small amount of CO, and thus pulmonary artery vessels are small

The ductus arteriosus remains patent in utero due to (1) prostaglandins (PGE2), (2) prostacyclin (PGI2) and (3) thromboxane A2

Blood gas parameters of in utero vessels

Vessel	pH	pCO$_2$	pO$_2$	O$_2$ Saturation
Uterine artery	7.40	32	95	98%
Uterine vein	7.34	40	40	76%
Umbilical vein	7.38	43	27	68%
Umbilical artery	7.35	48	15	30%

Modified from Cunningham FG, Gant NF, Leveno KJ, et al (eds): Williams Obstetrics. New York, McGraw-Hill Co, Inc. 2001, p 139.

Fetus tolerates lower pO$_2$ since:
1. Fetal hemoglobin with higher oxygen affinity
2. Increased O_2 carrying-capacity due to elevated hemoglobin concentrations in fetus
3. Increased ability to utilize glucose by anaerobic metabolism

Majority of fetuses not affected by congenital heart disease since:
1. Fetal oxygenation is not dependent on pulmonary blood flow (PBF)
2. Both RV and LV are important for systemic blood flow (SBF)
3. Communication between left and right sides of heart due to mixing at atrial and ductal levels

B. HEMODYNAMIC CHANGES AT BIRTH

At delivery

Umbilical arteries constrict soon after birth, preventing blood flow from infant to mother

In contrast, umbilical vein remains dilated, allowing blood to flow in the direction of gravity; thus, if infant held below placenta $\longrightarrow$ infant receives extra blood, while if infant held above placenta $\longrightarrow$ infant with blood loss

A delay in umbilical cord clamping will lead to an increase in infant's blood volume; by the 3rd day of life, this difference will be small

After delivery

Placental function of gas exchange becomes responsibility of lungs

Systemic vascular resistance (SVR) increases since low resistance placenta no longer involved

Ductus venosus closes since blood passage stopped

Expansion of lung with air leads to decreased pulmonary vascular resistance (PVR), increased PBF; with increased pulmonary venous return, the left atrial pressure increases and becomes greater than right atrial pressure, leading to functional closure of patent foramen ovale (PFO)

PDA closes as arterial O_2 saturation increases and ductus less responsive to prostaglandins

C. CARDIAC OUTPUT (CO)

$$CO = \frac{\text{systemic BP}}{\text{total peripheral vascular resistance}}$$

Factors affecting cardiac output
1. *Preload:* dependent upon volume within ventricle at end of diastole (influenced by blood volume, venous tone, atrial contractility, and intrapleural pressure)
2. *Afterload:* dependent upon the arterial pressure that the ventricle confronts during contraction; determined by end diastolic aortic pressure and aortic resistance

    Afterload is not as significant as preload since an increase in the afterload does not alter the CO until the blood pressure (BP) reaches a critical level

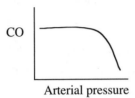

Modified from Guyton AC: Textbook of Medical Physiology. Philadelphia, WB Saunders Co, 1986, p 158.

3. *Inotropic ability of heart*
4. *Heart rate (HR)*—regulated by parasympathetic and sympathetic nervous system as well as hormonal system

Note: in neonate, CO more dependent on HR rather than stroke volume

D. STROKE VOLUME AND STROKE WORK

Definition of stroke volume (SV)
SV is the volume of blood ejected from ventricle during one heart beat
SV = end-diastolic volume (EDV)—end-systolic volume (ESV)

Definition of stroke work (SW)
Stroke work (SW) = work done by LV or RV during one heartbeat to increase BP
SW = MAP × SVP (MAP = mean arterial pressure)
LV stroke work = stroke volume output × (LV mean ejection pressure—left atrial pressure)
RV stroke work = stroke volume output × (RV mean ejection pressure—right atrial pressure)
RV stroke work is ~ 1/6 LV stroke work

Factors affecting SV and SW
Dependent on preload (end-diastolic V or initial fiber length), afterload (arterial BP) and inotropic ability of heart

E. FRANK-STARLING CURVE

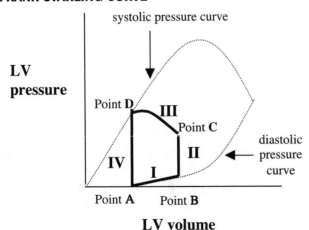

point A = mitral valve opens, volume =preload
point B = mitral valve closes
point C = aortic valve opens
point D = aortic valve closes
increased preload if II shifted to right
increased contractility if systolic pressure curve moves upward and to left, shifting IV to left
increased afterload if IV shifted to right
increased HR with increased contractility (IV to left slightly) and decreased preload (II to left)

Dotted loop represents Frank-Starling curve; inner circle represents LV pressure/volume loop of a single cardiac cycle; Roman numerals represent different phases of Frank-Starling curve; points represent intersection between these phases; Modified from Guyton AC: Textbook of Medical Physiology. Philadelphia, WB Saunders Co, 1986, p 159.

I = filling period
Begins at volume in LV based on amount of blood remaining from previous contraction (= end-systolic volume)
Ends at end-diastolic volume = preload

II = isovolumic contraction although volume of LV does not change, the intraventricular pressure increases until it equals the aortic pressure (or afterload) at end of diastole

III = ejection period due to further contraction of the heart, intraventricular pressure increases even more while the volume begins to decrease

IV = isovolumic relaxation at the end of the ejection period, the semilunar valves close and the ventricular pressure returns to the diastolic pressure; no change in volume

The Frank-Starling curve demonstrates the intrinsic ability of the heart to adapt to different blood volumes (or preload): as cardiac muscle is stretched with increasing amount of blood volume, contraction occurs with an increased force so that extra blood will be pumped out

As right atrium (RA) is stretched with increasing amount of blood volume, the HR is directly increased

Stroke volume = volume at point C–volume at point D

F. VENTRICULAR FUNCTION CURVES UTILIZING FRANK-STARLING LAW

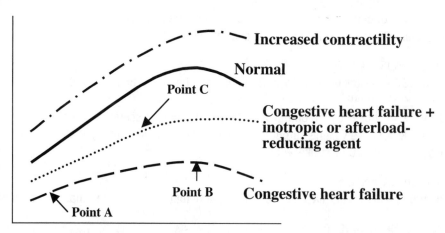

Modified from Beers MH and Berkow R (eds): The Merck Manual of Diagnosis and Therapy (17th ed). New Jersey, Merck Research Laboratories. 1999, p 1683.

Normal curve: demonstrates LV systolic pressure, SV, SW and CO increase quickly as the myocardial fiber is lengthened at the end of diastole

Congestive heart failure (CHF) curve: due to decreased inotropy, the ventricular function curve decreases in the presence of CHF (point A)
The ventricular function remains flatter prior to normal resting (from point A to point B)
If there are other reasons for decreased contractility (e.g. hypoxia, severe metabolic acidosis, β-blocker, increased systemic vascular resistance, cardiomyopathy), the ventricular function curve will appear similar to the CHF curve

CHF with inotropic or afterload-reducing agent curve: if a patient with CHF is treated with an inotropic or afterload-reducing agent, the ventricular function curve will improve (although still remains abnormal)

Increased contractility curve: due to increased catecholamines, increased thyroid hormone

G. Qp/Qs

Represents the ratio of PBF to SBF

[handwritten: Pulmonary / systemic]

Normal ratio $= 1$

Left-to-right shunt if Qp/Qs > 1 (large shunt if ratio >2 with PBF $2\times$ SBF)

Right-to-left shunt Qp/Qs < 1 (large shunt if ratio < 0.7)

$$\frac{Q\ pulmonary}{Q\ systemic} = \frac{pulm\ blood\ flow}{systemic\ blood\ flow} = \frac{aorta\ O_2\ saturation\ (sat)\ -\ SVC\ O_2\ sat}{left\ atrial\ or\ pulmonary\ venous\ O_2 sat\ -\ pulm\ art\ O_2\ sat}$$

H. RESISTANCE

$$PVR = \frac{mean\ PA\ pressure\ -\ mean\ LAP}{pulmonary\ blood\ flow} \qquad SVR = \frac{mean\ aortic\ P\ -\ mean\ RAP}{systemic\ blood\ flow}$$

LAP $=$ left atrial pressure; RAP$=$right atrial pressure

III. Overall Incidence of Congenital Heart Disease (CHD)

Overall incidence
    8 in 1000 live births with 2 in 1000 presenting less than 1 year of age
    ~25% of infants with CHD have additional non-cardiac anomalies

Recurrence risk
    2–5% risk of recurrence of CHD if one previous child with CHD; if two previous children with CHD, recurrence risk increases to 5–10%
    If mother has CHD, risk of child with CHD ~6.7% (range 2.5–18%)
    If father has CHD, risk of child with CHD 1.5–3%

Estimated incidence of specific defects

Congenital heart defect	Incidence
Ventricular septal defect (VSD)	16%; (VSD is the most common CHD)
Pulmonary stenosis with intact ventricular septum	7.5–12%
Tetralogy of Fallot (TOF)	8–10% (TOF is the most common cyanotic heart disease beyond infancy)
Atrial septal defect (ASD), ostium secundum type	6–11%
Transposition of the great arteries (TGA)	5–10% (TGA is the most common cyanotic heart disease in the first week of life)
Patent ductus arteriosus (PDA)	4–10% (in full-term infants)
Coarctation of the aorta (CoA)	5–8%
Atrioventricular (AV) septal defects (ostium primum ASD and AV canal)	2–5%
Total anomalous pulmonary venous return (TAPVR)	1–2.5%
Truncus arteriosus	1–4%
Hypoplastic left heart syndrome (HLHS)	~1.5% (HLHS is the 2nd most common cyanotic heart disease presenting in the first week of life and most common cause of mortality in the 1st week of life)

IV. Congenital Heart Disease

Cyanotic heart disease 5 "T's," "DO" and "ESP"	**T**ransposition of the great arteries, **t**etralogy of Fallot, **t**otal anomalous pulmonary venous return, **t**ricuspid atresia, **t**runcus arteriosus **D**ouble **o**utlet right ventricle **E**bstein's anomaly, **s**ingle ventricle, **p**ulmonary atresia
Left-to-right shunt	Ventricular septal defect, patent ductus arteriosus, atrial septal defect Complete atrioventricular canal Partial anomalous pulmonary venous return
Left and right-sided obstructive lesions	Coarctation of the aorta Pulmonary stenosis, aortic stenosis
Valvular disease	Aortic, mitral and tricuspid regurgitation
Other abnormalities	Hypoplastic left heart syndrome Cardiomyopathy Pulmonary hypertension

A. CYANOTIC HEART DISEASE

1. Transposition of the great arteries (TGA)

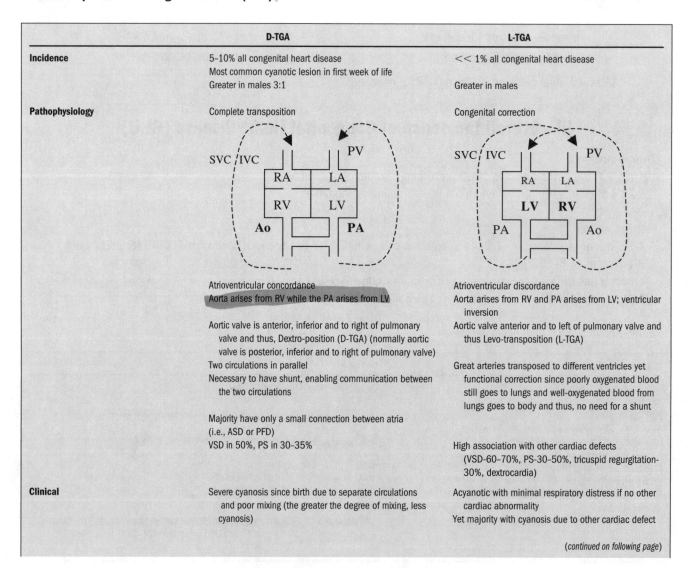

	D-TGA	L-TGA
Incidence	5–10% all congenital heart disease Most common cyanotic lesion in first week of life Greater in males 3:1	<< 1% all congenital heart disease Greater in males
Pathophysiology	Complete transposition	Congenital correction
	Atrioventricular concordance Aorta arises from RV while the PA arises from LV	Atrioventricular discordance Aorta arises from RV and PA arises from LV; ventricular inversion
	Aortic valve is anterior, inferior and to right of pulmonary valve and thus, Dextro-position (D-TGA) (normally aortic valve is posterior, inferior and to right of pulmonary valve) Two circulations in parallel Necessary to have shunt, enabling communication between the two circulations	Aortic valve anterior and to left of pulmonary valve and thus Levo-transposition (L-TGA) Great arteries transposed to different ventricles yet functional correction since poorly oxygenated blood still goes to lungs and well-oxygenated blood from lungs goes to body and thus, no need for a shunt
	Majority have only a small connection between atria (i.e., ASD or PFD) VSD in 50%, PS in 30–35%	High association with other cardiac defects (VSD-60–70%, PS-30–50%, tricuspid regurgitation-30%, dextrocardia)
Clinical	Severe cyanosis since birth due to separate circulations and poor mixing (the greater the degree of mixing, less cyanosis)	Acyanotic with minimal respiratory distress if no other cardiac abnormality Yet majority with cyanosis due to other cardiac defect

(continued on following page)

	D-TGA	L-TGA
	If restrictive PFO or ASD, O_2 sats will be lower The presence of VSD allows for better mixing If persistent PDA with decreased PVR, less cyanotic (aorta-to-pulmonary shunt) CHF (due to left-sided overload) No murmur unless VSD or PS Often with loud (anterior aortic valve below sternum) and single S2 (pulmonary valve further from chest wall and P2 not appreciated)	CHF if large VSD No murmur unless VSD, TR or PS *Single S2*
CXR	Heart size normal or slightly increased Increased pulmonary vascular markings (PVM) "Egg on a string" with narrow mediastinum (due to anterior-posterior aorta and MPA relationship) and involuted thymus	Straight left side of heart due to ascending aorta Other findings dependent on additional cardiac associations
EKG	Right QRS axis (between 90° and 160°) Right ventricular hypertrophy (RVH) Combined ventricular hypertrophy (CVH) if large VSD, PDA, PS, LVOT obstruction Can have right atrial hypertrophy (RAH)	Absence of Q waves in I, V5, V6 May have Q waves in V4R or V1 Varying degrees of AV block
Management	Prostaglandin (PGE1) Palliative Rashkind procedure if inadequate mixing Treat CHF Arterial switch (Jatene procedure) Mustard, Rastelli, or Senning if VSD and PS	Treat CHF (inotropic agents, diuretics, PA banding if uncontrollable) Surgery dependent on cardiac associations

Handwritten margin notes (CXR row): * single loud S2; If VSD – loud harsh systolic (M)

Handwritten note (Management row): Balloon septostomy

LVOT = left ventricular outflow tract; AV = atrioventricular; sats = saturations; PFO = patent foramen ovale; ASD = atrial septal defect; LAP = left atrial P; RAP = right atrial P; PVR = pulmonary vascular resistance; CHF = congestive heart failure; PS = pulmonary stenosis; TR = tricuspid regurgitation; WPW = Wolff-Parkinson-White; PA = pulmonary atresia.

2. Tetralogy of Fallot (TOF)

Incidence: 8–10% of all CHD

Most common cyanotic heart disease beyond neonatal period

Right aortic arch in 25%

Increased risk of coronary artery anomalies and extracardiac anomalies

Pathophysiology:

TOF = VSD + right ventricular outflow tract (RVOT) obstruction + overriding aorta + right ventricular hypertrophy (RVH)

VSD is typically perimembranous, always large and unrestrictive (thus, LVP=RVP)

The direction of shunting across VSD is dependent on the degree of RVOT obstruction and on relative differences between PVR and SVR

VSD defect often denoted as a malalignment defect because aortic root is overriding

RVOT obstruction can occur at the infundibular, valvar or supravalvar regions of the pulmonary artery

RVH develops due to RVOT obstruction

Handwritten margin notes:
1. Large VSD
2. Pulm Sten. OR RVOT obstruct
3. over ride aorta
4. RV hypertrophy

"BOOT" – concave pulm art. upturned apex

Mild RVOT Obstruction in TOF	Severe RVOT Obstruction in TOF
Shunt across ventricles is left-to-right	Decreased PBF, decreased pulmonary venous return to LA and thus LA and LV normal or slightly small
Acyanosis, *"pink Tet,"* may become cyanotic later in life (1–3 years of age)	Cyanosis, *"blue Tet"*
Typically, no CHF	Typically, no CHF
Systolic murmur at left lower sternal border that is usually transmitted upward along the entire left sternal border	PS murmur — note that the smaller the degree of PS, the louder the murmur due to greater amount of blood flowing through pulmonary valve; thus, if severe PS, there is a large right-to-left shunt (silent) and only a small amount of blood passes through pulmonary valves (thus, a softer murmur)
S2 often single and loud (since aorta is anterior)	S2 often single and loud (since aorta is anterior)
CXR: PVM vary depending on degree of RVOT obstruction	CXR: decreased PVM, normal heart size (may actually be smaller), boot-shaped later in life
EKG: RVH (in contrast to isolated large VSD), QRS axis may be normal	EKG: right axis deviation, RVH due to RV pressure overload, +/− RAE

Hypoxic spell

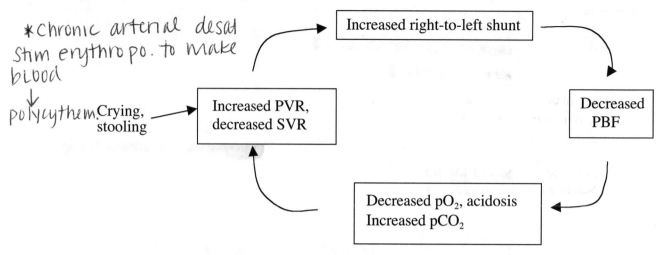

*chronic arterial desat
stim erythropo. to make
blood
↓
polycythem.*

Hyperpnea with rapid and deep respirations is the hallmark of the beginning of a spell
During a spell, there is decreased intensity to the murmur

Management of hypoxic spell
Knee-chest position
Morphine (effect probably on central nervous system and breaks cycle of hypoxia and agitation)
HCO_3 corrects acidosis and decreases respiratory drive
Vasoconstrictors to increase SVR
Propranolol—unclear mechanisms, decreases "spasm" of RVOT or stabilizes vasculature, preventing sudden
   decreases in SVR
Expand intravascular volume with fluid boluses

Management:
PGE1, palliative Blalock-Taussig (BT) shunt
Definitive complete repair with VSD closure and relief of RVOT obstruction

3. Pulmonary atresia (intact ventricular septum) *Need PDA*
Incidence:
   <1% of all congenital heart diseases *Ø communication btw. RV & PA*   *R→L shunt via ASD or PFO*
Pathophysiology:
RV typically hypoplastic with hypertrophied ventricular wall in 85%; pulmonary arteries typically well-developed due
   to in utero ductal flow
Requires ASD or PFO with PDA to survive
Clinical:
Severe cyanosis since birth
S2 single, typically no murmur; may have systolic murmur due to TR
CXR:
   Heart size normal or increased (due to RAE), MPA is concave, decreased PBF
EKG:
   Normal QRS axis (unlike TA-superior axis)
   LVH, can have RVH; RAH in 70% of cases
Management:
PGE1 immediately
   Angiography to determine coronary artery anatomy

If coronary circulation is not RV-dependent → RVOT reconstruction +/- BT shunt

If coronary circulation is RV-dependent → BT shunt

*Balloon atrial sep-
promote better
mixing*

Blalock Tussing shunt

4. Truncus arteriosus

Incidence:

1–4% of all congenital heart disease

Associated with DiGeorge Syndrome

Increased risk right aortic arch

Increased risk interrupted aortic arch

FISH for DiGeorge (22q11)

Pathophysiology:

Only one arterial blood vessel leaves the heart and gives rise to coronary, pulmonary and systemic arteries

Large VSD *always* present, leading to complete ventricular mixing

As PVR decreases, there is further increase in PBF

*Small infant c̄ ↑ pulm bl flow
& unresponsive CHF may
require pulm. artery
banding*

Types:

Main pulm. artery

Type I (50–70%) – MPA from truncus and then splits

Type II (30–50%)–each PA comes off posteriorly from truncus

Type III (10%) – each PA comes off laterally from truncus

Clinical:

Cyanosis and CHF (due to volume overload) – degree varies depending on degree of PBF (as PBF increases, greater degree of CHF and less cyanosis, while decreases in PBF lead to greater degree of cyanosis with less CHF)

Wide pulse pressure, bounding arterial pulses (due to diastolic runoff into PA)

Loud pansystolic murmur loudest at left lower sternal border

TV opening associated with a midsystolic ejection click

Single S2– Loud and loud ejection click

*PGE= if interrupted aortic
arch*

CXR:

Increased heart size, increased PVM, right aortic arch (50%)

EKG:

Normal axis initially, followed by CVH (70%), +/− LAE

Management:

Treat CHF

Early and complete surgical repair *Rastelli's
procedure*

*Maintain O2 Sat 75-85% to ↑PVR
& prevent excessive pulm. blood
flow*

5. Tricuspid atresia (TA) *Hypoplastic RV*

Pathophysiology:

Complete absence of tricuspid valve

TA with minimal VSD: leads to poor RV development due to lack of blood flow in utero; ductal-dependent; requires shunt

TA with VSD: size of VSD determines size of RV (the greater left-to-right shunt across VSD, greater RV size)

PA is common

Juxtaposed atrial appendages can be present; great arteries transposed in 30%

Clinical:

Cyanosis since birth

May develop CHF depending on anatomy

There is often a moderate systolic murmur and a single S2

CXR:

Heart size and pulmonary vascular markings are proportional to PBF

EKG:

Left superior QRS axis (between 0° and −90°) common (especially if no TGA)

*Hypoxemia worsens c̄ ↑
pulm stenosis & c̄ restriction
of L→R bl. flow @
the level of VSD*

*regurge 2-3/6 Ⓜ @LLSB
VSD*

Increased LV forces, decreased RV forces

RAH (typically with large P wave) or combined atrial hypertrophy

Management:

PGE1

Rashkind procedure if inadequate right-to-left shunting but not usually needed

If increased PBF → PA banding

If decreased PBF → shunt required

+/− other surgery depending on anatomy

→ pvlm bl. fl decreased

6. Ebstein's anomaly

ASD or PFO } R→L shunt

* In utero cardiac enlargement can cause Lung hypoplasia

Incidence:

<< 1% of all congenital heart defects

Suggested association with maternal Lithium use

High mortality

Increased risk for pulmonary hypoplasia due to large right heart in utero

Pathophysiology:

Tricuspid valve leaflets are displaced into RV

The portion of the RV wall that is above displaced leaflets becomes "atrialized"

TV regurgitation and/or tricuspid stenosis

Atrial communication in ~80% with right-to-left shunt

Clinical:

If severe, cyanosis due to decreased PBF (atrial shunting right-to-left) in first few days of life

Often without murmur

Hepatosplenomegaly, may develop CHF

CXR:

Usually dramatic cardiomegaly mostly because of severely dilated RA

Decreased PVM; no RVH

EKG: *SVT

RBBB, RAE, WPW (20%), occasional 1st degree AV block

Management:

If mild, no treatment

If severe, PGE1 to increase PBF

Treat CHF

Limited surgical options and surgery reserved for patients with severe symptoms

*place in O2 to ↓PVR ?improve pulm. bl. flow

7. Single ventricle

Incidence:

<1% of all congenital heart disease

Increased risk asplenia or polysplenia

Pathophysiology:

Both AV valves empty into a single ventricle

Most common form is a single LV with L-TGV (aorta arises from a small leftward RV)

No ventricular septum

Complete mixing of systemic and pulmonary venous blood with LVP = RVP

PBF dependent on PVR vs SVR and degree of PS

Clinical:

Symptoms dependent on PBF; if increased PBF, CHF, mild cyanosis and single or narrow S2 with systolic murmur; if decreased PBF, clinical presentation similar to TOF with moderate-severe cyanosis and minimal CHF

CXR:
  If increased PBF → heart is large and PVM increased
  If decreased PBF → heart is smaller and PVM decreased or normal
EKG:
  Abnormal QRS forces
  Often abnormal Q waves
Management:
  May require PGE1 if associated with severe coarctation and/or subpulmonary stenosis
  Treat CHF (PA banding if no PS and severe CHF)
  Palliative surgery (Glenn procedure); definitive surgery (Fontan procedure)

8. Total anomalous pulmonary venous return (TAPVR)

Incidence: *pulm veins → RA (normal to LA)*
  1–2.5% of all congenital heart disease
Pathophysiology:
  All pulmonary veins with fully oxygenated blood follow an abnormal route returning to RA via various paths *instead* of
    LA
  Secundum ASD of PFO is required for right-to-left shunt to provide systemic blood flow
  Supracardiac (most common) — PV via vertical vein to innominate, azygous or directly to SVC
  Cardiac — PV into RA directly or indirectly via coronary sinus
  Infracardiac = subdiaphragmatic — PV crosses the diaphragm and drains into portal vein or hepatic vein or IVC
  Mixed
Types:
  (1) obstructive and (2) nonobstructive
Clinical:

emergent surg.   *"snow-man"*

Obstructive TAPVR	Nonobstructive TAPVR
Infracardiac (subdiaphragmatic) almost always obstructive	Majority of *cardiac* and *supracardiac* are nonobstructive
Pulmonary venous hypertension, pulmonary edema, CHF	Increased PBF, may develop CHF
Cyanosis	Mild to moderate cyanosis (dependent on degree of mixing and streaming of blood across ASD)
Respiratory distress, often requires intubation soon after birth	Physiologically similar to large ASD except also cyanosis
Decreased systemic perfusion	
Typically without murmur	Systolic mumur at left upper sternal border and a diastolic murmur at lower sternal border
May have loud 2nd heart sound	Widely split and fixed S2 — quadruple rhythm
CXR: normal heart size, increased PVM due to increased pulmonary venous congestion; fluffy appearance — lung fields appear similar to aspiration pneumonia	CXR: increased heart size, prominent MPA segment, pulmonary congestion, increased PVM, snowman silhouette (if supracardiac type)
Oxygen sat PA = Ao due to complete RA mixing	Oxygen sat PA = Ao due to complete RA mixing
EKG: RVH	EKG: right axis deviation, RVH (rsR' in V1), RAE
Management: medical treatment of CHF	Management: medical treatment of CHF
Surgical repair urgent	Surgery not always needed immediately

9. Double outlet right ventricle

Incidence:
  <1% of all congenital heart disease
Pathophysiology:
  Aorta and pulmonary artery arise from RV
  VSD is required to provide an outlet from LV
  VSD can be subaortic, subpulmonic, doubly-committed or remote
  Great arteries can be normally related, side-by-side or transposed
  75% with some degree of PS:

If absence of PS → increased PBF
If presence of PS → decreased PBF, increased cyanosis

Clinical:
Clinical findings determined by the type and size of the VSD as well as the presence or absence of PS

CXR:
Varies depending on lesion

EKG:
RVH and right axis deviation
1st degree heart block is common

Management:
Treat CHF
Consider full repair if severe
Surgical repair dependent on location of VSD and presence or absence of PS

B. LEFT-TO-RIGHT SHUNTS

* Large defect dependant on PVR for amt of L→R shunt

1. Ventricular septal defect (VSD)

Incidence:
Most common congenital heart disease

* 1st days ∅(M)d↓↑ PVR

Most common cause of congestive heart failure (CHF) after the 2nd week of life

Types:
Perimembranous VSD—70%, membranous VSDs that can extend into inlet (e.g. AV canal), trabecular region (most common) or infundibular region (e.g. TOF)
Muscular VSD—25%, involves only muscular septum
Outlet VSD—5–7%, supracristal, conal, subpulmonary
Inlet VSD—5–8%, posterior and inferior to perimembranous VSD

* higher pressure in LV & higher SVR cause L→R

Clinical:
Symptoms dependent on degree of PVR and size of VSD since both will determine amount of shunting
Small VSD typically asymptomatic
Moderate-large VSD with CHF as PVR decreases (premature infants with lower PVR may develop symptoms sooner than full-term infants) leading to poor feeding, increased risk for pulmonary infections; if large VSD is not repaired, may lead to poor growth, developmental delay, and pulmonary vascular obstructive disease
In first few days of life, a murmur is not appreciated since there is minimal left-to-right shunting due to increased PVR
With decreased PVR, harsh holosystolic ejection murmur typically well-localized at left lower sternal border; the smaller the VSD, the louder the murmur; if large VSD, may be pansystolic and associated with apical diastolic rumble

CXR: palpable systolic thrill
Normal (if small VSD); if large VSD – increased PVM, increased heart size (dependent on degree of left-to-right shunt), LAE, LVE, possible RVH

EKG:
Normal (if small VSD), LVH due to LV volume overload (if moderate VSD) or CVH (if large VSD)

Management:
Spontaneous closure (especially if muscular VSD)
Treat CHF
Definitive surgery with direct closure when significant left-to-right shunt (Qp/Qs > 2:1) with severe CHF, poor growth or increased pulmonary artery pressure

surgery requires cardio-pulm bypass

2. Atrial septal defect (ASD), ostium secundum type

assoc. c̄ Mitral valve

Incidence:
6–11% of all congenital heart disease, greater in females (2:1)
May have anomalous pulmonary veins

Pathophysiology:

Since the (compliance of the RV > LV,) left-to-right shunting occurs across the ASD

*pulm or tricuspid stenosis can Reverse Shunt or Reduce it

The degree of shunting is dependent upon the size of the ASD and the compliance of the two ventricles

RV volume overload

Clinical:

Often asymptomatic; *widely split, fixed S2* (due to delayed RV depolarization and little change in venous return to RA with respiration)

Since there is minimal differences in pressure between the RA and LA, the blood flow through the ASD does not produce a murmur

Murmur due to relative pulmonary stenosis (upper left sternal border, systolic) and if larger ASD, relative tricuspid stenosis murmur (diastolic, right lower sternal border)

CHF is unusual

CXR:

Increased heart size, RAE, RVH, prominent MPA, increased PVM

No LAE (in contrast to VSD) since blood doesn't stay long in LA but rather, is shunted to RA

EKG:

If moderate or large, can lead to right axis deviation ($+90°$ to $+180°$), RVH or RV conduction delay (rsR' in V1)

Management:

Definitive closure if RV volume overload

Surgery usually at 2–5 years of age.

Untreated: can cause CHF & pulm. HTN
— can close spontaneously
Requires Bypass

3. Patent ductus arteriosus (PDA)

L → R shunt

Wide muscular connection btw pulm artery & aorta

Incidence:

4–10% of all full-term infants with CHD

Greater incidence in premature infants

Pathophysiology of ductus arteriosus closure:

Closure due to increased paO_2 with increased contracting mediators and decreased dilating mediators

Functional closure—occurs in most of full-term infants by 48 hours of age;

In contrast, premature infants may not have functional closure until days to weeks

Ductus arteriosus can re-open until anatomic closure occurs

Anatomic closure—complete at ~2–4 weeks of age

Following fibrosis, becomes the ligamentum arteriosum

Constrictors—PGF2α, acetylcholine, bradykinin, oxygen

Dilators—PGE1, PGI2 (prostacyclin), hypoxia, acidosis

In term: bl L→R Re-entering pulm circuit & ↑pulm. bl flow
* High pulm bl flow ↑PVR, pulm HTN & RV hypertrophy
In preterm: L→R d/t ↓PVR bl. Re-enter pulm circuit ↑pulm venous cong. → ↓ Lung compliance

Pathophysiology of PDA:

Similar to VSD

The degree of the left-to-right shunt is dependent on:

1. The diameter and length of PDA,
2. Pressure difference between aorta and PA, and
3. Difference between systemic and pulmonary vascular resistances

Left-to-right shunting increases as PVR decreases

Clinical:

(Machinery murmur) during systole (60%) or continuous (30%) (since left-to-right shunt during diastole and systole); loudest at left upper sternal border

If small PDA, usually asymptomatic

If moderate-large PDA, may have bounding peripheral pulses due to widened pulse pressure, hyperdynamic precordium, and symptoms of CHF

Premature infants with significantly increased left-to-right shunting may develop decreased lung compliance and intubated infants may have difficulty weaning from ventilator; in addition, significant left-to-right shunt may lead to abnormal cerebral hemodynamics; uncertain if increased risk NEC or pulmonary hemorrhage

CXR:

Normal if small PDA; if moderate to large PDA, increased heart size, increased PBF, LAE, LVH, large ascending aorta and large MPA

Cannot distinguish from VSD

EKG:

Often normal

If large PDA, may have LVH and perhaps combined ventricular hypertrophy

Management:

Early management improves outcome

Indomethacin (see section XC.) $0.2\,mg/kg$

Fluid restriction

Maintain adequate hematocrit

Surgical ligation

4. Complete AV canal (AVC) (endocardial cushion defect)

Incidence:

2–5% of all congenital heart disease

Majority of patients with AVC will have trisomy 21

Associated with PDA (10%) and TOF (10%)

Pathophysiology:

Developmental abnormality of endocardial cushion (normally leads to primum atrial septum, inlet ventricular septum, MV and TV)

Complete AVC = ostium primum ASD (lower part of atrial septum), inlet VSD, common atrioventricular valve

Partial AVC = primum ASD +/− cleft in MV (intact ventricular septum, usually normal TV)

Changes are due to combination of ASD and VSD as well as degree of AV valve insufficiency

Left-to-right shunt dept on PVR

Volume overload on left side due to left-to-right shunt across VSD and due to MR

Volume overload on right side due to ASD

Clinical:

CHF (secondary to volume overload on both ventricles) and cyanosis

Most patients will have systolic murmur, loudest at lower left sternal border (attributable to VSD); may appreciate murmur at the apex (due to MR)

May have apical diastolic murmur, accentuated P2 of second heart sound or gallop

CXR:

Increased PVM, increased heart size

EKG:

RVH; +/− LVH

Often with prolonged PR (i.e. 1st degree AV block)

Superior QRS axis (deep S wave in avF) due to anatomical abnormality of HIS bundle

Management:

Treat CHF

Surgical ASD and VSD closure

Surgical construction of two separate AV valves

Usually complete surgical repair

5. Partial anomalous pulmonary venous return (PAPVR)

Pathophysiology:

1 or more (not all) PV drain into RA via SVC, IVC or left innominate vein

Right pulmonary veins more often involved than left (twice as likely)

Right pulmonary veins drain into SVC (associated with sinus venosus defect), IVC (associated with scimitar syndrome), or RA

Left pulmonary veins drain most commonly into innominate vein

Hemodynamically, similar to ASD

The severity of increased PBF dependent on the number of anomalous pulmonary veins, presence and size of ASD and degree of PVR

Clinical:

Often asymptomatic

Usually ASD murmur with split, fixed S2

CXR:

Increased heart size, RAE, RVH, prominent MPA, increased PVM

EKG:

RVH, rsR' (RV conduction delay) or normal

Management:

Surgical correction if significant left-to-right shunt

C. LEFT AND RIGHT-SIDED OBSTRUCTIVE LESIONS

1. Coarctation of the aorta (CoA)

Incidence:

5–8% of all congenital heart disease; male > female (2:1)

30% of patients with Turner syndrome have coarctation

>50% also with bicuspid aortic valve, increased risk VSD

Types:

Usually coarctations are juxtaductal (opposite the entry point of ductus arteriosus)

Can be separated into two groups:

1. Presentation in infancy: if severe obstruction; this leads to CHF and decreased perfusion (when PDA closes); may develop LV failure
2. Presentation later in life: if coarctation is not significant; often asymptomatic initially and presents later in life with hypertension and decreased femoral pulses; coarctation usually more obstructive as patient grows; collaterals can develop

Clinical:

Blood pressure in upper extremities > lower extremities (if > 10 mmHg → abnormnal; if > 20 mmHg → significant obstruction)

Decreased femoral pulses

Systolic ejection murmur, loudest at left interscapular area in back (where descending aorta present) and at site of coarctation

May develop AR murmur due to bicuspid aortic valve

CXR:

If mild, normal heart size

Increasing heart size with increased severity of coarctation

"3 sign" on CXR

"E sign" on esophagram *(around 4mo.)*

Rib notching in older patients due to erosion of the undersurface of the ribs from the intercostal collateral circulation

EKG:

Usually normal

Management:

PGE1 if severe coarctation; treat CHF

Balloon angioplasty is controversial for native (unoperated) coarctation

Surgery with end-to-end anastomosis

Postoperative hypertension common in older children, less common in neonate

Handwritten margin notes:
* Severe coarc – loud single S₂
*most common Location: below origin of ℓ subclavian artery
~proximal to ductus = preductal
~postductal = collaterals may be asymptomatic

(handwritten top: ✓ critical stenosis ↓PVM)

2. Pulmonic stenosis (PS) and aortic stenosis (AS)

*(handwritten: *Noonan Syndrome)*

(handwritten right: "aortic knob" / valvular - most common)

	Pulmonic Stenosis	Aortic Stenosis
Incidence	5–8% of all congenital heart disease	5% of all congenital heart disease; >in males 4:1
Pathophysiology	Can be valvular (90%), subvalvular (infundibular, usually associated with TOF), or supravalvular (= peripheral pulmonic stenosis, associated with rubella and Williams syndrome)	Can be valvular (increased risk bicuspid aortic valve), subvalvular (e.g. idiopathic hypertrophic subaortic stenosis or IHSS), or supravalvular (associated with Williams syndrome) *(handwritten: "Elfin facies")*
	Often post-stenotic dilatation if valvular	Often post-stenotic dilatation if valvular
Clinical	If mild, asymptomatic	If mild, asymptomatic
	Typically no cyanosis (if severe PS may have some cyanosis due to right-to-left shunting at atrial level)	No cyanosis
	If severe PS, may develop RV failure	If critical AS, may develop CHF (due to pressure over load) and cardiogenic shock
	(handwritten: PPS) Systolic ejection murmur upper left sternal border (ULSB) radiates to back	Systolic ejection murmur upper right sternal border (URSB) and left midsternal border, radiates to neck and sometimes left lower sternal border (LLSB)
	Murmur loudness is proportional to degree of stenosis and lengthens with increasing degree of obstruction	Murmur loudness is not proportional to degree of stenosis; with more significant AS, there is a palpable thrill at 2nd right intercostal space
	Ejection click ULSB (site of pulmonary valve)	Systolic ejection click at apex
		Narrow pulse pressure
	May have widely split S2	May have paradoxical split of S2
CXR	Normal heart size (increased if CHF), prominent main pulmonary artery due to post-stenotic dilatation (valvular)	Normal heart size (increased if CHF)
	PVM normal (decreased if severe)	Post-stenotic dilated aorta if severe stenosis and valvular
EKG	Right axis deviation and RVH (proportional to degree of obstruction)	May observe increased LV forces with strain pattern in severe obstruction
Management	If critical PS—PGE1, balloon valvuloplasty	Neonate with critical AS—PGE1, treat CHF
		Balloon valvuloplasty (less successful c/w PS and may require aortic valvotomy)

(handwritten left margin: PPS–Rubella / William's Synd.)

D. Valvular Heart Disease

Aortic Valve Regurgitation (AR), Mitral Valve Regurgitation (MR) and Tricuspid Valve Regurgitation (TR)

In general, if severe valvular regurgitation, both proximal and distal chambers undergo volume overload and chamber dilatation

Typically, if neonate has valvular heart disease it is associated with other cardiac defects

	Aortic Valve Regurgitation	Mitral Valve Regurgitation	Tricuspid Valve Regurgitation
Pathophysiology	Volume overload of LV due to backflow of blood to LV	Volume overload of LA and LV leading to increased size of both chambers	Volume overload of RA and RV
	Aorta also becomes dilated due to > stroke volume		
	Increased systolic BP due to increased stroke volume		
	Decreased diastolic BP due to continuous backflow to LV during diastole		
Clinical	Wide pulse pressure	Systolic blowing murmur loudest over apex	Can be present in infants with perinatal depression and RV dysfunction
	Bounding pulses	Diastolic murmur at apex due to excess amount of blood across MV	Cyanosis if right-to-left at PFO
	Early diastolic blowing murmur loudest at LSB		Systolic blowing murmur at LLSB
			Diastolic rumble at LSB due to excess amount of blood across TV
			Severe TR → enlarged pulsatile liver and distended neck veins

(continued on following page)

	Aortic Valve Regurgitation	Mitral Valve Regurgitation	Tricuspid Valve Regurgitation
CXR	LVE, dilated ascending aorta	Increased LV size	Normal PVM
EKG	Increased LV forces	Increased LV forces	RAH
	In severe AR, may have ST wave depression and T wave inversions		Often unremarkable
Management	Treat CHF if develops	Treat CHF if develops	Conservative management unless surgery deemed necessary
	Valve repair and may need replacement; surgery reserved for cardiac symptoms, progressive increase in LV, or EKG changes	Valvuloplasty if possible; if not definitive MV replacement	

E. OTHER DISEASES

1. Hypoplastic left heart syndrome (HLHS)

Incidence:

Males greater than females

2nd most common CHD presenting with cyanosis in first week of life

Pathophysiology:

Severe stenosis or atresia of aortic or mitral valve, hypoplastic LV, and aortic arch hypoplasia

In utero RV can still provide systemic output due to ductal right-to-left shunting (PVR > SVR) but after delivery, CO is dependent on LV (secondary to closing PDA)

Lesion requires a patent ductus (necessary for systemic blood flow) and left-to-right atrial flow

Clinical:

Timing and severity of symptoms is dependent on (1) presence or absence of PDA, (2) adequacy of left-to-right atrial flow, and (3) relative PVR vs SVR

Immediately after birth, neonate with minimal symptoms (mild cyanosis and mild tachypnea) due to presence of PDA and elevated PVR providing right-to-left shunting across PDA

When PDA closes, infant develops CHF and decreased peripheral pulses, metabolic acidosis with renal, and gastrointestinal hypoperfusion (due to decreased SBF) progressing to shock

Murmur may be present

Single S2

CXR:

Increased PVM, increased heart size

EKG:

RVH, right axis deviation, decreased LV forces

Management:

PGE1 to maintain a patent ductus arteriosus and provide systemic perfusion (right-to-left shunting), minimal oxygen supplementation (to maintain elevated PVR), hypoventilation (since hypercarbia associated with elevated PVR), inotropic support, treat CHF

$+/-$ balloon atrial septostomy/septectomy

Staged surgical repair starting with Norwood

May require heart transplant

2. Cardiomyopathy (CM)

Type of CM	Hypertrophic	Congestive or Dilated	Restrictive
Incidence	Increased risk if Pompe disease, Hurler disease, and Noonan syndrome Of note – infant of diabetic mother and postnatal steroids may lead to hypertrophy but this is usually transient	Increased risk if abnormal myocardium (myocarditis, carnitine deficiency), abnormal coronary perfusion, or following arrhythmia	Least common of cardiomyopathies

(continued on following page)

Type of CM	Hypertrophic	Congestive or Dilated	Restrictive
Pathophysiology	Variable ventricular hypertrophy with increased inotropic function	Decreased ventricular inotropic function during systole associated with dilatation of left atria and left ventricle	Abnormal ventricular filling during diastole associated with stiff ventricles
	Can be global or localized; may be obstructive or nonobstructive; may have systolic anterior motion of MV		Normal initial systolic function
	Diastolic dysfunction is a prominent feature		Atrial dilatation out of proportion to ventricular dilatation
Clinical	May be asymptomatic with normal exam	CHF, poor distal perfusion	Typically without murmur
	May have harsh ejection murmur	May develop MR murmur	Later, exam may be consistent with pulmonary hypertension
	Neonates may have symptoms of CHF	S4 gallop may be appreciated	
	Thrill may be appreciated		
	In older patients: exercise intolerance, chest pain, palpitations, syncope	In older patients: exercise intolerance, fatigue, weakness	In older patients: exercise intolerance, fatigue, weakness, chest pain
CXR	Usually normal	Increased heart size	Normal or mild increase in heart size
	May have increased heart size	Pulmonary edema	
EKG	May be normal	Increased LV forces, ST and T wave changes	May have bilateral enlargement
	LVH, ST and T wave changes		
	Deep septal Q waves due to hypertrophied septum	Q waves	
	Increased risk of arrhythmias	Increased risk of arrhythmias	
Management	May require medical therapy	Treat CHF	Medical management and referral for heart transplant
	Treat CHF	Consider anticoagulation	
	If severe symptoms, consider myomectomy	Vasodilators	
	Want to ensure adequate preload to limit LVOT obstruction (prevent dehydration, avoid inotropes)	May need heart transplant	
	Digoxin contraindicated (since by increasing contractility, it may lead to increased obstruction)		

3. Eisenmenger's complex

Development of pulmonary vascular disease in patients with CHD

Presents in childhood with prolonged period of increased PVR (typically > 2 years) that is most often associated with left-to-right shunts

Smooth muscle hypertrophy of pulmonary vascular bed occurs and may lead to right atrial enlargement as well as right ventricular enlargement and hypertrophy

May require nifedipine, prostacyclin, nitric oxide, lung transplant

4. Cor pulmonale

RV disorder secondary to severe lung abnormality (e.g. severe chronic lung disease, upper airway obstruction)

Leads to increased RV afterload (from pulmonary vasoconstriction due to prolonged hypoxia, lung tissue destruction, or poor lung development)

RVH, RV dysfunction

Management includes treatment of underlying disease, diuretics, pulmonary vasodilators, oxygen therapy

Often irreversible if lung disease resolves

5. Pericardial effusion

Etiologies: pericarditis, severe anemia with CHF, post-cardiac surgery, leakage from central venous catheter

Clinical: if slow development of fluid, may have minimal symptoms; if rapid fluid accumulation, can develop pericardial tamponade with poor CO, tachycardia, hypotension; can have *pulsus paradoxus* (large decrease in BP with inspiration)

CXR: increased heart size

Diagnosis: confirm by echocardiogram

Management: if large effusion or hemodynamic instability perform pericardiocentesis; treat underlying etiology

6. Anomalous left coronary artery
Originates from pulmonary artery
CHF may develop due to LV dysfunction
Can lead to myocardial ischemia and/or infarction
EKG: deep Q wave in aVL and V4 to V6; increased LV forces as ventricle dilates

7. Cardiac tumors rare
In utero: asymptomatic, hydrops, fetal arrhythmia
Clinical: hemodynamics dependent on number of tumors, size of tumor(s) and location; increased risk for arrhythmias
Types
> *Rhabdomyoma*—most common primary cardiac tumor in neonates can be located anywhere in heart (often involves ventricle and septum); usually multiple; increased risk if tuberous sclerosis; can regress; surgery required if obstruction of flow
>
> *Fibroma*—usually well-circumscribed, single and fibrous; majority arise from LV and rarely involve septum; usually do not regress
>
> *Myxoma*—majority found in adulthood; located typically in left atrium; can develop inflow obstruction; tissue can embolize
>
> *Sarcoma*—very rare tumor arising from cardiac myocytes
>
> *Teratoma*—typically intrapericardial; can lead to pericardial effusion

8. Asplenia and polysplenia

Asplenia	Polysplenia
Absent spleen	Multiple splenic tissues—often with normal function
Sequence of bilateral right-sidedness	Sequence of bilateral left-sidedness
Always severe cardiac malformations	Less severe cardiac malformations
Cardiac: aorta and IVC juxtaposed (100%), TAPVR (90%), AVC (85%), TGA (75%), bilateral SVC (75%), PS/PA (75%), single ventricle (60%), dextrocardia (40%)	Cardiac: azygous return of IVC (70%), TAPVR (70%), bilateral SVC (50%), AVC (40%), dextrocardia (~40%), TGA (17%), PS/PA (10%), single ventricle (10%)
Respiratory: 2 right lungs (3-lobed)	Respiratory: 2 left lungs (2-lobed)
Gastrointestinal: midline liver, two gallbladders, right or left stomach, malrotation	Gastrointestinal: midline liver, right or left stomach, increased incidence of biliary atresia, malrotation
Hematology: Howell-Jolly and Heinz bodies	
Infection: increased risk of infection (especially Streptococcus pneumoniae)	
Cyanosis	Cyanosis
Poor prognosis	Poor prognosis (however, better than asplenia)

9. Cor triatriatum rare
Pathophysiology: LA is divided into two compartments by an abnormal fibromuscular septum; the proximal chamber communicates directly with the pulmonary veins and the distal chamber communicates with the mitral valve
Clinical: decreased peripheral pulses, tachypnea, poor weight gain, pulmonary edema, dyspnea, often with loud P2, +/− murmur
CXR: increased pulmonary vascular markings, prominent MPA segment
EKG: RAD, RVH, may have RAE
Management: treat pulmonary venous congestion, surgery

V. Clinical Manifestations of Congenital Heart Disease

A. CENTRAL CYANOSIS

1. Definition
Defined by the absolute amount of reduced Hb (not the O_2 saturation)

Observed if $> 3-5$ g of reduced Hb per dL of arterial blood

Anemia can decrease clinical detection of cyanosis while polycythemia may demonstrate clinical cyanosis sooner since level of reduced Hb easier to attain

2. Differential diagnosis of central cyanosis

Includes congenital heart disease, pneumonia, meconium aspiration syndrome, hyaline membrane disease, pulmonary hypertension with resulting right-to-left intracardiac shunting, pneumothorax, anatomical airway obstruction (e.g. choanal atresia, tracheomalacia), congenital cystic adenomatoid malformation, lobar emphysema, pleural effusion

Differential cyanosis: lower body more cyanotic than upper body due to right-to-left ductal shunting with increased PVR
e.g. critical CoA with PDA and increased PVR

Reverse differential cyanosis: upper body more cyanotic than lower body
e.g. TGA with intact ventricular septum and large PDA with PA to aorta shunting (observed if increased PVR or coarctation)

3. Hyperoxia test "Shunt Study"

Measure paO_2 following administration of 100% FiO_2; if there isn't a substantial increase in paO_2 consider cardiac etiology

Not always possible to rule out CHD with hyperoxia test

Most cardiologists consider a paO_2 during a hyperoxia challenge $> 100-150$ mm to be inconsistent with a cardiac defect

B. PHYSICAL EXAM

1. Heart sounds

S1 = closure of mitral and tricuspid valves

Loudest at apex or LLSB; occasionally can hear splitting since MV closure occurs before TV closure

Abnormal S1

Widely split S1: RBBB, Ebstein's anomaly

S2 = closure of aortic valve (A2) and closure of pulmonary valve (P2)

Heard best with diaphragm

Abnormal S2

Widely split, fixed S2: volume overload (ASD, PAPVR)

Single S2: pulmonary hypertension

One semilunar valve (PA, aortic atresia, HLHS, truncus arteriosus)

P2 not heard (TGA, TOF, severe PS)

Occasionally normal

Paradoxically split S2: aortic valve closure follows pulmonary valve closure

LV ejection delayed (severe AS)

Respiratory cycle A2P2 (expiration) and A2 P2 (inspiration)

The increased negative intrapleural pressure during inspiration leads to an increase in systemic venous return to right heart; the greater RV volume increases RV ejection time and delays pulmonary valve closure

2. Murmurs
Classification

Regurg Systolic Ⓜ 1.VSD 2.Mitral or 3. Tricuspid Regurg.

Systolic murmur

Holosystolic — begins with S1 and continues with similar intensity until S2; occurs with VSD

Ejection — crescendo-decrescendo or diamond-shaped due to low flow at the beginning and end of systole; occurs with stenotic aortic or pulmonic valves as well as obstructed outflow tracts

Early systolic — begins with S2 and disappears quickly before S2

Mid-to-late systolic — begins in the middle of systole; often with midsystolic clicks

Blowing murmur: valvular regurgitation

Diastolic murmur: ALWAYS pathologic; occurs with AR or PR (decrescendo), TS or MS (mid-diastole, diamond-shaped), and increased flow across TV or MV (mid-diastole, diamond-shaped)

Continuous murmur: during systole and part of diastole (can be throughout diastole); occurs with PDA, AV fistula, venous hum, collateral vessels, truncus arteriosus, aortopulmonary window

Gallops: occur with decreased ventricular compliance (CHF) and high-flow states

Systolic clicks: if > 24 hours of age, majority are abnormal and etiologies include AS, PS, truncus arteriosus

Localization of murmurs

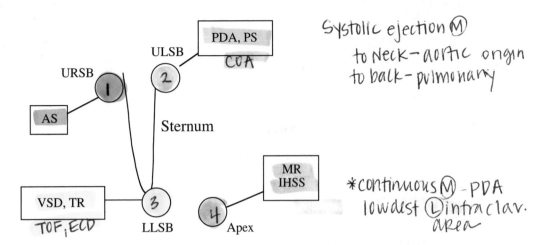

Systolic ejection Ⓜ
to Neck - aortic origin
to back - pulmonary

*continuous Ⓜ - PDA
lowdest Ⓛ intraclav.
area

3. Pulse pressure difference between systolic and diastolic BP

Narrow pulse pressure	Pericardial tamponade, AS, intravascular depletion
Wide pulse pressure	PDA (left-to-right), thyrotoxicosis, AV fistula, AR, truncus arteriosus (run-off by blood into pulmonary artery during diastole)

4. Blood pressure

Measurement:

If blood pressure cuff is too large → artificially lower BP

If blood pressure cuff is too small → artificially elevated BP

Blood pressure cuff width should be 2/3-3/4 circumference of extremity

Shock:

Blood flow to tissues is inadequate to meet tissue metabolic requirements leading to tissue hypoxia, metabolic acidosis, irreversible cellular changes, and subsequent cellular death

Early compensated shock: initial stage of shock due to catecholamine release leading to vasoconstriction, tachycardia and increased contractility

During this stage, blood flow to heart, brain, lungs, and kidneys is maintained while blood flow to skin, muscle, and gastrointestinal circulation is reduced

Late decompensated shock: tissue ischemia with cellular dysfunction and metabolic acidosis leading to subsequent cellular death

Hypovolemic Shock	Distributive Shock	Cardiogenic Shock
Decreased blood volume below a critical level	Inadequate relative intravascular volume due to vasodilation	Cardiac failure
Most common type of shock in neonate		
Decreased ventricular filling and decreased stroke volume	Normal circulating blood volume but insufficient for adequate cardiac filling	Impaired filling, impaired ventricular emptying, impaired contractility
Decrease in CO unless able to compensate with increased HR		
Presents initially with decreased urine output, decreased BP, increased HR (note: premature infants may actually have decreased HR), no CHF	Presents with decreased urine output, increased HR, decreased BP Often with bounding pulses	Presents with decreased urine output, increased HR, decreased BP CHF/pulmonary edema Often with hepatomegaly, cardiomegaly

(continued on following page)

Hypovolemic Shock	Distributive Shock	Cardiogenic Shock
Severe hemorrhage	Sepsis	Metabolic (e.g. hypocalcemia and hypoglycemia)
Severe fluid loss	Anaphylaxis	Congenital heart disease
Can also be associated with sepsis (capillary leakage into 3rd spaces and/ or interstitial spaces)	Vasodilators Toxins	Cardiac tamponade Severe perinatal depression Arrhythmias, myocarditis, cardiomyopathy, myocardial ischemia/infarction Can also be associated with sepsis (decreased contractility

Hypertension (see Renal chapter)

C. CONGESTIVE HEART FAILURE (CHF)

Signs and symptoms resulting from inability of heart to meet demands of body

Hydrops if severe fetal CHF, otherwise, symptoms can include tachypnea, tachycardia, hepatosplenomegaly, weak peripheral pulses, +/− gallop

CXR with increased heart size, increased PVM

Kerley B lines — short horizontal linear densities in lung extending to pleura due to interstitial edema; often difficult to see in neonates

Medical management with diuretics, inotropic agents

VI. Radiographic Findings in Cardiac Disease

Normal CXR
Cardiothoracic ratio often not helpful in neonate since it is altered with different lung expansions and by the presence of the thymic shadow; neonate with normal ratio < 0.65
AP view of heart on CXR:

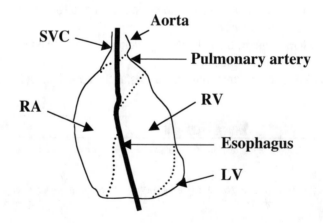

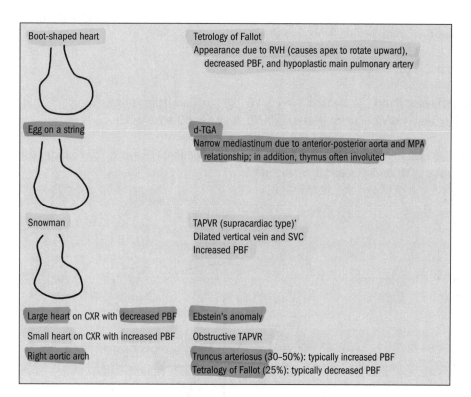

Boot-shaped heart	**Tetrology of Fallot** Appearance due to RVH (causes apex to rotate upward), decreased PBF, and hypoplastic main pulmonary artery
Egg on a string	**d-TGA** Narrow mediastinum due to anterior-posterior aorta and MPA relationship; in addition, thymus often involuted
Snowman	TAPVR (supracardiac type)' Dilated vertical vein and SVC Increased PBF
Large heart on CXR with decreased PBF	Ebstein's anomaly
Small heart on CXR with increased PBF	Obstructive TAPVR
Right aortic arch	Truncus arteriosus (30–50%): typically increased PBF Tetralogy of Fallot (25%): typically decreased PBF

VII. EKG and Arrhythmias

A. EKG RHYTHM

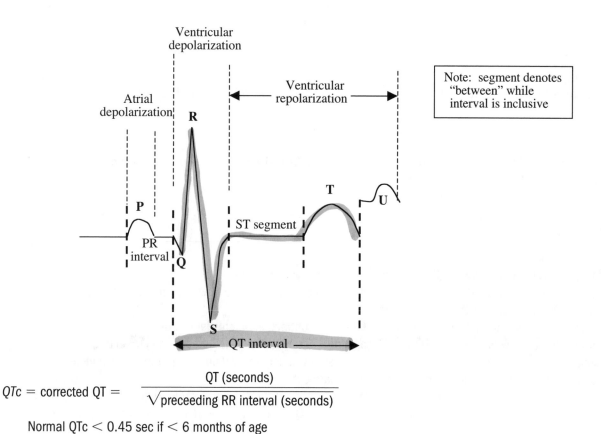

Ventricular depolarization

Atrial depolarization

Ventricular repolarization

Note: segment denotes "between" while interval is inclusive

R

P

ST segment

T

U

PR interval

Q

S

QT interval

$$QTc = \text{corrected QT} = \frac{\text{QT (seconds)}}{\sqrt{\text{preceeding RR interval (seconds)}}}$$

Normal QTc < 0.45 sec if < 6 months of age

RAE: peaked P wave (> 3 mm) in lead II

LAE: P wave duration > 0.1–0.12 sec, may have biphasic P wave

RV hypertrophy: increased R in V1, increased S in I or V6, right axis deviation; persistent upright T in V1 after 3 days of life; increased R/S ratio in V1 or decreased ratio in V6; may have Q wave in V1

LV hypertrophy: increased R in V6, increased S in V1; left axis deviation; Q wave in V5/V6 with peaked T waves; increased R/S ratio in V6 or decreased R/S ratio in V1

B. EKG AXIS

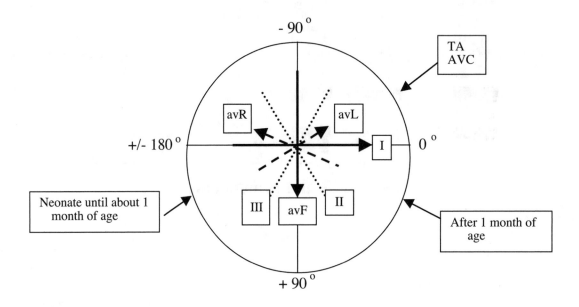

QRS axis: (represented in above vector diagram), neonate normally between 100° and 150°

P wave: normally upright in I and avF; normal P axis = 0° to 90°

T wave: normally upright in II, III, avF (inferior leads) and I, V5, V6 (lateral leads); T wave usually concordant with QRS axis
  Can be upright in V1 if less than 72 hours old
  If upright in V1 after 72 hours of age suggests RVH

C. ARRHYTHMIAS

1. Premature beats
  1. *Premature atrial contraction (PAC):* common in newborns; typically benign
     Early P waves that have a different axis and morphology compared to sinus P wave; usually normal QRS but may cause QRS aberration with change in morphology
     Due to premature beat originating in atrium that leads to contraction before sinus node
     May be associated with hyperthyroidism, CHD, cardiomyopathy, central line irritation of right atrium
  2. *Premature junctional contraction:* rare; premature beat originating from AV node or proximal HIS bundle; QRS morphology is normal; in general, does not require treatment
  3. *Premature ventricular contraction (PVC):* abnormal and prolonged QRS with ST slope away from QRS and without preceding P wave; T wave axis is usually directed opposite QRS; usually followed by a compensatory pause

Due to premature beat initiating from below AV node and bundle of HIS

May be unifocal (and thus uniform PVCs) or multifocal (different QRS complexes)

Bigeminy = alternating normal QRS wave with PVC

Couplet = two consecutive PVCs, less benign than bigeminy

Asymptomatic neonates with isolated PVCs and normal cardiac anatomy do not usually require treatment

Treat underlying cause (digoxin toxicity, infection, electrolyte abnormalities, hypoxemia, acidosis, CHD, excess aminophylline/caffeine, myocarditis)

2. Tachycardias

Reentry Tachycardia	Abnormal Automatic Focus	Triggered Activity
Begins and ends abruptly	Begins and ends gradually	Begins and ends gradually
Requires 2 pathways	Unclear etiology	
One route must be slower than other		
Majority of tachyarrhythmias		
e.g. WPW (observed when tachycardia resolved), atrial reentry (atrial flutter, atrial fibrillation), SVT (SA node or AV node reentry), ventricular tachycardia	e.g. junctional ectopic tachycardia, ectopic atrial tachycardia, ventricular tachycardia	Occurs with digoxin toxicity, excess catecholamines, electrolyte abnormalities
Typically stopped with DC cardioversion	Typically not stopped with DC cardioversion	

1. *Sinus tachycardia:* normal P wave and axis, atrioventricular conduction is normal; due to fever, hypovolemia, cardiac failure, severe anemia, medications (e.g. aminophylline/caffeine, isoproterenol, dopamine)
   HR usually < 250 with variability
2. *Ectopic atrial tachycardia:* abnormal atrial ectopic focus leads to rapid rate, abnormal P wave
   Can lead to cardiac dysfunction
   If treat, consider β-blocker or Class IC antiarrhythmic agents
3. *Junctional ectopic tachycardia:* rare, majority occur post-operatively; ectopic focus originates in AV node or proximal bundle of HIS; atrial and ventricular rhythms are often dissociated; narrow QRS in contrast to ventricular tachycardia
   RR faster than PP suggests junctional rhythm since ventricular rate faster than atrial rate
   Treatment includes normalization of electrolytes, minimization of inotropes, atrial pacing, +/− amiodarone and procainamide
4. *Atrial flutter:* ectopic atrial reentry with atrial rate 300–500, "sawtooth" configuration (best seen in II, III, avF and V1); QRS usually normal

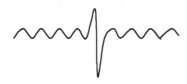

   Some AV block occurs since all atrial beats are not conducted and thus, variable RR intervals; starts and ends suddenly; may develop CHF
   If stable, treat with digoxin to block ventricular rate and procainamide or other anti-arrhythmic medications to block atrial response
   If unstable, DC cardioversion or esophageal pacing followed by digoxin
5. *Atrial fibrillation:* multiple atrial reentry sites leading to irregular atrial waves and an abnormal atrial rate of 350–600
   QRS complex predominantly normal but irregular RR intervals
   Treat with DC defibrillation, digoxin to slow ventricular rate
6. *Supraventricular tachycardia (SVT):* rhythm arising from atrium, AV junction or accessory pathways (see VIID.)

7. *Ventricular tachycardia (V tach):* 3 or more ventricular premature beats at 120–200, widened QRS (note: if wide QRS tachycardia, need to assume due to V tach until further information); inverted T waves; may have VA dissociation

Rhythm arises below bundle of HIS

Neonates may present with CHF

Etiologies include CHD, electrolyte abnormalities, hypoxemia, myocarditis, cardiac tumors, digoxin toxicity, prolonged QT syndrome, and cardiomyopathy; most often idiopathic and self-resolving in neonates

If stable, typically treat with lidocaine; if unstable, treat with DC cardioversion

Anti-arrhythmic chronic therapy

8. *Ventricular fibrillation:* abnormal QRS complexes with rapid irregular rate

Etiologies include CHD, prolonged hypoxia, hyperkalemia, myocarditis, medications, cardiomyopathy, tumors

Treat by DC defibrillation, lidocaine, amiodarone

3. Atrioventricular conduction abnormalities

1. *First degree AV block:* PR interval prolonged due to AV node delay

Associated with myocarditis, digoxin toxicity, hyperkalemia, hypothyroidism, CHD; treatment not usually needed

2. *Second degree AV block:* atrial impulses are not consistently conducted to ventricle

Mobitz type I = Wenckebach – increasing PR interval until an atrial impulse not conducted and then no QRS; due to AV node block; usually well-tolerated and no therapy required

Mobitz type II = abrupt atrial beat that is not conducted; no change in PR interval; may progress to complete AV block; may require pacemaker

3. *Complete AV block* = 3rd degree AV block: complete AV dissociation, ventricular and atrial rates are independent with atrial rate faster than ventricular rate

Due to block of conduction in AV node or HIS Purkinje system

Often with associated CHD (L-TGA, AVC), maternal lupus or following cardiac surgery

Clinical—symptoms dependent on (1) presence or absence of underlying structural heart disease and (2) the ventricular escape rate – the lower the rate, the more likely to be symptomatic

May develop CHF (secondary to decreased cardiac output), possible hydrops in utero

Risk factors for poor outcome – HR < 55/min (in neonates), prolonged QT, wide QRS, ventricular premature beats, abnormal ventricular function

Management – if asymptomatic, no treatment required; pacemaker if symptomatic or thought to have risk factors for poor outcome

4. *Right bundle branch block:* right axis deviation, prolonged QRS and slurring of S in I, V5 and V6

Increased risk with Ebstein's anomaly and post-op cardiac surgery; however, may *not* be associated with congenital heart disease

5. *Left bundle branch block:* left axis deviation, prolonged QRS, loss of Q waves in I, V5 and V6; wide S waves in V1 and V2

4. Other arrhythmias

Prolonged QT syndrome: due to abnormality of ventricular repolarization leading to QT interval > 0.45 sec in neonates (note that newborns < 1 week of age may have increased QTc that later normalizes)

Etiologies can be congenital or acquired (drugs, electrolyte abnormalities – low calcium or magnesium)

Can lead to ventricular tachycardia

Has been associated with sudden infant death syndrome

Treat with anti-arrhythmic medication (propranolol is first-line), may require pacemaker

Sick sinus syndrome: due to injury of SA node; typically following cardiac surgery

Slow, irregular sinus rate; often associated with atrial flutter or atrial fibrillation

5. Electrical management of arrhythmias

Use largest paddle size that allows maximal contact with chest and good separation between the 2 paddles (infants: 4.5 cm size until 1 year of age or 10 kg)

Electrical cardioversion: 0.25–0.5 joules/kg for SVT and atrial dysrrhythmias, increase 50–100% each time an electrical charge is delivered and fails; maximum 2 joules/kg

Electrical defibrillation: optimal dose not established for infants — current recommendation is to use a starting dose of 1–2 joules/kg and if arrhythmia is still present, increase to 4 joules/kg; if still unsuccessful, again use 4 joules/kg

D. SUPRAVENTRICULAR TACHYCARDIA (SVT)

Incidence

Most common pediatric symptomatic arrhythmia

Increased risk CHD (e.g.. Ebstein's anomaly, L-TGA), medications (e.g. caffeine, epinephrine), cardiomyopathy, myocarditis, cardiac tumors, fever, hyperthyroidism

Diagnosis

Typically narrow QRS complex (if wide, treat as if V tach)

P waves may be difficult to identify

Neonatal SVT	Sinus Tachycardia in Neonate	Neonatal Ventricular Tachycardia
Rate 220–330 (usually > 240)	Rate < 230	Rate 120–210
Little variation in rate	Variation in rate	
Begins and ends abruptly	Begins and ends slowly	
Abnormal P wave axis (~85°)	Normal P wave axis	P wave may be dissociated from QRS
Absent P wave in 40%		
QRS wave normal in >90%	QRS normal	Wide QRS
3% with wide complex SVT		
If > 1–2 days of SVT, may lead to CHF	Associated with anemia, hypovolemia, shock, fever, medications (e.g. epinephrine, dopamine, isoproterenol, aminophylline)	Associated with CHD, electrolyte abnormalities, myocarditis, hypoxemia, digoxin toxicity, and shock
		Greater risk for cardiovascular collapse

Wolff-Parkinson-White (WPW) (a type of SVT)

(1) Prolonged QRS, (2) shortened PR interval, and (3) initial slurring of QRS (= delta wave, often present since ventricular myocardium is activated early)

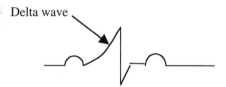

Delta wave

Due to electrical pathway between atrium and ventricle, bypassing AV node (which is faster than travelling through AV node); associated with SVT

Can be associated with Ebstein's anomaly or L-TGA although most commonly found in patients with structurally normal heart

Management of SVT

Short-term therapy: assess if patient is hemodynamically stable

If unstable → synchronized DC cardioversion; consider esophageal overdrive pacing

If stable → vagal maneuvers (bag of ice to face, gagging reflex); adenosine if no change

After SVT resolved, repeat EKG and determine if underlying rhythm abnormal

Medication for SVT	Characteristics
Adenosine Short-term therapy	Transiently blocks AV node and can interrupt AV node limb of re-entry (thus not effective if SVT doesn't involve AV node) Very short 1/2 life (about 10 seconds) Administer by rapid intravenous administration
	(continued on following page)

Medication for SVT	Characteristics
Digoxin Long-term therapy	Monitor EKG and BP during administration May need higher doses if patient receiving aminophylline/caffeine Not used if WPW (unless premature infant)
Propranolol Long-term therapy	First-line if WPW and full-term infant
Other	Other anti-arrhythmic medications (e.g.. procainamide)
Verapamil	Calcium-channel blocker (slows AV node conduction) CONTRAINDICATED in neonates due to associated sudden death

In utero SVT: diagnosis by rapid HR on prenatal echo; need to rule out CHD; treatment if sustained or develops hydrops

E. ELECTROLYTE ABNORMALITIES

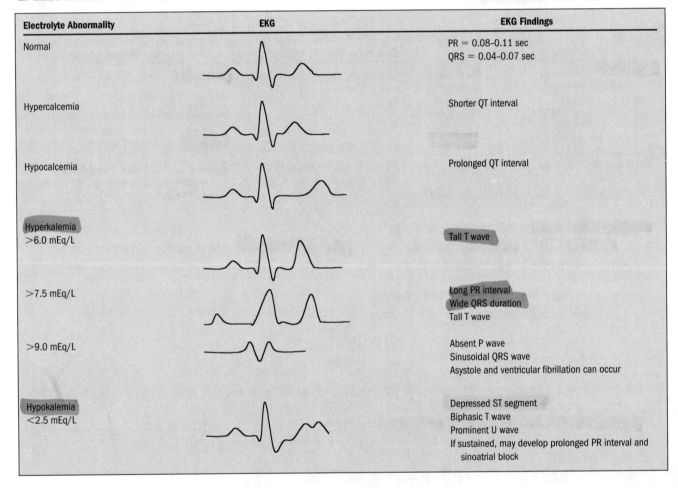

Electrolyte Abnormality	EKG	EKG Findings
Normal		PR = 0.08–0.11 sec QRS = 0.04–0.07 sec
Hypercalcemia		Shorter QT interval
Hypocalcemia		Prolonged QT interval
Hyperkalemia >6.0 mEq/L		Tall T wave
>7.5 mEq/L		Long PR interval Wide QRS duration Tall T wave
>9.0 mEq/L		Absent P wave Sinusoidal QRS wave Asystole and ventricular fibrillation can occur
Hypokalemia <2.5 mEq/L		Depressed ST segment Biphasic T wave Prominent U wave If sustained, may develop prolonged PR interval and sinoatrial block

VIII.   Echocardiography

A. M-MODE = "ice pick" view of heart

Transducer is placed on left sternal border and positioned toward part of heart to be examined

This mode is important for assessing
1. Size of chambers, ventricular wall thickness
2. LV systolic function — fractional shortening
3. Valve movements and interventricular septum wall motion

4. Pericardial fluid

Shortening fraction (SF)
Normal SF = 28–40%

$$SF (\%) = \frac{LV \text{ diastolic dimension} - LV \text{ systolic dimension}}{LV \text{ diastolic dimension}} \times 100$$

B. 2-DIMENSIONAL IMAGING = cross-sectional view, transducer positioned along several cross-sections through heart with 4 views:

1. *Parasternal*
   Long axis: excellent imaging of left side of heart with images of LV inflow and outflow tracts, MV, LA, LV, AV, ascending aorta
      Best for viewing the great artery relationship to the interventricular septum (e.g. overriding aorta)
   Short axis: cross-sectional view of heart and great arteries at different levels
      Semilunar valves, MV, papillary muscles aortic and pulmonary valves well-visualized, PA and branches, RVOT, coronary arteries, LV
      Best for viewing PDA

2. *Apical*
   Shows all four chambers simultaneously, AV valves seen well, can also visualize the LVOT and aortic valve
   Best for viewing AVC

3. *Subcostal*
   A subxyphoid view in which one can view all four chambers, atrioventricular valves, septum, LVOT, aortic valve, RVOT, pulmonary valve, pulmonary veins, systemic veins
   Best for viewing ASD

4. *Suprasternal notch*
   Best for aortic arch

C. DOPPLER ECHO

The Doppler effect is created by a change in the sound frequency with motion

Color flow mapping ideal for identifying shunts and abnormal blood flow through valves

D. FETAL ECHO

Indications: arrhythmia, congenital anomalies, chromosomal abnormalities, nonimmune hydrops, suspected heart disease based on screening ultrasound, parental or sibling history of CHD, maternal diabetes or collagen vascular disease, maternal drug exposure (e.g. alcohol, lithium), genetic disorder in family

Difficult to diagnose: CoA (since may not have obstruction until PDA closes), minor valve abnormalities, and small VSDs

IX. Pressure Tracings

Catheter from umbilical vein advanced through the heart

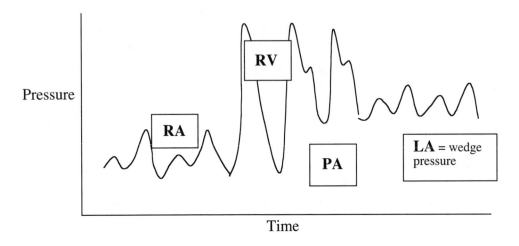

X. Therapeutic Agents in Cardiac Disease

A. SYMPATHETIC RECEPTORS

Receptor	Locale	Effect
α1	Arterial and venous smooth muscle	Smooth muscle contraction (vasoconstrictor) by increasing Ca entry No change in cAMP Increases contractility (inotrope) Gluconeogenesis Decreases insulin release
α2	Sympathetic nerves CNS	Blocks norepinephrine release Inhibits sympathetic output No change in cAMP
β1	Sinoatrial node Atrial and ventricular muscle AV node and Purkinje system	Increases HR with action on SA node Increases conduction velocity with action on AV node Increases contractility Increased renin secretion All above by activating adenylate cyclase, leading to increased cAMP
β2	Arterial and venous smooth muscle	Smooth muscle relaxation (vasodilator) Bronchial relaxation Increases HR and contractility Decreased intestinal motility and tone Induces glycogenolysis Increases insulin secretion

B. INOTROPIC AGENTS

Drug and α or β Effect	Chronotrope (HR), Inotrope and SVR	Characteristics
Amrinone and Milrinone Phosphodiesterase inhibitors	++ good chronic inotrope Decreases SVR	Inhibits cAMP breakdown This increase in cAMP leads to increased Ca cellular entry, increased contractility, relaxation of vascular smooth muscle cells (leading to vasodilation and decreasd afterload) Independent of receptors and thus no tolerance Decreases afterload
Digoxin Inhibits N/K ATPase pump in cardiac myocytes leading to increased Ca influx	*CV dimin. sens. to Dig R/T Receptor affinity* − chronotrope (due partly to vagal effect and also effect of SA node) + inotrope Decreases SVR	Ideal inotrope for CHF Anti-arrhythmic by decreasing atrioventricular conduction Note: other medications may alter digoxin levels Toxicity: GI symptoms, decreased HR, prolonged PR interval, AV block, monitor K$^+$ and Ca levels
Dobutamine *∅UAC* β1 >> β2 Very little α activity 2–20 μg/kg/min More similarities to isoproterenol than dopamine	+ chronotrope (less of an increase in HR compared with dopamine and isoproterenol) + inotrope May decrease SVR	Synthetic catecholamine Good for cardiogenic shock or myocardial dysfunction since no increase in afterload Less effective than dopamine for septic shock No effect on renal blood flow May decrease coronary perfusion due to decrease in SVR
Dopamine Endogenous catecholamine Precursor of epinephrine and norepinephrine (NE) Its effect is partly attributable to release of endogenous NE and thus, with prolonged use, decreased effectiveness 2–20 μg/kg/min	++ chronotrope + inotrope SVR effect is dose- dependent (increases with increased alpha activity)	Inhibits Na/K ATPase and Na/hydrogen pump at low doses, uniquely dilates renal vasculature 2 μg/kg/min (and perhaps lower): dopaminergic receptors (renal, splanchnic, coronary and cerebral) Increases renal blood flow, increases GFR and increases FENA 2–6 μg/kg/min: β1 and dopaminergic >6–20 μg/kg/min: β1 and some α1 >20 μg/kg/min: α1 (controversial if this effect occurs in neonates)
Epinephrine Most potent vasopressor Endogenous catecholamine β1 and β2, α < 0.3 μg/kg/min: β1 and β2 > 0.3 μg/kg/min: α	++ chronotrope + inotrope SVR effect is dose-dependent (increases with increased alpha activity)	Adverse effects include: hypokalemia, local tissue ischemia, renal vascular ischemia, severe hypertension
Isoproterenol Synthetic catecholamine β only (1 and 2) 0.05–1.0 μg/kg/min (usually > 0.5 not required)	+++ chronotrope and thus, helpful for complete heart block + inotrope Decreases SVR leading to peripheral vasodilation	May decrease coronary blood flow due to vasodilation of muscular regions Not helpful in shock since leads to vasodilation in skin and muscle vascular beds May lead to hypoglycemia since induces insulin secretion
Nitroprusside	Decreases SVR	Vasodilator (arterial greater than venous) Increases cGMP levels Rapid onset, short duration Increases intracranial pressure Light-sensitive May lead to cyanide toxicity Extravasation may lead to tissue sloughing/necrosis
Norepinephrine α > β1 > β2	+ chronotrope + inotrope Increases SVR	Epinephrine preferred in neonates Profound vasoconstriction Renal vasoconstriction May lead to hypocalcemia and hypoglycemia

C. DIURETICS (see Respiratory chapter)

D. INDOMETHACIN

Cyclooxygenase inhibitor that blocks prostaglandin synthesis and leads to closure of PDA; greater clearance with increasing postnatal age and weight

Contraindications: PDA with right-to-left shunt, evolving intraventricular hemorrhage, necrotizing enterocolitis, creatinine > 1.8, renal abnormalities that inhibit renal function, thrombocytopenia

Complications: gastrointestinal bleeding, transient oliguria due to decreased glomerular filtration rate, increased serum creatinine, hyponatremia (due to fluid retention), decreased platelet aggregation

With conventional indomethacin regimen, successful closure of PDA in 60–80% of clinically significant PDAs in premature infants with ~30% relapse rate

E. PROSTAGLANDIN (PGE1)

Action: effect within 30 minutes of initiating a continuous infusion; functions to maintain patency of ductus arteriosus for ductal-dependent CHD; vasodilator

Common side effects (6%–15%): apnea (usually less than 6 hours after initiation), fever, cutaneous flushing, bradycardia

Less common side effects (1–5%): hypotension, seizures, tachycardia, cardiac arrest, edema, infection, disseminated intravascular coagulation

Chronic effects: may develop cortical bone proliferation

F. ENDOCARDITIS PROPHYLAXIS

To prevent bacteria from adhering to damaged endocardium

Required during dental and other invasive procedures

Prophylaxis Recommended	Prophylaxis NOT recommended
Most CHD	Isolated secundum ASD
Prosthetic valves	Innocent murmurs without CHD
Previous bacterial endocarditis	Post-surgery after 6 months for:
Rheumatic heart disease with valve disease	Secundum ASD
Hypertrophic cardiomyopathy	VSD
Mitral valve prolapse with regurgitation	PDA
	Mitral valve prolapse without regurgitation
	Pacemakers/defibrillators
	Previous rheumatic heart disease without valve disease

XI. Surgical Repair of Cardiac Defects

Repair	Procedure	Cardiac Defect
Rashkind balloon septostomy (atrial mixing)	Balloon catheter is threaded from IVC to RA, crosses PFO or ASD and enters LA Balloon is then inflated and pulled back to the RA so that the atrial septum is torn	d-TGA with VSD and PS Severe MS HLHS if inadequate left-to-right flow
Blalock-Taussig shunt	Shunt between subclavian artery and ipsilateral pulmonary artery Creates a left-to-right shunt to increase PBF	TA, PA, TOF with severe PS

(continued on following page)

Repair	Procedure	Cardiac Defect
Glenn	SVC connected to PA A bidirectional Glenn allows flow to both RPA and LPA Goal: to increase PBF without increasing volume load on RV	TA Single ventricle with severe PS
Mustard (atrial inversion)	Atrial septum is removed and an intra-atrial baffle is created This allows blood from SVC/IVC to be routed across LA to LV to PA Blood from PV flows over the baffle to the aorta Later in life, may develop RV dysfunction, TR, arrhythmia	d-TGA
Senning	Rerouting similar to Mustard but instead of using avascular pericardium, the baffle is created by atrial septum and RA free wall	d-TGA
Rastelli	Patch VSD allowing LV connection to aorta and conduit/homograft from RV to PA	d-TGA with VSD and PS (Note: cannot do Jatene since PS would become AS)
Jatene (arterial switch)	Arterial switch so that RV connects to PA and LV connects to aorta Coronary reimplantation to aorta	d-TGA (ideal surgery for this lesion)
Fontan (single ventricle repair)	Rerouting of SVC and IVC to PA bypassing the ventricles to create separate systemic and pulmonary circulations Must have normal PVR to allow for adequate blood flow to lungs (unsuccessful in infants with elevated PVR)	TA Single ventricle
Norwood	*Stage I* 1. Atrial septectomy to prevent pulmonary venous congestion 2. MPA divided; proximal PA is connected to ascending aorta 3. Possible reconstruction of hypoplastic aorta 4. Systemic-pulmonary artery shunt to provide pulmonary blood flow *Stage II* (bidirectional Glenn) This is an intermediary procedure to decrease the volume overload on the RV until stage III can be done 1. Shunt removed 2. Connect SVC directly to PA *Stage III* (modified Fontan) Requires normal PVR, adequate-sized pulmonary arteries and good ventricular function	HLHS

XII. Associations with Congenital Heart Disease

A. SYNDROMES ASSOCIATED WITH HEART DISEASE

Syndrome and Approximate Incidence of CHD	Characteristic Cardiac Defect
Carpenter syndrome (50%)	PDA, VSD, ASD, PS, TOF, TGA
Cat eye syndrome (> 33%)	TAPVR, persistent left SVC
CHARGE association (50–70%)	TOF, DORV, VSD, ASD, PDA, right-sided aortic arch
Cornelia de Lange syndrome (occasional)	VSD most common
Cri du chat syndrome (5p-) (30%)	Variable
DiGeorge syndrome	Aortic arch abnormalities (right-sided aortic arch, interrupted aorta, truncus arteriosus)
Ehlers-Danlos syndrome	Aortic root dilatation, mitral valve prolapse
Ellis-van Creveld syndrome (50%)	Common atrium
Glycogen storage IIa (Pompe disease)	Hypertrophic cardiomyopathy (due to glycogen deposition)
Goldenhar syndrome (occasional)	VSD > PDA > TOF > coarctation of aorta

(continued on following page)

Syndrome and Approximate Incidence of CHD	Characteristic Cardiac Defect
Holt-Oram syndrome (>50%)	ASD most common
Homocystinuria	Arterial and venous thromboses, medial degeneration of aorta and elastic arteries
Hurler syndrome	Thickened valves (especially mitral), coronary artery disease, hypertrophic cardiomyopathy
Klippel-Feil sequence	VSD
Marfan syndrome	Dilated aorta and aortic root, aortic aneurysm, MV prolapse
Meckel-Gruber syndrome (occasional)	ASD, VSD, PDA, CoA, PS
Noonan syndrome (>50%)	Dysplastic or thickened pulmonary valve, left ventricular hypertrophy (most often due to local anterior septal wall hypertrophy; less often diffuse hypertrophy), ASD, VSD, PDA, branch stenosis of pulmonary arteries
Rubenstein-Taybi syndrome (25%)	PDA, VSD, ASD
TAR syndrome (thrombocytopenia, absent radius) (30%)	TOF, ASD
Trisomy 13 (Patau syndrome) (80–90%)	80–90% with VSD or PDA < 50% with other cardiac anomalies
Trisomy 18 (Edward syndrome) (95–99%)	VSD, PDA, PS, CoA
Trisomy 21, (40–50%)	Complete AVC > VSD > PDA
Turner syndrome 45, X (35%)	Bicuspid aortic valve (30%), CoA (10%), aortic stenosis Mitral valve prolapse, aortic dissection and hypertension later in life
VACTERL association (50%)	VSD > TOF, CoA
Williams syndrome (50–70%)	Supravalvular subaortic stenosis > peripheral pulmonary artery stenosis, PS

B. INFECTIOUS DISEASES ASSOCIATED WITH CONGENITAL HEART DISEASE

In Utero Exposure	Cardiac Defect
Coxsackie B virus	Myocarditis
Parvovirus B19	Myocarditis
Rubella	PDA, peripheral pulmonic stenosis, PS, AS, TOF, myocarditis

C. MATERNAL MEDICATIONS ASSOCIATED WITH CONGENITAL HEART DISEASE

Medication	Cardiac Defect
Aspirin	Pulmonary hypertension
Ethanol	VSD, ASD, TOF, CoA
Hydantoin or phenytoin	ASD, VSD, CoA, PDA, PS, TOF
Indomethacin	Premature closure of PDA
Lithium	Ebstein's anomaly
Retinoic acid	TGA, TOF, DORV, truncus arteriosus, aortic arch abnormalities, HLHS
Thalidomide	Conotruncal malformations
Trimethadione	VSD, ASD, TGA, TOF, HLHS, TA
Valproic acid	ASD, VSD, AS, PA/IVS, CoA, TOF
Warfarin	PDA, PPS

D. MATERNAL DISEASES ASSOCIATED WITH CONGENITAL HEART DISEASE

Lupus erythematosus	Increased risk for congenital heart block Maternal anti-Ro and anti-La autoantibodies that belong to IgG class and thus can cross placenta and deposit on fetal myocardium and lead to conduction abnormalities

(continued on following page)

	The risk for heart block in the fetus is independent from the severity of maternal illness (often, fetal heart block can be the first sign of maternal lupus)
	In utero symptoms of lupus-related heart block are rare (if present, typical with CHF)
	30–60% of mothers with an infant who has complete heart block will have lupus
Diabetes mellitus	Increased risk for d-TGA, VSD, ventricular hypertrophy
	Risk for congenital heart disease is lower in mothers with normal HbA1C levels
	Poor glucose control even in 3rd trimester still increases the risk for CHD due to associated ventricular hypertrophy (probably due to insulin functioning as a growth factor for fetal cardiomyocytes)

We would like to thank Dr. Karen Altmann for her extremely thorough editing of this chapter; her knowledge of cardiology and her friendship have been invaluable as we put this book together.

References

Beers MH and Berkow R (eds): The Merck Manual of Diagnosis and Therapy (17th ed), New Jersey, Merck Research Laboratories. 1999.

Berger S (ed): Pediatric cardiology. *Pediatric Clinics of North America.* Volume 46(2), 1999.

Cloherty JC and Stark AR (eds): Manual of Neonatal Care (4th edition), Cardiac Disorders Section. Philadelphia, Lippincott-Raven Publishers, 1998.

Cunningham FG, Gant NF, Leveno KJ, et al. (eds): Williams Obstetrics (21st edition). New York, McGraw-Hill Co, Inc. 2001.

Dubin AM. Arrhythmias in the newborn. *NeoReviews* 2001; (8):e146–151.

Fanaroff AA and Martin RJ (eds): Neonatal-Perinatal Medicine (6th edition). St Louis, Mosby–Year Book Inc, 1997.

Fink BW. Congenital Heart Disease: A Deductive Approach to its Diagnosis. St Louis, Mosby–Year Book, Inc (3rd ed), 1991.

Fyler DC (ed): Nadas' Pediatric Cardiology. Philadelphia, Hanley & Belfus, 1992.

Gillette PC. Congenital heart disease. *Pediatric Clinics of North America.* Volume 37 (1), 1990.

Guyton AC and Hall JE: Textbook of Medical Physiology (10th ed). Philadelphia, WB Saunders Co, 2000.

Hansen TN, Cooper TR and Weisman LE (eds): Neonatal Respiratory Disease (2nd edition). Pennsylvania, Handbooks in Health Care Co, 1998.

Jones KL: Smith's Recognizable Patterns of Human Malformations (5th ed). Philadelphia, WB Saunders Co, 1997.

Long WA (ed): Fetal and Neonatal Cardiology. Philadelphia, WB Saunders Co, 1990.

Nathan DG and Orkin SH (eds): Nathan and Oski's Hematology of Infancy and Childhood (5th edition). Philadelphia, WB Saunders Co, 1998.

Park M: Pediatric Cardiology for Practitioners (3rd edition). St Louis, Mosby, 1996.

Young TE and Mangum OB. Neofax: A Manual of Drugs Used in Neonatal Care (15th edition). Raleigh, NC, Acorn Publishing, Inc., 2002.

CHAPTER 4

Neurology and Development

TOPICS COVERED IN THIS CHAPTER

I. Development of the Nervous System and Selected Disorders
- A. Anencephaly
- B. Encephalocele
- C. Myelomeningocele
- D. Arnold-Chiari malformation
- E. Aprosencephaly
- F. Holoprosencephaly sequence
- G. Agenesis of corpus callosum

II. Cerebral Blood Flow and Vasoreactivity
- A. Vascular supply
- B. Cerebral vasoreactivity

III. Neurological Evaluation and Abnormalities
- A. Head
  - 1. Growth
  - 2. Shape
  - 3. Fontanels
- B. Cranial nerves
  - 1. Bilateral facial paresis = Mobius syndrome
- C. Tone
  - 1. Hypertonia
  - 2. Hypotonia
- D. Patterns of weakness
- E. Reflexes

IV. Neurological Studies
- A. Cerebrospinal fluid (CSF)
- B. Electroencephalogram (EEG)
- C. Imaging
  - 1. Ultrasound (US)
  - 2. CT scan
  - 3. MRI scan

V. Hydrocephalus
- A. Obstructive
- B. Communicating

VI. Hypoxic-Ischemic Encephalopathy (HIE)
- A. AAP-ACOG definition of perinatal asphyxia
- B. Changes in substrate metabolism and neurotransmitters
- C. Neurological presentation: Sarnat stages
- D. Multisystem effects (when injury is severe and diffuse)
- E. Management

VII. Patterns of Cerebral Injury
- A. Selective neuronal necrosis
- B. Parasagittal cerebral injury
- C. Focal or multifocal ischemia
- D. Periventricular hemorrhagic infarction
- E. Periventricular leukomalacia (PVL)

VIII. Intracranial Hemorrhage
- A. Subdural
- B. Subarachnoid
- C. Cerebellar
- D. Intraventricular

IX. Birth Trauma
- A. Extracranial hemorrhage
  - 1. Caput succedaneum
  - 2. Cephalohematoma
  - 3. Subgaleal
  - 4. Extradural
- B. Nerve injury
  - 1. Brachial plexus injuries
  - 2. Spinal cord injury
  - 3. Facial nerve (VII) palsy (distal)

X. Neuromuscular Disorders
- A. Lower motor neuron path
- B. Disorders of lower motor neuron
  - 1. spinal muscular atrophy, type I (Werdnig-Hoffmann disease)
  - 2. acquired transient neonatal myasthenia gravis
  - 3. congenital neonatal myasthenia gravis
  - 4. congenital myotonic dystrophy
- C. Disorders with hypotonia and weakness
  - 1. Riley-Day syndrome or "familial dysautonomia"
  - 2. Prader-Willi syndrome
  - 3. arthrogryposis multiplex congenita

XI. Seizures

XII. Vein of Galen Malformation

XIII. Congenital Intracranial Tumors

XIV. Neurocutaneous Syndromes

XV. Cerebral Palsy (CP)

XVI. Mental Deficiency

XVII. Hearing Loss

XVIII. Learning Disability

I. Development of the Nervous System and Selected Disorders

Developmental Process	Gestational Age of Development	Associated Abnormalities (conditions in bold discussed further)
Primary/secondary neurulation (dorsal induction)	Primary: 3–4 weeks Secondary: 4–7 weeks	**Primary neurulation:** brain, spinal cord (except lower sacral segment) **Anencephaly** Myeloschisis **Encephalocele** **Myelomeningocele (MM)** **Arnold-Chiari malformation** **Secondary neurulation:** spinal cord, lower sacral segments Spinal cysts, tethered cord, lipoma, teratoma, Myelocystocele, meningocele-lipomeningocele
Prosencephalic development (ventral induction)	2–3 months	Formation: **aprosencephaly** Cleavage: **holoprosencephaly** Midline development: **agenesis of corpus callosum,** agenesis of septum pellucidum, septo-optic dysplasia
Neural and glial proliferation	3–4 months	Micrencephaly Macrencephaly
Neuronal migration	3–5 months	Schizencephaly (no cortex) Lissencephaly (smooth brain) Pachygyria (broad gyri) Polymicrogyria
Neuronal organization	Axonal outgrowth and proliferation: 3 months to birth Dendritic and synapse: 6 months to 1 year Synaptic rearrangements: birth to several years	Disorders of organization found in: Mental deficiency Trisomy 21 Fragile X syndrome Autism Angelman syndrome Prematurity
Myelination	Birth to years (some aspects not complete until adulthood) Corticospinal tract: 38 weeks' gestation to 2 years The last pathway to myelinate is the association bundle, which connects the prefrontal cortex with the temporal and parietal lobes (complete ~ 32 years)	Disorders of myelination found in: Cerebral white matter hypoplasia Prematurity Malnutrition

A. ANENCEPHALY

= abnormal development during primary neurulation within first 26 days of gestation; failure of anterior tube closure and subsequent degeneration of the forebrain (i.e., absence of major amount of brain tissue, skull and scalp; may have sparing of brainstem and cerebellum)

Incidence
0.2 to 0.3/1000; female > male; Hispanic women greater risk
Increased risk with maternal hyperthermia, and maternal folate, copper, and zinc deficiencies
Recurrence risk is 2% to 5%
13% to 33% have other abnormalities, including congenital heart disease, congenital diaphragmatic hernia, renal malformation, hypoplastic adrenal glands, omphalocele, trisomy 13 or 18 (prenatal evaluation should include a karyotype analysis)

Clinical
Elevated maternal α-fetoprotein
Detected by fetal ultrasound by 14 to 15 weeks' gestation (note: must distinguish from ruptured encephalocele and amniotic bands with scalp-covered lesions)

Karyotype

Often associated with polyhydramnios

65% with spontaneous abortion

Physical examination of neonate shows absence of large part of skull, absent scalp over skull abnormality, and exposed hemorrhagic, fibrotic tissue; unconscious but varying degrees of brainstem function; have spontaneous extremity movements and startle myoclonus; often with increased tone and reflexes

Legal issue

Organ transplantation remains controversial because of the persistence of brainstem function and, therefore, difficulty in establishing brain death

B. ENCEPHALOCELE

= abnormal development during primary neurulation; failure of closure of rostral neural tube, resulting in herniation of meninges and brain tissue through a skull defect

Incidence

~0.15/1000 live births

40% with associated anomalies (e.g., neural tube defect, microcephaly)

Observed in patients with Meckel-Gruber syndrome

Clinical

Occipital location (~70%) > frontal, parietal or nasofrontal region

Increased risk for spontaneous abortion

Because most are covered by skin, usually normal maternal serum α-fetoprotein

Management

Assess for other anomalies; send chromosomes

Surgery if expect good prognosis

Prognosis

Mostly determined by amount of brain tissue within sac

Also depends on presence or absence of hydrocephalus, microcephaly, and other anomalies

Frontal encephalocele with better prognosis

Delivery route depends on size of sac

C. MYELOMENINGOCELE

= abnormal development during neurulation in which there is failure of posterior neural tube closure; open defects are not covered by skin and thus cerebrospinal fluid (CSF) leakage of α-fetoprotein can occur *in utero* into amniotic fluid and maternal circulation

Incidence

0.2 to 1.0/1000 live births

Worldwide geographic distribution; in the United States, increased frequency in the east and south regions, and lowest frequency in the west region

Maternal folic acid supplementation decreases the risk for neural tube defect by 60% to 70% in first child

Increased risk if mother has diabetes, or is taking certain medications (e.g., valproate, carbamazepine)

General classification cystic dilation of meninges & defect in overlying skin
1. Meningocele —

   Meninges herniate through bony abnormality (spina bifida) and form a cystic sac filled with spinal fluid

The spinal cord is not involved, and nerve roots are normal

2. Myelomeningocele

The spinal cord, with meninges, herniates through a defect in the spinal canal; the cord may abnormally progress distally

Neurologic deficit is below level of lesion

Increased risk for another affected child

Clinical

Specific clinical features depend on level of lesion (see chart below)

Level of Lesion	Segmental Innervation	Reflex present	Ambulation Potential
Cervical/Thoracic	Variable	None	Poor
Thoracolumbar	T12 to L2	None	Full braces; long-term ambulation unlikely
Lumbar	L3 to L4	Knee jerk	May ambulate with braces and crutches
Lumbosacral	L5 to S1	Ankle jerk	Ambulate with or without short braces
Sacral	S2 to S4	Anal wink	Ambulate without braces

T=thoracic; L=lumbar; S=sacral; note that ~80% of lesions are in the lumbar area, which is the last segment to close; Modified from Cloherty, JP and Stark AR (ed): Manual of Neonatal Care (4th edition). Philadelphia, Lippincott-Raven, 1998, p. 537.

Management

In utero: experimental procedures include surgical resection and coverage of defect to prevent ongoing exposure to amniotic fluid (which is thought to be toxic to the neural tissue)

Karyotype

Postnatal: cover lesion with warm normal saline by sterile, nonlatex technique; cover sac with sterile dressing, saran wrap, or both; assess for other abnormalities (e.g., scoliosis, hydrocephalus, Arnold-Chiari malformation); determine level of neurologic function; MRI or CT scan to evaluate associated central nervous system (CNS) abnormalities and hydrocephalus; surgical repair of lesion; may require ventriculoperitoneal shunt if hydrocephalus

Monitor for hydrocephalus (occurs in 80%; may develop postsurgical repair of lesion)

Monitor neuromuscular function, urologic function, and development of orthopedic abnormalities

Prognosis

Depends on level of lesion (the lower the lesion, better the outcome) and presence of other anomalies

Increased risk for mental deficiency and learning disability

D. ARNOLD-CHIARI MALFORMATION: caused by a primary neurulation defect

Types:

Type I: caudal displacement of cerebellar tonsils below foramen magnum; fourth ventricle always in normal position; often associated with hydromelia; can also be associated with skeletal anomalies (scoliosis most common)

Type II: more extensive; elongation and caudal displacement of cerebellar tonsils, fourth ventricle, choroid plexus, and medulla; these descend into the cervical spinal canal; often associated with hydrocephalus

Type III: similar to a cervical meningocele yet with displacement of cerebellum and lower brainstem into sac

E. APROSENCEPHALY

= abnormal development during prosencephalic stage in which there is absence of telencephalon and diencephalon with porencephalic remnant

Clinical

Minimal cranial volume but because maldevelopment occurs late, will have intact skull, hair, and dermal coverings (unlike those with anencephaly)

Cyclopia, or absence of eyes
Associated anomalies with external genitalia and limbs

F. HOLOPROSENCEPHALY SEQUENCE

= abnormal development during prosencephalic stage in which there is a primary defect in cleavage

Incidence
1/15,000 to 20,000
Recurrence risk of 6% if sporadic, nonchromosomal, and nonsyndromic

Associations
~30% to 50% with chromosomal abnormality (especially trisomy 13)
Increased risk in offspring of diabetic mothers
Familial recurrences have been described (family members may have subtle features such as ocular hypotelorism,
   midfacial abnormalities, microcephaly, mental deficiency, single maxillary central incisor)

Clinical
Grossly abnormal brain evident by a single-shaped cerebral structure with a common large central ventricle, absence of
   the corpus callosum, a membranous roof over the third ventricle, absence of the olfactory bulbs, optic nerve
   hypoplasia, no development of the supralimbic cortex, presence of cyclops, and variable dysmorphic facies (e.g.,
   cleft lip, palate, rudimentary nasal structures)
Extremely lethal during fetal life
50% have extracranial abnormalities (e.g., myelomeningocele, renal malformations, congenital heart disease, polydactyly)
Positive transillumination (as in hydranencephaly)
Apnea, seizures, abnormalities in hypothalamic functions (temperature instability, diabetes insipidus, syndrome of
   inappropriate antidiuretic hormone secretion), mental deficiency if long-term survival

Management
Consider elective termination
Karyotype, family history
If mild form and infant survives, conduct endocrine assessment

Prognosis
Extemely poor unless very mild form

G. AGENESIS OF CORPUS CALLOSUM

= abnormal development during prosencephalic stage in which there is a defect in midline development

Incidence
0.3% to 0.7% (higher in people with developmental delay)

Associations
Neurologic malformations (e.g. Dandy-Walker malformation, holoprosencephaly); facial anomalies, congenital heart
   disease; metabolic disorders (e.g., nonketotic hyperglycinemia, pyruvate dehydrogenase deficiency), *in utero*
   infections; trisomy 8, 13, and 18

Management
Confirm diagnosis with MRI

Assess for other fetal anomalies (intracranial and extracranial)
Karyotyping

Prognosis
Increased risk for neurodevelopmental abnormalities (especially if there are neurologic malformations or presence of
seizures)
If isolated, unclear risks (often with normal developmental outcome)
Increased risk for seizures later in life

II. Cerebral Blood Flow and Vasoreactivity

A. VASCULAR SUPPLY

1. Anterior cerebral artery: from internal carotid artery; supplies medial frontal, parietal lobes, and caudate

2. Middle cerebral artery: from internal carotid artery; supplies lateral hemispheres

3. Posterior cerebral artery: from basilar artery, which is from the vertebral artery; supplies midbrain, occipital lobes,
   inferior temporal lobes

B. CEREBRAL VASOREACTIVITY

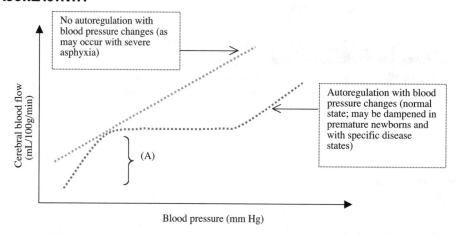

(A) with decreasing gestational age, mean arterial blood pressure approaches the lower limit of the autoregulation plateau; this predisposes the premature brain to decreased
cerebral blood flow with changes in blood pressure. Modified from Volpe JJ: Neurology of the Newborn (4th edition). Philadelphia, W.B. Saunders, 2001, p. 253, 258.

Cerebral perfusion pressure (CPP)
= mean arterial pressure (MAP)–intracranial cerebral pressure (ICP)

Cerebral blood flow (CBF)

Increased CBF	Decreased CBF
Increased blood pressure in asphyxiated infant	
Increased $PaCO_2$	Decreased PaO_2
Decreased $PaCO_2$	Increased PaO_2
Dopamine	
Decreased hemoglobin concentration	Increased hemoglobin concentration
Increased proportion of fetal hemoglobin	Decreased fetal hemoglobin
Hypoglycemia	
Seizures	

III. Neurological Evaluation and Abnormalities

A. HEAD

1. Growth
In utero: head growth usually preserved and is the last growth parameter to be adversely affected

Postnatally: week 1: decrease in head circumference (HC)

> week 2: increase ~0.5 cm
>
> week 3: increase ~0.7 cm
>
> thereafter: increase ~1.0 cm/week

Slow head growth: assess for brain abnormalities and neurologic impairment

Fast head growth: assess for hydrocephalus

Microcephaly: (decreased HC > 2 to 3 standard deviations below mean)

> Associated with chromosomal abnormalities (e.g. trisomy 13, 18, and 21; deletion 13q; CHARGE association, Meckel-Gruber syndrome; Smith-Lemli-Opitz syndrome), *in utero* or postnatal infections; *in utero* drug exposure (e.g., alcohol, isoretinoin); prenatal exposure to radiation; maternal phenylketonuria and phenylketonuria

Macrocephaly (increased head circumference > 3 standard deviations above mean and absence of hydrocephalus or cranial masses)

> Associated with benign familial macrocephaly (~50%; usually autosomal dominant; male > female), Beckwith-Wiedemann syndrome, neurofibromatosis, Soto syndrome, fragile X syndrome, achondroplasia

2. Shape

Cranial sutures

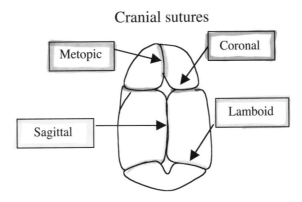

Craniosynostosis = premature closure of cranial sutures

> Growth of sutures occurs parallel to the affected suture and decreased growth perpendicular to the fused suture

> Although etiology usually occurs prenatally, craniosynostosis is rarely observed at birth (it is almost always observed before age 6 months)

> Possible etiologies include hypophosphatemia, rickets, idiopathic hypercalcemia, associated syndrome (e.g., Crouzon and Apert syndrome)

> Surgical goals: improve skull and facial appearance, prevent increase in intracranial pressure, ensure normal brain growth, and prevent compromise of visual and auditory function

Abnormal head shapes seen in craniosynostosis

Type of craniosynostosis	Characteristics	Skull shape
Scaphocephaly or dolichocephaly 56% Premature closure of the *sagittal* suture	Most common craniosynostosis Males > females Least often associated with other lesions Small to absent anterior fontanel Forehead broader than occipital region Palpable ridge Brain growth normal Surgery for cosmetic improvement If no other lesions and early surgical repair, not associated with increased intracranial pressure (ICP) or other neurologic complications	
Frontal plagiocephaly 25% Premature closure of unilateral *coronal* suture	Frequency of unilateral form = bilateral form Greater in girls High incidence of developmental abnormalities and mental deficiency Associated with Crouzon's syndrome and Apert's syndrome Early correction to prevent neurologic sequelae	
Brachycephaly 13% Premature closure of bilateral *coronal* sutures	Can be observed in Carpenter syndrome	
Trigonocephaly 4% Premature closure of *metopic* suture	More often in boys Correction purely cosmetic Associated with hypotelorism	
Occipital plagiocephaly 2% Premature closure of the unilateral *lamboid* suture	Least common	
Multiple suture involvement	Increased risk for increased ICP Increased risk for mental deficiency Surgery as soon as possible	Combination of above skull shapes

Other clinical scenarios in which abnormal head shape is seen:
   Plagiocephaly = oblique head
     Asymmetrical, flattened skull with compensatory changes in the remaining skull
     Associated with torticollis, constant resting position of head
   Dolichocephaly = elongated head with flat sides
     Often seen in growing, premature infants

3. Fontanels *3rd font → cong. anom.*
Wide variation in size of fontanels
Useful to assess for increased ICP

anterior closes 8-16 mo.

Closed fontanels at birth are associated with immobile, ridged sutures; may be associated with premature synostosis
Anterior fontanel completely closed by age 2 years; posterior fontanel can be closed at birth in a sizable portion of normal full-term newborns
Enlarged anterior fontanel can be caused by hydrocephalus, CNS infection, hypothyroidism, trisomy 13, trisomy 18, trisomy 21, Zellweger syndrome, and bone disorders (e.g., hypophosphatasia)

B. CRANIAL NERVES

I	Olfaction
II	Vision, optic fundi
III	Pupils
III, IV, VI	Extraocular movements
V	Facial sensation, masticatory power
	V1: ophthalmic
	V2: maxillary
	V3: mandibular
VII	Facial movements
VIII	Auditory
V, VII, IX, X, XII	Sucking and swallowing
XI	Sternocleidomastoid function
XII	Tongue
VII, IX	Taste

1. Bilateral facial paresis = Mobius syndrome
Secondary to hypoplasia or absence of cranial nerve nuclei
Leads to expressionless face
There is no effective treatment and no recovery

C. TONE

1. Hypertonia
Less common than hypotonia
Results from injury to the corticospinal tract or extrapyramidal system
Etiologies include
  Hypoxic ischemic encephalopathy
  Meningeal inflammation
  Hemorrhage
  Bilateral cerebral injury
  Basal ganglia injury

2. Hypotonia (see Section X for specific disorders)
Normal full-term infants have legs flexed and elevated, but infants with hypotonia have "frog-leg" posture and legs flat
May have prenatal history of decreased fetal movements and polyhydramnios (caused by decreased swallowing ability)
Possible etiologies: chromosomal (e.g., trisomy 21, Prader-Willi syndrome, Angelman syndrome), infection, hyperbilirubinemia, some metabolic disorders (e.g., urea cycle defects, isovaleric academia), hypothyroidism, hypermagnesemia, medication (e.g., phenobarbital), hypoxic-ischemic encephalopathy, see other neurologic diseases in Section X
Clinical signs: infant slips through fingers when held under the armpits
  Abnormal Dubowitz examination
  Difficult to differentiate hypotonia from weakness in the newborn

D. PATTERNS OF WEAKNESS

Region of injury	Clinical presentation
Focal cerebral	Contralateral hemiparesis Eye deviation to side of lesion Full-term infants: weakness in upper extremity > lower extremity Preterm infants: weakness in lower extremity > upper extremity
Parasagittal cerebral	Weakness in proximal limbs Upper extremity > lower extremity
Periventricular cerebral, bilateral	Symmetric weakness Lower extremity > upper extremity
Spinal cord	Initial flaccid weakness in all extremities with facial sparing Evolving spasticity in weeks to months
Lower motor neuron	Flaccid weakness in all extremities Facial sparing Fasciculations
Nerve roots	Specific patterns of focal weakness as dictated by which roots are affected
Peripheral nerve	Generalized weakness
Neuromuscular junction	Generalized weakness Hypotonia
Muscle	Generalized weakness and hypotonia Proximal > distal Face, eye, and specific muscles can also be affected

E. REFLEXES

Deep tendon reflexes (DTRs)
  Upper motor neuron lesion (cerebrum, spinal cord)
    DTRs normally present at birth and become brisk weeks or months later
  Lower motor neuron lesion with nerve involvement
    DTRs absent and asymmetric plantar response present
  Neuromuscular junction injury
    DTRs unaffected and significant muscular weakness present
  Muscle injury
    DTRs associated with decrease in muscular strength

Clonus
  5 to 10 beats can be normal in newborns; abnormal if present > age 3 months

Moro
  Appears at gestational age (GA) 28 to 32 weeks, established by GA 37 weeks, and disappears by age 6 months
  Should be symmetric
  If asymmetric, suggests peripheral injury (root, plexus, or nerve)
  If nonhabituating, suggests cerebral injury

Palmar grasp
  Appears at GA 28 weeks, established by GA 32 weeks, disappears by age 2 months
  If asymmetric, suggests peripheral injury (root, plexus, or nerve)
  If nonhabituating, suggests cerebral injury
  Persistence of palmar grasp characteristic of athetoid cerebral palsy

Tonic-neck reflex
Appears at GA 35 weeks, established by age 1 month, disappears by age 7 months
Persistence may suggest focal cerebral abnormalities

Placing and stepping
Appears at GA 37 weeks

IV. Neurological Studies

A. CEREBROSPINAL FLUID (CSF)

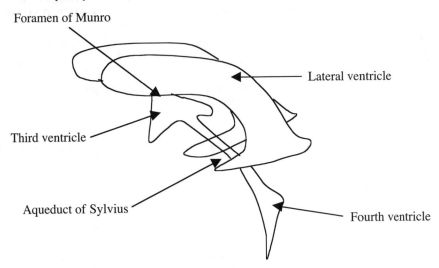

CSF produced in lateral ventricles by *choroid plexus* (constant rate of 0.37 mL/min) → intraventricular foramen of Munro → third ventricle → cerebral aqueduct of Sylvius→ fourth ventricle → lateral foramens of Luschka and Magendie → subarachnoid space→ brainstem, cerebellum, spinal cord

Choroid plexus
Mass of special cells located in the atrium of the lateral ventricles
These cells regulate the intraventricular pressure by secreting or absorbing CSF

Choroid plexus cysts
Neuroepithelial folds filled with CSF and debris
Detected by fetal ultrasound as early as 11 weeks gestation and usually disappears by 26 weeks gestation
Occurs in ~0.5% of normal fetuses
Majority are normal and without clinical significance
Although choroid plexus cysts can be an isolated finding, a small percentage of fetuses may have trisomy 18
   (additional ultrasound findings are typically observed in fetuses with trisomy 18)
Further evaluation (i.e., chromosome analysis) is not necessary unless there are other abnormal findings

CSF metabolism
CSF remade every 5 to 7 hours
Volume: 10 to 30 cc for premature infants; 40 cc for full-term infants
99% water, Na major cation

CSF abnormalities
1. Low glucose (hypoglycorrhachia): found in meningitis, systemic hypoglycemia, and some patients with intracranial hemorrhage

2. Xanthochromic (yellow discoloration): found in cerebral hemorrhage, hyperbilirubinemia, increased protein or can be an isolated finding; if xanthochromia with increased CSF red blood cells and increased CSF protein, suggests intracranial hemorrhage (low glucose may also be present)

Increased intracranial pressure
Increased extracerebral volume: blood, CSF, exudates, effusion
Increased intracerebral volume: blood, edema, mass
Increased intraventricular volume: blood, CSF

B. ELECTROENCEPHALOGRAM (EEG)

useful in confirming or denying SZ. & provide info about permanency of prior asphyxial insult

As gestational age increases, EEG demonstrates refinement of organization

Gestational age (weeks)	EEG findings
27–28	Discontinuous Long periods of quiescence occasionally interrupted by synchronous bursts No EEG response to external stimuli
29–30	Discontinuous Asynchronous activity Appearance of "delta brushes" in central region and temporal theta bursts
31–33	Continuous activity Predominantly asynchronous with synchrony during active sleep "Delta brushes" over occipital and temporal areas
34–35	Improved continuity and synchrony in awake and active sleep "Delta brushes" with increased voltage and speed Temporal theta bursts disappear Transient frontal shape waves appear EEG changes with external stimuli
36–37	Continued improvement in continuous and synchronous activity Able to differentiate between awake state and sleep "Delta brushes" disappear from central region
38–40	Continuous activity in quiet and active sleep and during awake state Synchrony activity predominates "Delta brushes" of occipital region disappears

Specific EEG findings and their significance
  Disordered development: if EEG findings (as described in the above table) are delayed > 3 weeks, this may suggest an underlying disturbance
  Background depression: occurs after generalized insults, such as hypoxic-ischemic encephalopathy, meningitis, encephalitis, metabolic disorders
    If unilateral, suggests one-sided cerebral lesion caused by ischemia, hemorrhage, or abnormal development
  (★) Persistence of this pattern is a poor prognostic sign
  Burst suppression: intermediate stage between depression and electrocerebral silence
    No EEG response to external stimuli
    Poor prognosis
  Electrocerebral silence: persistence > 72 hours indicates cerebral cortical death; not always accompanied by brainstem death
    If brainstem activity, patient may survive, but in a persistent vegetative state
  Periodic discharges: in premature infants, may be associated with various insults in prematurity
    In full-term infants, usually associated with infarction in the distribution of the middle cerebral artery

burst supression OR extrem. low voltage pattern or initial near or total isoelectric tracing } poor neuro prognosis

Multifocal sharp waves: high voltage for long periods
  Multiple potential etiologies
Central positive sharp waves: characteristic pattern in premature infants with periventricular leukomalacia (PVL)
Hypsarrhythmia: observed in infantile myoclonic spasms
  Typically observed after age 2 months

C. IMAGING

1. Ultrasound (US)
Advantages: easily done at bedside; serial imaging readily available for indications such as monitoring evolving
    posthemorrhagic hydrocephalus
  Can use Doppler technology to assess cerebral blood flow velocity
Disadvantages: poor ability to detect posterior fossa lesions

2. CT scan
Advantages: offers greater information compared with US for most parenchymal processes and fluid collections
    (including blood) in the subdural and subarachnoid spaces and in the posterior fossa
  Superior to MRI for identifying intracranial calcifications
Disadvantages: transport required, exposure to ionizing radiation

3. MRI scan
Advantages: high-resolution imaging; no radiation
  Superior for assessing migration and myelination disorders, myelination, ateriovenous malformations, ischemia, PVL,
    spinal cord
Disadvantages: longer time to acquire images
  Poor identification of calcifications

V. Hydrocephalus

Presenting clinical signs include increased anterior fontanel, increased head circumference, and separated cranial
  sutures

A. OBSTRUCTIVE (Non-communicating)

1. Intraventricular hemorrhage (IVH): post-hemorraghic (most common) IVH

2. **Aqueductal stenosis:** because of congenital obstruction of the aqueduct (duct connecting the third and fourth
    ventricles), leading to third and lateral ventricular dilatation
Incidence: ~1/3 of patients with obstructive hydrocephalus
Possible etiologies:
  May be caused by an unrecognized viral disease (e.g., mumps, rubella, parainfluenza)
  Can be associated with Arnold-Chiari malformation
  X-linked with associated adducted thumbs, agenesis of corpus callosum, mental deficiency
  Autosomal recessive (most nonfamilial) with associated VACTERL

3. Agenesis of corpus callosum (see section IG)

4. Dandy-Walker malformation
Incidence: accounts for 5% to 10% of congenital hydrocephalus

70% of affected infants will have other CNS abnormalities, including agenesis of the corpus callosum and abnormal neuronal migration

Features:

    a. cystic dilatation of the fourth ventricle

    b. Cerebellar vermis hypoplasia or aplasia

    c. Hydrocephalus (75%): may not be clinically evident until months or years later

Management: includes ventriculoperitoneal shunt with possible need for shunt placement in the posterior fossa cyst

Prognosis: long-term outcome related to the severity of malformation and associated defects

    Greater mortality and morbidity if symptomatic early in neonatal period compared with later in life

5. **Congenital hydrocephalus:** onset *in utero* and presentation in the first days of life

    Often accompanied by severe congenital anomalies

    Etiology: Dandy-Walker malformation (5% to 10%), teratogenesis (e.g., radiation exposure, intrauterine infection (e.g., toxoplasmosis, cytomegalovirus), maternal malnutrition, genetic factors (e.g., X-linked aqueductal stenosis), tumor, intrauterine intraventricular hemorrhage, vein of Galen malformation

    Management: assess for other anomalies, karyotyping, MRI or CT, determine if there is an underlying cause, ventriculoperitoneal shunt placement

6. Masses

B. COMMUNICATING

1. IVH
2. Arnold-Chiari malformation (see section ID)
3. Lissencephaly
4. Encephalocele (see section IB)
5. Leptomeningeal inflammation
6. Group B streptococcus ventriculitis
7. Congenital absence of arachnoid granulation
8. Oversecretion of CSF (e.g., choroid plexus papilloma)
9. Acquired hydrocephalus

VI. Hypoxic-Ischemic Encephalopathy (HIE)

A. AAP-ACOG DEFINITION OF PERINATAL ASPHYXIA

1. Profound umbilical arterial metabolic or mixed acidemia with pH < 7
2. APGAR score < 3 for > 5 minutes
3. Neonatal neurologic sequelae: seizures, hypotonia, coma
4. Multiple organ dysfunction

B. CHANGES IN SUBSTRATE METABOLISM AND NEUROTRANSMITTERS

Hypoxic effect

    Changes that are increased:

        An initial increase in cerebral blood flow

        Increase of glucose influx to brain

        Increase in glycogenolysis (increase cAMP)

        Increase in glycolysis (increase cAMP)

        Increased lactate and hydrogen ions

    Changes that are decreased:

        Decreased oxidative phosphorylation

Decreased brain glucose

Decreased phosphocreatinine (PCr), adenosine triphosphate (see graph below)

Changes are more pronounced in white matter compared to gray matter

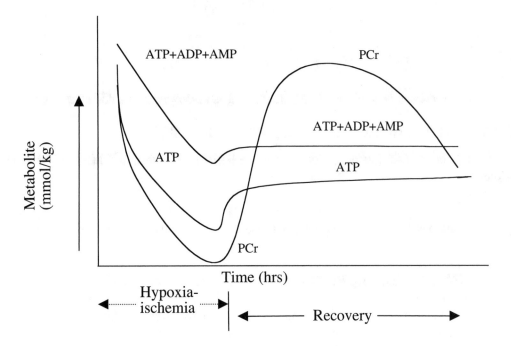

ATP = adenosine 5'-triphosphate; ADP = adenosine 5'-diphosphate; AMP = adenosine 5'-monophosphate; PCr = phosphorcreatine. Printed with permission from Polin RA and Fox WW (ed): Fetal and Neonatal Physiology (2nd Edition). Philadelphia, W.B. Saunders, 1998, p. 2131.

C. NEUROLOGICAL PRESENTATION: SARNAT STAGES

Characteristic	Stage 1	Stage 2	Stage 3
Level of consciousness	Hyperalert	Lethargic	Stuporous
Muscle tone	Normal	Mild hypotonia	Flaccid
Posture	Mild distal flexion	Strong distal flexion	Intermittent decerebration
Tendon reflexes	Overactive	Overactive	Depressed
Myoclonus	Present	Present	Absent
Complex reflexes:			
Suck	Weak	Weak or absent	Absent
Moro	Strong	Incomplete, weak	Absent
Tonic neck	Slight	Strong	Absent
Oculocephalic	Normal	Overreactive	Weak or absent
Autonomics:			
Pupils	Dilated	Constricted	Variable, often unequal
Heart rate	Tachycardia	Bradycardia	Variable
Secretions (bronchial and salivary)	Sparse	Profuse	Variable
Seizures	Absent	Present	Uncommon
EEG	Normal	Low voltage	Periodic, isolelectric, burst suppression

(continued on following page)

Characteristic	Stage 1	Stage 2	Stage 3
Prognosis	100% normal	80% normal Typically abnormal if symptoms > 5-7 days 20% mild to moderate risk for long-term deficits	Almost 100% with severe sequelae

Modified from Sarnat HB, Sarnat MS. "Neonatal encephalopathy following fetal distress." *Arch Neurol* 33, 1976, p. 700.

A normal neurologic examination and a normal EEG after 1 week is associated with a normal outcome

D. MULTISYSTEMIC EFFECTS (WHEN INJURY IS SEVERE AND DIFFUSE)

Acute asphyxia elicits *diving reflex* (preferred blood flow to the brain, heart, and adrenal glands with vasoconstriction to other organs)

Seizures
  Often resistant to anticonvulsant therapy (possibly because of a lack of cortical inhibition vs. excessive cortical activity)
  50% of seizures are subtle, focal, multifocal, or myoclonic
  Typically, seizures are first noted at age 12 to 24 hour and often resolve by age 5 to 7 days as the underlying acute encephalopathy resolves
  Must also assess for other metabolic derangements (e.g., hypoglycemia, hypocalcemia, hypomagnesemia)
  Phenobarbital is the first-line agent followed by dilantin; may also consider lorazepam

Hypotonia, possible coma

Cardiac manifestations include transient myocardial ischemia, congestive heart failure, left or right ventricular dysfunction, tricuspid regurgitation murmur within first 24 hours of life

Renal dysfunction leading to oliguria and possibly acute tubular necrosis

Pulmonary hypertension may occur (especially after meconium aspiration)

E. MANAGEMENT

Maintain O_2 and CO_2 in normal ranges
Hyperventilation not recommended and may be detrimental
Monitor arterial blood pressure because cerebral perfusion pressure is dependent on MAP (CPP=MAP-ICP)
Administer volume slowly; overall fluid restriction
Monitor electrolytes and glucose
Control seizures

VII. Patterns of Cerebral Injury

A. SELECTIVE NEURONAL NECROSIS (most common injury after hypoxic-ischemic encephalopathy)

Pathogenesis
  Oxygen deprivation; potential role of excitatory amino acids
  Changes occur 24 to 36 hours after injury

Distribution
  1. Diffuse
  2. Cerebral cortex-deep nuclear structures
  3. Deep nuclear structures (basal ganglia, thalamus, globus pallucidum)

Clinical outcome
  Mental deficiency
  Feeding difficulties, seizures, ataxia
  Pyramidal cerebral palsy

B. PARASAGITTAL CEREBRAL INJURY (mostly an ischemic lesion of full-term neonates)

Pathogenesis
  Disturbance in cerebral perfusion secondary to systemic hypotension, hypoxemia, acidosis (severe perinatal depression)
  Areas of necrosis fall between border areas perfused by the anterior, middle, and posterior cerebral arteries
  These border areas are susceptible to decreases in cerebral perfusion pressure

Distribution
  Usually bilateral and symmetrical; however, one side can be more affected
  Parasagittal supermedial areas, with posterior cerebral hemisphere more often involved

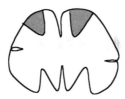

Clinical outcome
  Weakness in proximal limbs, upper > lower (spastic quadriplegia)
  Weakness in shoulder girdle
  If posterior artery is affected, deficits in auditory, visual, spatial, and language abilities may be present
  Cognitive deficits

C. FOCAL OR MULTIFOCAL ISCHEMIA (mostly an ischemic lesion of the full-term neonate)

Distribution
  Unilateral (~90%) > bilateral (~10%)
  Left hemisphere is three times more likely to be affected, left middle cerebral artery is the most common site; left MCA (~60%) > right MCA (~20%) > bilateral MCA (~10%) > other arteries (~5%)

Etiology
  Unknown (~50%), perinatal asphyxia (~33%)
  Remaining etiologies (each ≤ 2%): trauma, meningitis, polycythemia, hypernatremia/dehydration, postnatal hypotension, congenital heart disease, protein C deficiency, protein S deficiency, antithrombin III deficiency, antiphospholipid antibodies, cocaine exposure *in utero*

Neonatal presentation
  Decreased level of consciousness
  Periodic breathing or respiratory failure
  Intact papillary response and oculomotor response
  Hypotonia, minimal movement
  Seizures: 12 to 24 hours of life; may be associated with apnea
  Feeding dysfunction is common, including abnormalities in sucking, swallowing, and tongue movements
  Hypotonia/hypertonia: proximal limbs, upper> lower

Clinical outcome
  Hemiplegia or quadriplegia
  Cognitive deficits
  Seizure disorder

D. PERIVENTRICULAR HEMORRHAGIC INFARCTION

Risks
  Prematurity, IVH, severe illness

(handwritten note: periventric-intraventric ~90% have hemorrhage within 1 wk)

Location
  Typically large, asymmetric, majority unilateral
  Located dorsal and lateral to the external angle of the lateral ventricle(s)

(handwritten note: presence of ventric. dilation optim. ascertained @ 2 wks)

Pathogenesis
  Caused by hemorrhagic necrosis of periventricular white matter
  Directly related to IVH because:
    1) ~80% are associated with a large, typically asymmetric IVH
    2) Lesion typically on same side as IVH
    3) Develops after IVH occurs (peak time ~fourth day of life)
  IVH obstructs blood flow in terminal vein, leading to venous infarction in distribution of medullary veins (drain the cerebral white matter into the terminal vein)

Diagnosis
  US ideal because of high sensitivity and resolution

Clinical outcome
  Spastic hemiparesis or asymmetric quadriparesis with upper extremities affected as much as lower extremities

E. PERIVENTRICULAR LEUKOMALACIA (PVL) (mostly a lesion of premature neonates)

Risks
  Prematurity (rarely found > GA 32 weeks), severe illness, IVH, maternal-fetal infection, prolonged period of hypoxia
    (e.g., postnatal systemic hypotension)

Pathogenesis
  Caused by focal injury and necrosis of periventricular white matter
  Three main physiologic features that predispose premature infants:
    1) Periventricular vascular anatomic factors
    2) Cerebral perfusion pressure dependent on systemic blood pressure
    3) Increased vulnerability of actively differentiating or myelinating periventricular glial cells

Insult (vascular, inflammatory) leading to oligodendroglial cell death and myelin deficiency
May develop lateral ventricular dilation in presence of myelin deficiency

Ultrasound findings
Bilateral, linear echodensities adjacent to external angles of lateral ventricles
Findings on US may not be evident until 1 month or later

Clinical outcome
Spastic diplegia (with lower extremities more affected than upper extremities) is the most common clinical sequela
Cognitive and visual deficits

VIII. Intracranial Hemorrhage

A. SUBDURAL ✱ Hydrocephalus ↑ risk
Uncommon hemorrhage in neonates (full-term infants > preterm infants)
Caused by trauma and tearing of veins and venous sinuses

Clinical
Symptoms depend on severity and location of bleed
Hemorrhage in posterior fossa (infratentorial):
Severe hemorrhage with acute signs: stupor, lateral eye deviation, unequal pupils, abnormal light response, nuchal rigidity, opisthotonos, bradycardia, respiratory abnormalities, apnea, or death
Insidious onset: may be clinically silent for days, followed by lethargy, full fontanel, irritability, respiratory abnormalities, apnea, bradycardia, eye deviation, facial paresis
Hemorrhage over convexities:
May have minimal or no symptoms
Severe hemorrhage with acute signs: seizures, lateral eye deviation, nonreactive dilated pupil on side of hematoma, hemiparesis
Insidious onset: may be clinically silent for months with initial presentation of increasing head circumference (may occur if chronic subdural effusion)

Diagnosis
CT scan: safe, quick, able to detail injury
MRI can provide further views of posterior fossa
US not very effective at identifying subdural hemorrhage
Avoid lumbar puncture because it may provoke herniation

Management
Close monitoring
If severe neurologic signs, requires surgical evacuation

Prognosis
Severe infratentorial hemorrhages have an extremely poor prognosis
Less severe posterior fossa hemorrhages have a variable prognosis: if recognized and treated, ~80% to 90% will have normal outcomes; ~10% to 15% may have serious sequelae including hydrocephalus requiring shunt placement; ~5% mortality
Convexity subdural hemorrhages generally have a favorable outcome, although there is a increased risk for focal cerebral signs and hydrocephalus

B. SUBARACHNOID

* Most frequent bleed
Premature infants > full-term infants
Rarely of clinical significance and often asymptomatic
May have early onset refractory seizures (usually on the second postnatal day)
Diagnosis by CT scan
Prognosis very good

C. CEREBELLAR

Premature infants > full-term infants
Uncommon
Can be serious
May have symptoms of brainstem compression and irritation evident by respiratory irregularities, apnea, bradycardia,
   lateral deviation of eyes
Diagnosis can be made by US yet CT scan more definitive
Many have long-term neurodevelopmental deficits

D. INTRAVENTRICULAR

Hemiparesis on side contralateral to bleed is most common abnormality

Common
Premature infants > full-term infants
Premature newborns
   Incidence (may vary between centers): < 750 g = 32%; 751–1000g = 30%; 1001–1250g = 15%; 1251–1500g =
      8%; 1551–2250g = 1.4%
   Location: germinal matrix, subependymal germinal matrix
   Risks: multifactorial (developmental fragility, vulnerability and vascularity of germinal matrix, fluctuating cerebral blood
      flow, increase in central venous pressure, coagulation disturbance)
   Clinical: 50% occur within first 24 hours of life; 90% by 72 hours of life; variable presentation from clinically silent to
      catastrophic
   Diagnosis: serial US

80% c̄ severe manifest major neurodevelop disab.

   Management: monitor for development of posthemorrhagic hydrocephalus and PVL
   Prognosis: depends on severity, presence of parenchymal injuries, and presence of complications (e.g., hydrocephalus,
      PVL)

Full-term newborns
   Incidence: in one series, observed in 2.0% of healthy newborns
   Location: germinal matrix, subependymal germinal matrix
   Risks: trauma and asphyxia, although a significant proportion may have no definable cause
   Clinical: irritability, lethargy, apnea, seizures
   Diagnosis: US or CT scan
   Management: monitor for development of posthemorrhagic hydrocephalus
   Prognosis: 55% neurologically normal, 40% with severe neurologic sequelae, 50% require shunts, 5% mortality

IX. Birth Trauma

A. EXTRACRANIAL HEMORRHAGE

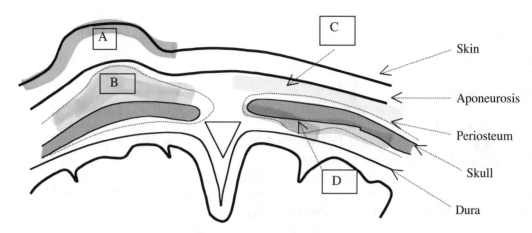

Printed with permission from Fletcher, MA: Physical Diagnosis in Neonatology. Philadelphia, Lippincott-Raven, 1998, p. 184.

1. Caput succedaneum (A)
Common
Hemorrhagic edema
   Soft, superficial, pitting
   Crosses suture lines
At vertex of head with associated cranial molding
Spontaneously resolves over several days

2. Cephalohematoma(B)
1% to 2% of all births
Boys > girls increased risk if primiparous mother and delivery by forceps
Subperiosteal
   Confined by suture lines
Firm and tense
Underlying skull fracture in 10% to 25%
Spontaneously resolves in few weeks to months
Monitor for hyperbilirubinemia

3. Subgaleal (C)
Less common
Beneath galae aponeurotica
Blood beneath the scalp can dissect through subcutaneous tissue of the neck and behind the ear; up to 30% of blood
   volume can be sequestered (may even require blood transfusion)
Monitor for hyperbilirubinemia
Can be firm or fluctuant
Spontaneously resolves over 2 to 3 weeks

4. Extradural (D)
Rare
Superiosteal bleeding on the inner surface of the skull
Caused by a disruption of the middle cerebral artery or vein and venous sinuses
Linear skull fractures and cephalohematomas may coexist

Early signs of increased intracranial pressure

Diagnosis by emergent CT scan with image of convex-shaped hemorrhagic lesion

Management includes evacuation (aspiration or surgical)

B. NERVE INJURY

1. Brachial plexus injuries
0.5 to 2.0/1000 births

Stretching of plexus and nerve roots

Upper roots most vulnerable (traction occurs first on C5, then on C6, and so on)

90% unilateral, right > left

Can have *total brachial plexus* injury, which has features of both Erb's and Klumpke's palsy

Risks: large for gestational age, complications of labor and delivery process

Management: prevent contractures, physical therapy, further evaluations if no recovery by 3 months of age

Prognosis: in one series, 88% normal by 4 months; 92% normal by 1 year

Infants with full recovery show improvement by age 2 weeks and recover by age 6 months

If residual impairment is observed at age 15 months, it usually persists

Potential morbidity: impaired function and strength, muscle atrophy, contractures, and impaired growth

	Erb-Duchenne palsy (proximal)	Klumpke's palsy (distal)
Nerve roots	C5-C7	C8-T1
Clinical signs and symptoms	Most common (90%)	Least common
	"Waiter's tip" position with arm adducted and internally rotated, extension of elbow, pronation of forearm, flexed wrist and fingers	Rare to be isolated (often upper roots involved as well, leading to total palsy)
	Biceps reflex absent	Weakness of flexors of wrist and fingers as well as weak finger abduction
	Intact palmar grasp	Wrist and fingers extended, digits in neutral position
	Absent shoulder moro while hand moro is present	Biceps reflex absent
	C4/5: phrenic nerve paralysis, respiratory distress, decreased diaphragm movement, chest x-ray (CXR) with elevated hemidiaphragm	Grasp reflex absent
		Complete moro absent
	C7: flexion deformity of the hand, winging of the scapula, absent moro, intact grasp reflex, cutaneous sensory loss over the deltoids and radial aspect of upper arm, decreased temperature and perspiration	T1: unilateral Horner's syndrome with miosis, ptosis, anhidrosis, decreased pigmentation of the iris

2. Spinal cord injury
Associated with traction and excessive rotation during delivery

Clinical presentation:

Flaccid weakness, lower extremities > upper extremities

Sensory level at lower neck to upper trunk

Paradoxical respirations

Paralyzed abdominal muscles with rounded, distended appearance

Atonic anal sphincter

Distended bladder

Initial diagnosis can be made by US; MRI provides better delineation of the lesion

3. Facial nerve (VII) palsy (distal)
Most common cranial nerve to be injured during birth (~0.75% of live births)

Caused by nerve compression with hemorrhage and edema of the nerve sheath

Usually unilateral, left (~75%) > right

Clinical signs:

Weakness of lower and upper facial muscles

Asymmetric cry

Lack of normal lower facial muscle contraction on the paretic side, including lack of complete eyelid closure, inability to wrinkle brow, and flat nasolabial fold

Prognosis: good; most recover within 1 to 3 weeks

Management: protection of involved eye with drops; tape paralytic eyelid

X. Neuromuscular Disorders

A. LOWER MOTOR NEURON PATH

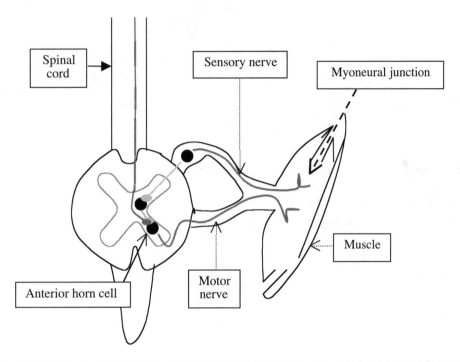

Printed with permission from Fanaroff AA, Martin RJ (eds): Neonatal and Perinatal Medicine: Diseases of the Fetus and Infant (6th edition). St. Louis, Mosby, 1997, p. 822.

B. DISORDERS OF LOWER MOTOR NEURON

Location	Disorders (abnormalities in bold discussed further in chapter)
Anterior horn cell	Hypoxic-ischemic myelopathy **Spinal muscular atrophy, type I (Werdnig-Hoffmann Disease)** Neurogenic arthrogryposis Congenital motor and sensory neuropathy Congenital hypomyelinating neuropathy Charcot-Marie Tooth disease

Neuromuscular junction	**Acquired transient neonatal myasthenia gravis**
	Congenital myasthenia gravis
	Diseases involving a defect in acetylcholine release:
	    Clostridium tetani infection
	    Clostridium botulinum infection
	    Hypermagnesemia
	    Aminoglycoside toxicity

Congenital myopathy	Myotubular myopathy Congenital fiber type disproportion myopathy Muscular dystrophy

(continued on following page)

Location	Disorders (abnormalities in bold discussed further in chapter)
Muscular dystrophy	**Congenital myotonic dystrophy**
	Duchenne dystrophy (Xp21 linked)
	Congenital muscular dystrophy
	Muscle-eye-brain disease
	Early infantile facioscapulohumeral dystrophy
Metabolic and multisystem disease	Mitochondrial disorder
	Peroxisomal disorder (e.g., neonatal adrenoleukodystrophy, cerebrohepatorenal syndrome, or Zellweger syndrome)
	Pompe disease (acid maltose deficiency)
	Phosphofructokinase deficiency
	Phosphorylase deficiency
	Debrancher deficiency
	Carnitine deficiency

Printed with permission from Fanaroff AA, Martin RJ (eds): Neonatal and Perinatal Medicine: Diseases of the Fetus and Infant (6th edition). St. Louis, Mosby, 1997, p. 912.

1. Spinal muscular atrophy, type I (Werdnig-Hoffmann disease)

Genetics: autosomal recessive, chromosome 5

Pathogenesis: degeneration of *anterior horn cell*

History: decreased fetal movements, may have affected siblings

Clinical: onset < 6 months of age

Presents with severe generalized hypotonia

Classic posture with "frog-leg" position and upper extremities abducted, rotated ("jug handle" appearance)

Legs more affected than arms; proximal more affected than distal

Marked head lag

Bulbar weakness evident by poor suck and swallow, weak cry, tongue fasciculations

Facial sparing

Areflexia (absent deep tendon reflexes)

Bell-shaped chest with abdominal breathing

Normal functions include extraocular movements, sensory examination results, sphincter function, and diaphragmatic function (thus, ventricular support less likely)

Death < 2 age years

Diagnostic studies

CPK normal

EMG with nonspecific denervation, fasciculations, and fibrillations

Muscle biopsy demonstrating atrophy of motor units

Nerve conduction velocity normal

2. Acquired transient neonatal myasthenia gravis

Incidence: 10% to 20% infants born to mothers with myasthenia gravis (no correlation to severity or duration of maternal disease)

Recurrence risk ~75%

Pathogenesis: immune process involving the *neuromuscular junction*

Neonate is affected by maternally transmitted antiacetycholine receptor antibodies from mother with myasthenia gravis

Clinical

In utero hypotonia and weakness may lead to decreased fetal movements, arthrogryposis, polyhydramnios, and pulmonary hypoplasia

2/3 may have respiratory failure caused by weak respiratory muscles and poor ability to handle secretions

Facial weakness, swallowing and feeding difficulties (up to 1/3 may need gavage feedings), weak cry, ptosis, oculomotor disturbance, no fasciculations, intact deep tendon reflexes

Mean duration of illness is 18 days

Most require anticholinesterase therapy

Diagnostic studies: readily apparent if known maternal history; less obvious if maternal history unknown

CPK normal

EMG demonstrates progressive decline in amplitude with repetitive nerve stimulation, which returns to baseline after a period of rest or administration of neostigmine

Muscle biopsy results normal

Nerve conduction velocities normal

Responsive to anticholinesterase treatment (neostigmine)

3. Congenital neonatal myasthenia gravis

Pathogenesis: genetic defect of the *neuromuscular junction*

Types: congenital myasthenia is autosomal recessive and caused by a deficiency of endplate acetylcholine receptors

Familial infantile myasthenia is a rare autosomal recessive disorder caused by presynaptic deficiency in acetylcholine synthesis or packaging into vesicles

Clinical

Congenital myasthenia

Less severe; symptoms in the first few weeks of life can include ptosis, ophthalmoplegia, facial weakness, poor suck and cry

Familial infantile myasthenia

Can be severe; neonate may have hypotonia, respiratory failure, apnea, severe feeding difficulties, facial weakness, or ptosis

Oculomotor function less affected than congenital type

Typically, improvement with age

Diagnostic features

Congenital myasthenia

Similar to acquired transient neonatal myasthenia gravis

Familial infantile myasthenia

Demonstrates fatigue on EMG with prolonged stimulation of faster rates

4. Congenital myotonic dystrophy

Genetics: autosomal dominant, chromosome 19, caused by expanded CTG repeat ("triple repeats") with severity determined by number of repeats

Inherited almost entirely from mother

Risks: the more severe and the earlier the onset of maternal disease, the greater the risk for congenital myotonic dystrophy

Pathogenesis: inherited disorder of muscle caused by altered protein, which leads to dysfunctional sodium and potassium channels

Maternal and pregnancy history: polyhydramnios (caused by disordered fetal swallowing), prolonged labor (caused by uterine dysfunction in affected mother; may be the only sign in the mother because many mothers are undiagnosed)

Maternal symptoms may include inability to open eyes completely after tightly shutting them and delayed release of hand grip

Clinical: symptoms typically in the first hours or days of life

Facial diplegia: "tent-shaped" mouth, poor oral-motor function, respiratory failure, hypotonia and weakness, arthrogryposis, areflexia or hyporeflexia, muscle atrophy

Mental deficiency later in life

Neonatal mortality can be as high as 40%

Diagnosis

CPK normal

EMG with "myotonic" changes eliciting a "dive-bomber" sound (can be difficult to obtain in newborn)

Abnormal muscle biopsy (small and round muscle fibers with large nuclei and sparse myofibrils)

Nerve conduction velocities normal

C. DISORDERS WITH HYPOTONIA AND WEAKNESS

1. Riley-Day syndrome or "familial dysautonomia"

Genetics: rare, autosomal recessive disorder that is prominent in Ashkenazi Jewish population; defective gene is at the 9q31–33 locus

Pathogenesis: disorder of the peripheral nervous system; reduced number of small unmyelinated nerves that carry pain, temperature, taste, and mediate autonomic functions; reduced large myelinated afferent nerve fibers

Clinical: symptoms evident in first year of life

Poor suck and swallow with increased risk for aspiration

Emesis, abdominal distention, loose bowel movements, irritability

Pale, blotchy skin

Hypotonia, absent corneal reflexes, decreased or absent deep tendon reflexes, hypersensitive pupillary denervation

Decreased tongue papillae

Temperature and blood pressure instability

Diagnosis: can confirm by pupil constriction in response to metacholine eye drops or pilocarpine (normal pupil without response)

No flare with intradermal histamine

2. Prader-Willi syndrome

Genetics: ~70% with deletion of 15q 11q13; ~25% caused by maternal uniparental disomy; ~5% caused by maternal methylation at several loci within 15q11–13 region

Deleted piece is always of *paternal origin*

Prenatal history: may have decreased fetal movements, breech presentation, or both

Clinical triad: hypotonia, cryptorchidism (and hypogonadism), and poor feeding

Other clinical findings: small hands and feet, almond-shaped palpebral fissures, thin upper lip, light-colored hair

Mild to severe mental deficiency, dolichocephaly, increased risk for scoliosis

Failure to thrive during infancy followed by obesity that typically presents between age 6 months to 6 years

3. Arthrogryposis multiplex congenita

Fixed joints with limitation of movement

Can be associated with numerous disorders, including any disease process that affects the motor system

Manage infant by stretching, serial casting, and tendon or ligament release procedures

XI. Seizures

Etiology (very broad differential)

Hypoxia-ischemia

Cerebral hemorrhage

Metabolic (e.g., hyponatremia, hypoglycemia, hypocalcemia, metabolic disorders)

Infection

handwritten at top: ∠48hrs p̄ birth = poor prognosis
> 4days = good prognosis

handwritten at top right: Clonic sz. have better prognosis than other types

Developmental cerebral anomalies

Drug withdrawal (e.g., maternal use of heroin, methadone, barbiturates)

Clinical presentation and seizure types

Subtle *(handwritten: Most common in neonate (partic: preterm))*

Most frequent neonatal type

Oral, facial, or ocular activity (e.g., blinking, tonic horizontal eye deviation, sustained eye opening, lip smacking, tongue-thrusting)

"Swimming" or "pedaling" limb movements

May have associated apnea or changes in heart rate, blood pressure, or respiration

Multifocal clonic

Clonic activity and movements of one limb with migration to another part of the body in a non-ordered fashion (non-Jacksonian)

May resemble "jitteriness"

Not usually associated with apnea or eye movements

Primarily in full-term infants

Focal clonic

Well-localized; repetitive

One limb or area

Not usually unconscious

Usually represents focal disease but can also reflect more diffuse disease such as metabolic disorders

Full-term infants > premature infants

Tonic

Tonic defined as an abrupt change in tone that leads to a change in posture

Often described as "posturing," "stiffening," and "rigidity"

If generalized, may appear to be decerebrate posturing but will also have changes in respiration, eye movements, and apnea

Primarily in premature infants

Myoclonic *(handwritten: uncommon in term infants, rarely in preterm)*

Rapid, sudden shock-like jerks of flexion of both arms +/− legs

Individually or in brief series

Both premature and full-term infants

Diagnosis

EEG *(handwritten: better prognostic in term than preterm)*

General management principles

Treat underlying etiology

Correct metabolic abnormalities (abnormal Na, Ca, glucose, or Mg levels)

Control seizure activity with anticonvulsants: phenobarbital, phenytoin, lorazepam

Head imaging

Rule out infection

Consider pyridoxine to rule out inherited deficiency

Phenobarbital vs. phenytoin pharmacokinetics

Phenobarbital

Initial drug of choice for neonatal seizures

Desired therapeutic level of 20 to 40 mg/L

Metabolism in the cytochrome P_{450} system in liver

Decreased cerebral metabolic rate

$t_{1/2}$ 0 to 7 days of life = 100 hours
$t_{1/2}$ > 28 days of life = 60 to 70 hours
May be given orally or intravenously

Phenytoin

Maternal use may cause embryopathy (see Maternal-Fetal Medicine chapter)

Desired therapeutic level 10 to 20 mg/L

Metabolism in the cytochrome P_{450} system in the liver and excretion in the urine

Preferred route is intravenous; oral administration not ideal because of poor gastrointestinal absorption

Monitor for cardiac arrhythmias

XII. Vein of Galen Malformation

Pathogenesis

Recent evidence suggests that the venous malformation is probably a persistent median prosencephalic *vein of Markowski* (*in utero,* this vein drains into the vein of Galen and usually regresses by 2 weeks of fetal life)

Mechanism of brain injury

Intracranial steal secondary to diastolic run-off

Hemorrhagic infarction after thrombosis of dilated vein

Cerebral ischemia caused by decreased cardiac output after high-output congestive heart failure

Brain atrophy secondary to compression

Clinical

Symptoms depend on size of aneurysm (the greater the size, the greater the amount blood shunted through the lesion) ~44% present in neonatal period

Congestive heart failure (the larger the degree of shunting, the earlier the presentation of failure; usually presents in first few hours of life and tends to worsen during first 3 days of life; typically refractory to medical management)

Continuous cranial bruit

Hydrocephaus (~15%, not usually observed in neonatal period, possibly secondary to aqueductal obstruction or elevated venous pressure)

Increased risk for developmental delay and seizures

If small aneurysm, may present later in life with headaches, focal neurologic deficits, and syncope

Diagnosis

Ultrasound doppler, CT scan, or MRI and angiography

Management

Timing and approach of treatment depends on age of patient, severity of congestive heart failure, and architecture of lesion

Main therapy goal is to minimize congestive heart failure

Embolization (transvenous or transarterial approach, better survival compared with surgical technique)

Prognosis

Outcome dependent on severity of congestive heart failure and degree of brain injury

Increased risk for neurologic deficits

Despite therapeutic techniques, morbidity and mortality remain high

XIII. Congenital Intracranial Tumors

Incidence
  Rare
Types
  Teratomas > neuroepithelial tumors (e.g., medulloblastoma, astrocytoma, choroid plexus papilloma)
  Usually supratentorial (in older children, usually infratentorial)
Clinical
  Most common presentation is increasing head circumference with bulging fontanel; may also have seizures, vomiting, abnormal eye movements, irritability, associated hemorrhage
Diagnosis
  Neuroimaging
Management
  Major modalities include surgery, chemotherapy, and radiation
Prognosis
  Very poor

XIV. Neurocutaneous Syndromes

Disorder	Genetics	Clinical features
Sturge-Weber syndrome	Unknown or sporadic	Pink-purple, flat, hemangiomata (port-wine stain) in distribution of first division of trigeminal nerve that is present at birth Typically unilateral CNS ipsilateral "tramline" intracortical calcifications Glaucoma and visual deficits Macrocephaly: hyperplasia of the endothelium Seizures (grand mal, present at age 2 to 7 months), mental deficiency Hemiparesis contralateral to facial lesion Worse with age
Tuberous sclerosis	Autosomal dominant Implicated chromosomes: 9, 16	50% with hypopigmented "ashleaf" macules (use Wood's lamp) present at birth or soon after, variable in number, greatest on trunk and buttocks CNS tumors Eye involvement Seizures, mental deficiency Enamel pits in teeth Cardiac rhabdomyomas Worse with age

Neurofibromatosis syndrome	Autosomal dominant
	Chromosome 17
		1/3500
		Café-au-lait spots
		  Do not cross the midline, have sharp borders
		  Multiple, > 1.5 cm
		  Rarely present at birth, 80% by one year, 100% by 4 years
		Freckling in axilla, inguinal folds, and perineum
		Associated macrocephaly, aqueductal stenosis
		Associated tumors: cutaneous neurofibroma, schwanoma, and pheochromocytoma
		Mildly short stature
		Seizures, mental deficiency

McCune-Albright syndrome	Sporadic	Irregular brown-pigmentations Fibrous dysplasia of bones

(continued on following page)

Disorder	Genetics	Clinical features
		Precocious puberty
		Hyperthyroidism
		Hyperparathyroidism
		Pituitary adenomas
Von Hippel-Lindau disease	Autosomal dominant Short arm chromosome 3	Caused by overexpresion of transcription factor hypoxia-inducible factor, which leads to increased tumor growth CNS tumors: hemangioblastoma, most commonly in cerebellum Multiple systemic hemangiomata Retinal angiomas Pheochromocytomas

XV. Cerebral Palsy (CP)

Incidence
2 to 5/1000
Greater incidence with decreasing gestational age and birth weight
~5% to 20% of premature infants < 1500 g develop CP
< 32 weeks 5% to 10%; 34 weeks < 1%, ≥ 36 weeks < 0.1%
40% of all patients who develop cerebral palsy are < 37 weeks gestation

Risks
Extreme prematurity (most common type is spastic diplegia)
Symptomatic congenital infection
Bilirubin encephalopathy (increased risk for athetoid CP)
Severe perinatal depression
APGAR score is poor indicator of infants at risk for brain damage:
Majority of full-term infants who develop CP have normal APGAR scores
If neonate with APGAR score of 0 to 3 at 5, 10, and 20 minutes of life, the risk of developing CP is ~1%, 9%, and 57%, respectively
High percentage of infants who develop CP do not have any of the above risk factors

Classification by neurologic dysfunction
1. *Spastic (pyramidal)* (most common)
   Increased tone
   Increased deep tendon reflexes
   Gross motor affected
   Fine motor usually not affected
   Cognitive function usually not affected (although may be affected if quadriplegia is present)
2. *Athetoid (extrapyramidal)*
   Mixed tone in same muscle
   Both gross and fine motor affected
   Cognitive function usually not affected
   Hearing deficits
   Speech abnormalities
3. *Mixed*
   Mixed tone in various muscles
4. *Ataxic (atonic)* (least common)
   Decreased tone, poor coordination
   Decreased reflexes
   Severe cognitive delay

Classification by extremities involved
  Quadriplegia: involvement of all four limbs
  Hemiplegia: involvement of one side (e.g., right arm and right leg)
  Diplegia: involvement of legs only or legs more affected than arms

Clinical
  Hypotonia, inability to suck, and weak cry > 24 hours of life each carry a 10 to 20-fold increased risk for CP
  May also have hypertonia
  Non-progressive motor disorder
  Recognized at 6 to 18 months corrected age
  Increased risk for seizures, cognitive dysfunction, sensory impairments, orthopedic deformities, emotional and
    behavioral disorder

Interventions
  Physical therapy and occupational therapy; provide assistive devices
  May require orthopedic surgery, rhizotomy, bracing, or botulism toxin injections

XVI. Mental Deficiency

Incidence
  ~3% of population functions 2 standard deviations below mean intelligence quotient (IQ) of general population (IQ <
    70 to 75)

Etiology

Onset	Incidence (%)	Etiology

Prenatal	44	Single brain defect (14%) caused by:
		  Microcephaly
		  Hydrocephalus
		  Hydranencephaly (absent cerebral hemispheres)
		  Neural tube defect
		Multiple defects (including brain) caused by:
		  Chromosomal abnormality (12%, e.g., trisomy 21 and fragile X syndrome)
		  Other (6%; e.g., congenital hypothyroidism)

Perinatal	~3	Trauma Perinatal depression Metabolic: kernicterus, severe neonatal hypoglycemia Infection: meningitis Other: intracranial hemorrhage
Postnatal	~12	Environmental: trauma, lead encephalopathy Metabolic: hypernatremia, severe hypoglycemia, inborn errors of metabolism Infection: meningitis, encephalitis Other: severe hypoxemia
Unknown	41	Metabolic Chromosomal Other

The most common inherited etiology of mental deficiency is fragile X syndrome; **language development is the best predictor of mental deficiency;** Modified from Jones KL: Smith's Recognizable Patterns of Human Malformations (5th edition). Philadelphia, WB Saunders Co, 1997, p. 683

Classification
Previously classified by intelligence quotient:

Intelligence quotient (IQ)	Degree
52 to 68	Mild
36 to 51	Moderate
20 to 35	Severe
< 20	Profound

Above classification has been replaced by level of support required:
   Intermittent: constant support not needed; limited: ongoing support but of varying intensity; extensive: consistent ongoing and daily support; pervasive: high support for all activities

Clinical
   Low IQ accompanied by limitations in social, language, and self-adaptive functions
   May have seizures, psychiatric disorders, or behavioral abnormalities
   Often develop depression

Management
   Early intervention program as soon as mental deficiency is recognized
   Family support or counseling
   Attempt to identify cause
   Consultation with neurologist, speech pathologist, social worker, and occupational or physical therapist
   Educate to maximize social and occupational skills
   Determine support that is needed

Prognosis
   The greater the degree of deficiency, the greater the immobility and the higher the mortality

XVII. Hearing Loss

Incidence
   Profound, bilateral hearing loss: 1/1000
   Mild to moderate hearing loss: 2/1000
   Unilateral hearing loss: 1/1000 (left ear affected more than right ear)

Etiology
   Genetic (Pendred syndrome, Waardenburg syndrome, Treacher Collins syndrome, CHARGE association, Klippel-Feil sequence, trisomy 8, Stickler syndrome)
   Acquired [infections, severe hyperbilirubinemia, complications of prematurity, ototoxicity of medications (e.g., gentamicin, vancomycin, furosemide)]
   Ear malformations
   Unknown

Classification of hearing loss
   1. Range

Hearing category	Range (decibel)
Normal	−10 to 20
Mild	21 to 40
Moderate	41–55
Moderate severe	56–70
Severe	71–90
Profound	> 90

2. *Type*
   Conductive
   Sensorineural
   Other (including cortical hearing impairment and perceptual disorders)

Diagnosis
   90% of cases should be detected in the newborn period
   Most newborn screening programs use an automated brain-stem response (ABR)
      In the ABR test, an evoked potential is used to estimate an audiogram
      A change in EEG is detected at the midbrain level in response to sound
      Most screening programs use a lower limit level of 35 db

Management
   If infant refers (did not pass at the 35 db range), rescreen within 10 days of original test with an ABR at an audiology
      center that is capable of performing an expanded audiogram with complete decibel ranges
   If remains positive for hearing loss, the following is recommended:
      Otolaryngologist consult
      Hearing aid, possible cochlear implant
      Specialized early intervention

Outcome
   On average, 7% of infants screened will refer
   Of the referrals, 80% rescreen as normal hearing; 20% have a true hearing deficit

XVIII. Learning Disability

Definition
   A deficit in the psychological process with an imperfect ability to listen, speak, read, write, spell, or do math
   There is a significant discrepancy between learning potential and actual academic achievement
   Must exclude mental deficiency, deafness, lack of opportunity

Incidence
   Two peaks: early elementary (reading, spelling, math) and late elementary (concept classes)

Clinical
   Must be at least 1 standard deviation or a 15-point difference between the scores on a standardized intelligence test
      (higher) and a standardized achievement test (lower)
   Can present at any age

References

Beers MH, Berkow R (eds): The Merck Manual of Diagnosis and Therapy (17th edition), Whitehouse Station, NJ, Merck Research Laboratories, 1999.

Bianchi DW, Crombleholme TM, D'Alton ME. Fetology. New York, McGraw-Hill, 2000.

Cargan AL. Review of hypoxic-ischemic encephalopathy. Pediatric Residency Conference, Babies & Children's Hospital of New York, January, 1995.

Cloherty, JP, Stark AR (ed). Manual of Neonatal Care (4th edition). Philadelphia, Lippincott-Raven, 1998.

Fanaroff AA, Martin RJ (eds): Neonatal-Perinatal Medicine (6th edition). St. Louis, Mosby 1997.

Fletcher MA. Physical Diagnosis in Neonatology. Philadelphia, Lippincott-Raven Publishers, 1998.

Jones KL: Smith's Recognizable Patterns of Human Malformations (5th edition). Philadelphia, WB Saunders, 1997.

Neault, M. Newborn screening update. Division of Newborn Medicine Clinical Conference Series. Children's Hospital, Boston, MA, 2002.

Polin RA, Fox WW (eds): Fetal and Neonatal Physiology (2nd edition). Philadelphia, WB Saunders, 1998.

Volpe JJ. Neurology of the Newborn (4th edition). Philadelphia, WB Saunders, 2001.

Volpe JJ. "Brain injury in the premature infant—current concepts." Current Concepts in Neonatology Conference, Children's Hospital, Boston, MA, 1996.

Volpe JJ. Current concepts: neonatal seizures. *N Engl J Med*. 1973; 289(8):413–416.

CHAPTER 5

Genetics

TOPICS COVERED IN THIS CHAPTER

I. Molecular Genetics

A. DNA AND RNA

DNA (deoxyribonucleic acid): a double helix compound that contains four nitrogen bases (adenine-A, cytosine-C, guanine-G and thymine-T) and a sugar (deoxyribose)-phosphate backbone
DNA bases contain the code for mRNA

RNA (ribonucleic acid): a single-stranded compound that contains four nitrogen bases (adenine-A, cytosine-C, guanine-G and uracil-U) and a sugar (ribose)-phosphate backbone
Types of RNA
 Messenger RNA (mRNA): RNA that is formed from the transcription of DNA; primary mRNA is formed first and undergoes splicing (removal of introns) to form mature mRNA
 Ribosomal RNA (rRNA): RNA that is part of the ribosome and helps bind mRNA and tRNA to the ribosome
 Transfer RNA (tRNA): RNA that transports amino acids and assists in translation of mature mRNA; the anticodon portion of the tRNA (contains a specific amino acid at the 3′ end) binds to a complementary mRNA codon

Transcription: the process by which a mRNA sequence is synthesized from a DNA template

DNA polymerase: an enzyme that is important in DNA replication by utilizing a complementary DNA strand as a template to synthesize a new strand

RNA polymerase: an enzyme that binds to a promoter region and synthesizes mRNA from a DNA template

Reverse transcriptase: an enzyme that transcribes RNA into DNA (i.e. reverses transcription)

Restriction endonuclease: a bacterial enzyme that breaks a DNA sequence at a specific site

B. GENE

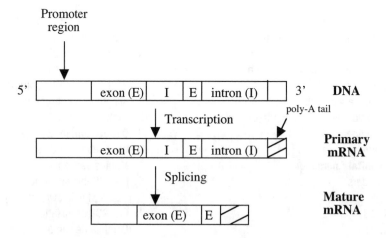

Gene: the unit of heredity that contains DNA sequences with exons and introns

Intron: the DNA sequence of a gene located between 2 exons that is transcribed into messenger RNA (mRNA) but *spliced out* during the formation of mature mRNA; function is unknown

Exon: the DNA sequence of a gene located between 2 introns that is transcribed into mRNA and *retained* after the primary mRNA is spliced
= the ultimate gene product

Promoter: a DNA sequence located 5′ to a specific gene; RNA polymerase binds to this region so that transcription (DNA into mRNA) can occur

Enhancer: a DNA sequence that interacts with specific transcription factors and leads to increased transcription of the gene

Polyadenylation sequence (poly-A tail): 100–200 adenine nucleotides that are located at the 3′ end of primary mRNA; this sequence may be important in mRNA stabilization

Allele: different DNA sequences that a gene may have in a population

Locus: the location of a specific gene within a chromosome

Polymorphism: a locus in which 2 or more alleles have gene frequencies greater than 1% in a population and thus cannot be explained by recurrent mutations
Polymorphisms allow for multiple combinations of alleles at different loci and thus a large degree of genetic diversity
Since polymorphisms are markers of genetic diversity, they are often used as tools for mapping the human genome
e.g., loci coding for ABO blood group

C. PROTEIN

Translation: the process by which an amino acid sequence is assembled utilizing the mature mRNA sequence; tRNA is required for translation since this is the only RNA that can bind directly to amino acids

Post-translational protein modification: alterations (e.g., hydroxylation, glycosylation, cleavage) of a polypeptide sequence that occurs after translation

D. GENETIC TECHNIQUES

Polymerase chain reaction (PCR)
Technique: amplification of a specific DNA sequence without requiring isolation of that sequence from genomic DNA
Using 2 oligonucleotide primers located on either end of the DNA sequence of interest, the DNA is heated and cooled in the presence of DNA polymerase and numerous free nucleotides
During this reaction, the specific DNA sequence is denatured (i.e. single-stranded), hybridized with primers and then extended
Advantages: can work with very small amount of DNA
Disadvantages: 1. Must know DNA sequence that flanks the region of interest
2. Due to its high sensitivity, there is a high risk of contamination
3. Difficult to utilize PCR if sequence is longer than a few kilobases

Southern analysis (or blot or transfer): DNA is digested by restriction enzymes that recognize specific DNA sequences
DNA is then loaded onto an agarose gel and undergoes electrophoresis, allowing the fragments to be separated by size
The gel pattern is transferred to filter paper and then exposed to a labeled *DNA probe* to identify which fragment is homologous to the probe

Northern analysis (or blot or transfer): analagous to Southern analysis yet hybridization of a *labeled DNA probe* to digested RNA

Western analysis (or blot): proteins are separated based upon size and charge by electrophoresis on a gel and a specific antibody is used as a probe to identify the protein of interest

Linkage studies: provide an indirect method to diagnose genetic diseases
  Analysis using 2 loci that are located near each other on the same chromosome (i.e. "linked") to determine if an individual has inherited a chromosome containing a disease gene
  While these loci are physically linked, they are not functionally related
  DNA polymorphisms can be used as markers
  Advantages: can be used to diagnose any genetic disease that is mapped
    The sequence of the gene for the disease does not need to be precisely identified
  Disadvantages: risk of recombination, requires testing of many family members to establish linkage, not all markers are helpful in all families, can have mutations of marker or disease gene leading to unsuccessful study

FISH (fluorescent in situ hybridization)
  Technique: synthesis of a single-stranded DNA probe that is complementary to the sequence of interest
    This probe is then tagged with a fluorescent marker
    Cultured cells are then exposed to the fluorescent probe, which will hybridize to its complementary sequence
    The fluorescent signal is easily identified using ultraviolet light
  Application: used to identify the presence or absence of a specific sequence in a cell
    Available for trisomy 13, 18 and 21, Prader-Willi syndrome, Angelman syndrome, cri du chat, DiGeorge sequence/velocardiofacial syndrome, Miller-Dieker (congenital lissencephaly), Williams syndrome, 4p deletion

Mass spectrometry: detection of very small differences in mass of PCR products due to variations in DNA sequence

Prenatal diagnosis: available for numerous diseases including cystic fibrosis, Duchenne muscular dystrophy, fragile X syndrome, all gangliosidoses, galactosemia, glycogen storage disease type II, hemophilia A and B, Huntington disease, maple syrup urine disease, methylmalonic acidemia, all mucopolysaccharidoses, myotonic dystrophy, sickle cell disease, phenylketonuria, Smith-Lemli-Opitz syndrome, Tay-Sachs disease, α and β thalassemia, Zellweger syndrome
  This group continues to be expanded each year

II. Morphogenesis

A. NORMAL MORPHOGENESIS

Requirements include: Proper cell migration
  Control over cellular mitotic rate
  Appropriate interaction between adjacent tissues
  Aggregation of similar cell types
  Controlled cell death
  Normal hormonal influence
  Appropriate mechanical factors

B. ABNORMAL MORPHOGENESIS

MALFORMATION: abnormal tissue formation; e.g., renal agenesis, micrognathia, cleft palate
  Incidence
    Major malformations: 2–3% of neonates with major malformations
      The most common major congenital malformations in the US are neural tube defects
    Minor malformations: 85% of all newborns without any minor malformations, 13% of newborns with 1 minor malformation, 0.8% with 2 minor malformations, and 0.5% with 3 minor malformations

As the number of minor malformations increase, there is a greater risk of major malformations (i.e. if 3 minor malformations are observed, there is ~90% risk of a major malformation; in contrast, if 1 minor malformation is observed, there is a ~3% risk of a major malformation)

Etiologies: Environmental
  Genetic—Chromosomal (10%)
    Single gene (4%)
    Multifactorial (genetic and environmental) (~25%)
    Mitochondrial
  Unknown (most common ~40-45%)

Deformation: associated with altered mechanical forces (extrinsic or intrinsic) on normal tissue; mechanical
  e.g., arthrogryposis due to external in utero constraints

Disruption: breakdown of normal tissue; destructive
  e.g., amniotic bands, limb reduction defects due to vascular anomalies, porencephaly

Dysplasia: abnormal organization of cellular formation into tissue; deregulation
  e.g., hemangioma, ectodermal dysplasia

Syndrome: a pattern of many primary malformations due to one etiology   Down's Syndrome

Sequence: a primary defect with secondary effects
  e.g., Pierre Robin sequence due to primary mandibular maldevelopment with secondary findings of micrognathia, cleft palate and glossoptosis

III. Inheritance of Genetic Diseases

A. CHROMOSOMAL DISORDERS

1. Chromosomal maldistribution
Normally there are 22 pairs of autosomes and 1 pair of sex chromosomes = 23 pairs
Chromosome: composed of a short arm (p) and a long arm (q); the central region or centromere is where the microtubules attach to assist in cell division
  The distal regions of the chromosome contain the *telomere,* which maintains the integrity as well as the stability of the chromosome
An error in assortment can lead to *aneuploidy* (an abnormal number of chromosomes) due to *polyploidy* (extra number of chromosomes), or *monosomy* (decreased number of chromosomes)
Etiology: majority due to nondisjunction (inability of chromosomes to disjoin during meiosis)
Examples: trisomies (13, 18, 21), Turner syndrome (45, X), Klinefelter syndrome (47, XXY)

2. Chromosomal rearrangements
Deletions: loss of chromosomal material
Microdeletions: deletion that is too small to be detected using a microscope
  e.g., DiGeorge syndrome, Prader-Willi syndrome
Duplication: an extra copy of chromosomal material
Mutation: a change in the DNA sequence (e.g., point mutation occurs when one base pair is substituted for another)
Translocations: exchange of genetic material between 2 different chromosomes
  Balanced—typically no abnormality due to balance of genes yet risk of offspring with abnormality
    e.g., the Philadelphia chromosome is a balanced translocation in which most of chromosome 22 translocates onto the long arm of chromosome 9; this is associated with chronic myelogenous leukemia

Unbalanced—the chromosomal rearrangement leads to a gain or loss of chromosomal material

Reciprocal translocation: a type of translocation in which there is a break in 2 different chromosomes and the material is exchanged; normal phenotype

Robertsonian translocation: a type of translocation which occurs when the long arms of 2 different chromosomes fuse at the centromere and the very small short arms are lost; only involves chromosomes 13, 14, 15, 21 and 22

Since the short arms contain very few genes, the phenotype is normal; however, the offspring can have monosomy or trisomy of the long arms

Most common type is between chromosome 21 and 14

Responsible for 3–5% of trisomy 21

Inversion: a piece of a chromosome is broken and reinserted in the opposite direction; if the centromere is included → pericentric inversion; if the centromere is not involved → paracentric inversion

Isochromosome: abnormal division or breakage at a centromere during mitosis leading to a chromosome with either two long arms or two short arms

Ring chromosome: if a deletion occurs at both tips of a chromosome, the remaining chromosome fuses to form a ring

Usually these chromosomes are lost, resulting in monosomy

B. SINGLE-GENE DISORDERS (MENDELIAN INHERITANCE)

The most common single-gene disorder in Caucasian population is cystic fibrosis

1. Autosomal dominant

Incidence: observed in 1/200 individuals

Each autosomal dominant disease is rare in a population

Characteristics: wide variation of expression

Vertical transmission of the disease phenotype

No skipped generations (affected children have at least one affected parent unless spontaneous mutation)

Approximately equal number of males and females affected

Males and females are equally likely to transmit the disease to offspring

Father to son transmission can be observed

Recurrence risk: for offspring of one carrier parent is 50%

If both parents are affected, recurrence risk is 75%

2. Autosomal recessive

Incidence: rare in population

Characteristics: less variation in expression than autosomal dominant diseases

Clustering of the disease among siblings but not usually in parents or other ancestors

Approximately equal number of males and females affected

Males and females are equally likely to transmit the disease to offspring

Recurrence risk: for offspring of two carrier parents recurrence risk = 25% (e.g., cystic fibrosis)

If an affected homozygote mates with a heterozygote, recurrence risk is 50%

If both parents are affected homozygotes, recurrence risk is 100%

3. X-linked

Lyon hypothesis: one X chromosome in each female cell is inactivated *randomly* early in embryonic development and is unable to be reactivated (i.e. *fixed*)

This leads to an equal # of X-linked genes in males and females

Females will then have 2 populations of cells: one population with an active X chromosome that is paternally derived and another population with an active X chromosome that is maternally derived

The inactive X chromosome forms a *Barr body;* normal females will have 1 Barr body per cell while normal males will not have any Barr bodies; females with Turner syndrome will not have any Barr bodies

Female patients with 45, X (Turner syndrome) will be affected since X inactivation is *incomplete* so that some regions of the X chromosome are active in all copies

	X-linked Recessive	X-linked Dominant
Characteristics	Since females have 2 copies of the X chromosome and males only have one, X-linked recessive diseases are usually clinically evident in males	Rarer than X-linked recessive diseases
		2x as common in females as males
	Fathers cannot transmit the disease to son(s)	Fathers cannot transmit the disease to son(s)
	A heterozygote female who is phenotypically normal can transmit disease to offspring (i.e. "skipped generation")	Rare to have skipped generations
	An affected father will transmit the disease to all his daughters who will be carriers and pass the disease on to ~1/2 of their sons	Heterozygote females may be less severely affected than affected males
	Since X-inactivation is random, heterozygote females may be phenotypically abnormal since the majority of active X chromosomes may be abnormal	
Recurrence risk	Dependent on genotype of each parent and the sex of their offspring	Dependent on genotype of each parent and the sex of their offspring

4. Examples of single-gene disorders

Autosomal recessive majority	Metabolic: *cystic fibrosis, majority of inborn errors of metabolism*
	Hematology: α-and β-thalassemia, sickle cell disease
	Endocrine: 21-hydroxylase deficiency
	Neurology: congenital muscular dystrophy
Autosomal dominant	Hematology: Protein C and S deficiency, spherocytosis (majority, minority due to autosomal recessive inheritance), Gilbert disease, von Willebrand disease (majority)
	Neurology: congenital myotonic dystrophy, neurofibromatosis
	Genetic: Apert syndrome, Crouzon syndrome, Holt-Oram syndrome, Marfan syndrome, Noonan syndrome, Stickler syndrome, Treacher Collins syndrome
	Dermatology: aplasia cutis, bullous ichthyosis and ichthyosis vulgaris, epidermolysis bullosa simplex, keratosis pilaris, partial albinism, Peutz-Jegher syndrome, *Waardenburg syndrome*
	Renal: adult polycystic kidney disease
	Gastrointestinal: familial polyposis, Gardner syndrome
	Opthalmologic: retinoblastomas (some with variable penetrance, sporadic in 60%)
	Orthopedic: achondroplasia, postaxial polydactyly, osteogenesis imperfecta, thanatophoric dysplasia
X-linked recessive	Metabolic: Fabry disease, Hunter disease, Menkes disease
	Hematology: *glucose-6-phosphate dehydrogenase deficiency, Wiskott-Aldrich* syndrome, *hemophilia A and B*
	Neurology: red-green color blindness, Duchenne muscular dystrophy
	Dermatology: hypohidrotic ectodermal dysplasia, X-linked ichthyosis
	Renal: nephrogenic diabetes insipidus
X-linked dominant	Dermatology: incontinentia pigmentosa
	Genetics: fragile X syndrome

Words in italics represent commonly recognized disorders in these categories.

5. Variations of single-gene disorders

In some cases, the distinction between dominant and recessive may not be rigid
   e.g., heterozygotes for the autosomal dominant disease achondroplasia will have reduced stature, while homozygotes for achondroplasia are more severely affected and often die in infancy
In some cases, a disease can be *either* autosomal dominant or recessive due to different mutations that alter the gene product
New mutation: may result in different inheritance patterns
   e.g., achondroplasia is an autosomal dominant disease in which 7/8 cases are due to new mutations; thus despite dominant inheritance, a patient with achondroplasia may not have a family history of the disorder and the recurrence risk for siblings is low; however, this patient will transmit disease to future offspring
Mosaicism: 2 or more genetically different cell lines in the same person
   This may lead to a phenotypically normal parent transmitting a mutation to offspring who may express the mutation
   e.g., type II osteogenesis imperfecta, achondroplasia, Duchenne muscular dystrophy, hemophilia A

Reduced penetrance: a person with a genotype for a disease may not exhibit the phenotype (an *all or none* phenomenon) but can transmit the disease to offspring; e.g., retinoblastoma

Variable expression: severity of expression of a disease may vary; e.g., neurofibromatosis I

Genomic imprinting: some genes may be expressed differently depending on whether the gene is inherited from the mother or the father

  e.g., Beckwith-Wiedemann syndrome, Prader-Willi syndrome, and Angelman syndrome (if deletion of a specific region within the long arm of chromosome 15 is inherited from the father, the offspring will have Prader-Willi syndrome; however, if the deletion is inherited from the mother, the offspring will develop Angelman syndrome)

Uniparental disomy: if offspring inherits 2 copies of a chromosome from one parent and none from the other

  e.g., can occur following attempted self-correction of a trisomic chromosome by elimination of 1 chromosome; this may lead to 2 copies of the chromosome from the same parent

Expansion of trinucleotide repeats: can lead to genetic diseases

  Often increased # of repeats with each generation

  e.g., congenital myotonic dystrophy is an autosomal dominant disease that is due to an expanded CTG repeat

    If 5–30 copies→ unaffected

    If 50–100 copies → may be mildly affected

    If 100–several thousand copies → severely affected

  Also in fragile X syndrome

C. MULTIFACTORIAL DISORDERS

Definition: due to a combination of genetic abnormalities and environmental influences

Characteristics: most affected children have unaffected parents

Recurrence risk: risk changes between populations

  Greater risk with increasing # of affected family members

  Greater risk with increased severity of expression of the disease

  Risk is proportional to closeness or relatedness

Examples: cleft lip and/or cleft palate, anencephaly and spina bifida, clubfoot, congenital hip dysplasia, pyloric stenosis

D. MITOCHONDRIAL DISORDERS

Definition: a small number of diseases that are due to alterations in the mitochondrial chromosome

Characteristics: mitochondrial DNA (does not contain introns) have a high mutation rate ($\sim$10x greater than nuclear DNA) due to limited DNA repair mechanisms in the mitochondrial DNA and perhaps due to damage from oxygen free radicals

Mitochondrial DNA are inherited *maternally;* thus, transmission only occurs from affected females

Mitochondrial diseases have a large degree of phenotypic variability due to *heteroplasmy* (within one cell may have different ratios of normal and mutated mitochondrial DNA)

  i.e., one family may have very different manifestations of the same mitochondrial disease or an individual may manifest a change in phenotype with increasing age

Recurrence risk: offspring of affected males are not at risk of acquiring disease

All offspring of affected females will have some degree of abnormal mitochondrial mutations but not all will manifest disease

IV. Associations with Congenital Anomalies

A. ADVANCED MATERNAL AND PATERNAL AGE

Genetic Disorders Associated with Advanced Maternal Age	Genetic Disorders Associated with Advanced Paternal Age (Increased Risk of NEW Mutations—Especially Autosomal Dominant)
Klinefelter syndrome	Achondroplasia
Trisomy 13	Apert syndrome
Trisomy 18	Marfan syndrome
Trisomy 21	Treacher Collins syndrome
	Osteogenesis imperfecta
	Waardenburg syndrome

B. MALE VS FEMALE

Male (Male: Female)	Female (Female: Male)
Respiratory: laryngomalacia (2:1)	Respiratory: choanal atresia (2:1)
Cardiac: ventricular septal defect, transposition of the great arteries (3:1), coarctation of the aorta (2:1), hypoplastic left heart disease, subdiaphragmatic total anomalous pulmonary venous return (4:1) (note: if drainage into portal veins, male = female), pulmonic and aortic stenosis	Cardiac: atrial septal defect (2:1), patent ductus arteriosus (3:1)
	Neurology: anencephaly (3:1)
	Endocrine: congenital hypothyroidism (2:1)
Gastrointestinal: pyloric stenosis (5:1), Hirschsprung disease (4:1), imperforate anus, omphalocele (3:1)	Gastrointestinal: choledochal cysts (2.5:1)
	Hematologic: thrombocytopenia with absent radii (2:1)
Orthopedic: clubfoot (2:1)	Orthopedic: congenital hip dysplasia (5.5:1)
Renal: unilateral multicystic dysplastic kidney disease	Renal: uterocele (5–7:1)
Dermatology: acne	Dermatology: hemangioma
Genetics: cleft lip (with or without cleft palate) (2:1), Poland sequence (3:1)	Genetics: trisomy 18 (3:1)

C. RECURRENCE RISK

Disorder	Recurrence risk
Cardiac defect	If one previous child with congenital heart disease → 3–4% risk to next child
	If two previous children with congenital heart disease → 10% risk to next child
Cleft lip	If one child with cleft lip and normal parents → 4–5% risk to next child
	If one child with cleft lip and one parent affected → 10% risk to next child
Cleft palate	If one child with cleft palate → 2–6% risk to siblings
Congenital hip dysplasia	If one child with hip dysplasia → 3–4% risk to next child (0.5% if male, 6.3% if female)
Club foot	If one child with club foot → 2–5% risk to next child (2% if first child is male, 5% risk if first child is female)
	If one parent with club foot and one affected child → 25% risk to next child
Hirschsprung	If one child with Hirschsprung → 3–5% risk to next child
Neural tube defects	If one child with neural tube defect → 3–5% risk to next child
Pyloric stenosis	If mother with pyloric stenosis → 19% risk of affected son, 7% risk of affected daughter
	If father with pyloric stenosis → 5.5% risk of affected son, 2.4% risk of affected daughter
	If one child with pyloric stenosis → 3% risk to next child (4% if male, 2.4% if female)
Trisomy 21	If mother has balanced translocation → 10–15% risk of affected child
	If father has balanced translocation → 5% risk of affected child
	Prior child with trisomy 21 and no parent with translocation→ 1 % risk to sibling until risk due to advanced maternal age is higher than 1% (typically after 37 years of age)

Modified from: Jones KL: Smith's Recognizable Patterns of Human Malformations (5th edition). Philadelphia, WB Saunders Co, 1997, p 722.

D. CALCULATIONS

1. Hardy-Weinberg equilibirum

Hardy-Weinberg equilibrium: relates allele frequency to genotypic frequency in a population at equilibrium

e.g., assume a single autosomal locus with two alleles (A and a)

Thus, there are 3 possible genotypes (AA, Aa and aa)

Assume the population frequency of A is "p" and of a is "q"

Since there are only two alleles "p + q =1"

Random mating of Aa mother and Aa father will lead to a genotype frequency of "p^2" for AA, "2pq" for Aa and "q^2" for aa

Must assume a large population, random mating, lack of mutations, no migration, and no selection

2. Calculation of allele and gene frequencies

Calculation of allele frequency of an autosomal recessive disorder given the population incidence of that disease

e.g., if cystic fibrosis (CF) occurs in 1 of 1700 Caucasian neonates, the frequency of CF homozygotes is 1/1700 or 0.00059, which is "q^2"; the CF allele frequency (or q) will be the square root of "q^2" = 0.024, since p + q =1; then p (the normal allele) = 1-q, which is 0.976

Calculation of genotype frequency of an autosomal recessive disorder given the population incidence of that disease

e.g.,. to continue using above CF example, the frequency of CF carriers (heterozygotes or 2pq) is then 2 × 0.976 × 0.024 = 0.047

The frequency of homozygote normals is then "p^2," which is 0.093

The frequency of CF is then "q^2," which is 0.00059

3. Cystic fibrosis recurrence risk

1 in 25 Caucasians is a heterozygote carrier of the CF gene

CF is autosomal recessive

Question: if a pregnant woman has a sister with CF, what is risk to offspring of having CF?

Answer: father risk of carrier state is 1/25

Mother's parents both were carriers and thus the chance of mother being a carrier is 2/3 (know that she does not have CF)

The chance that both parents can pass on the gene to offspring is 1/4

Thus, 1/25 × 2/3 × 1/4 = 1/150 chance that offspring will have CF

V. Specific Congenital Anomalies

A. TRISOMY DISORDERS

1. Trisomy 8

Etiology

Rare, majority are mosaic since complete trisomy 8 typically lethal in utero

Clinical

Extremities—deep creases of palms and soles, *camptodactyly*

Facial—*thick lips, deep-set eyes, prominent cupped ears,* prominent forehead, hypertelorism, micrognathia, short or webbed neck

Neurology—mild to severe mental deficiency

Other—pelvic dysplasia, hip dysplasia, uteral-renal anomalies, may have cardiac abnormalities

2. Trisomy 13

Etiology

= Patau syndrome, 1 in 5–10,000 live births

>90% die within first year of life

80% with complete trisomy (extra chromosome of *maternal* origin) and remainder due to translocation

95% of trisomy 13 conceptions lead to spontaneous abortions

Clinical (features found in >50% of patients with trisomy 13)

High number of *midline abnormalities*

Cardiac (80-90%)—ventricular septal defect > patent ductus arteriosus

Dermatology—*aplasia cutis*

Extremities—*polydactyly*, transverse palmar crease, *narrow hyperconvex fingernails*

Facial—*cleft lip, cleft palate*, small eyes, colobomas (iris), retinal dysplasia, sloping forehead

Gastrointestinal—umbilical or inguinal hernia

Genitourinary—cryptorchidism, abnormal scrotum, bicornate uterus

Neurology—microcephaly, *holoprosencephaly*, seizures (often with hypsarrhythmia), severe mental deficiency if survive, deafness

Other—pelvic dysplasia, apnea in neonatal period, *persistence of fetal hemoglobin* (increased Gower hemoglobin), increased neutrophils with nuclear projections; triple screen not helpful

3. Trisomy 18

Etiology

= Edward syndrome; 1 in 6000; 90% mortality within 1st year of life

> 95% with complete trisomy 21 (extra chromosome of *maternal* origin in ~90%)

Small percentage with mosaicism

95% of trisomy 18 conceptions lead to spontaneous abortions

Females > males (3:1)

Clinical (below features found in >50% patients with trisomy 18)

Cardiac (95-99%)—ventricular septal defect, patent ductus arteriosus > bicuspid aortic valve, pulmonary stenosis, coarctation of the aorta

Extremities—*clenched hand*, overlapping of 2nd finger over 3rd or 5th finger over 4th, hypoplastic nails, small pelvis, rocker-bottom feet (in 10-50%)

Facial—micrognathia (may be associated with Pierre Robin sequence), *small mouth*, small eyes, small palpebral fissures, malformed low-set ears, occipital prominence   *omphalocele*

Gastrointestinal—umbilical or inguinal hernia

Genitourinary—cryptorchidism

Neurology—hypertonia after neonatal period, narrow biparietal diameter, choroid plexus cyst, mental deficiency if survive

Other—short sternum, one umbilical artery, intrauterine growth restriction, *short sternum;* triple screen with low β-human chorionic gonadotropin, low unconjugated estriol, low maternal α-fetoprotein; 1/3 are premature and 1/3 are postmature

4. Trisomy 21 = Down syndrome

Etiology

1 in 800 live births

In a large majority, extra chromosome is *maternal* (mostly due to nondisjunction)

94% complete trisomy, ~3-5% Robertsonian translocation (usually chromosome 13, 14 or 15), 2% due to mosaicism (associated with milder phenotype)

Increased risk with advanced maternal age due to increased risk nondisjunction with increasing age:

Maternal Age	Risk of Trisomy 21 Full-Term Infant
20 years old	1 in 1667
25 years old	1 in 1250
30 years old	1 in 952
35 years old	1 in 385
40 years old	1 in 106
45 years old	1 in 30
Modified from Bianchi DW, Crombleholme TM and D'Alton ME: Fetology. New York, McGraw-Hill, 2000, p 12.	

Although increasing risk with increased maternal age, ~3/4 of children with trisomy 21 are born to mothers <35 years old since this age group has a higher reproduction rate

Clinical

Cardiac (40–50%)—most common type is *endocardial cushion defect* > ventricular septal defect > patent ductus arteriosus > anomalous subclavian artery, mitral valve prolapse, aortic regurgitation

Endocrine—hypothyroidism

Extremities—*transverse palmar crease* (~45% compared with ~3% of normals), *5th finger with hypoplastic middle phalanx, 5th finger clinodactyly*, wide gap between 1st and 2nd toes, *hyperflexibility of joints,* broad and short hands and feet

Facial—*upslanting palpebral fissures,* small ears, *flat facies,* Brushfield spots (speckled iris), inner *epicanthal folds,* large protruding tongue, flat maxillary and malar region, *short neck with redundant posterior folds,* flat occiput

Gastrointestinal—duodenal atresia, increased risk of Hirschsprung disease

Genitourinary—hypogonadism, infertile male, most females are infertile

Neurology—*hypotonia,* mild microcephaly, moderate to severe mental deficiency (IQ typically 25–60 yet may be more functional than IQ suggests)

Other—small stature, *pelvic dysplasia,* increased risk immunologic dysfunction, leukemia (15–20x compared with general population), and Alzheimer's disease

B. DELETIONS

1. Cri du chat

Etiology

Partial deletion of the short arm of the 5th chromosome (deleted portion is of *paternal* origin in 80% of de novo events)

Majority are de novo events

Clinical

Cardiac (30%)—ventricular septal defect, patent ductus arteriosus, tetralogy of Fallot

Extremities—transverse palmar crease

Facial—*hypertelorism, downward slant of palpebral fissures,* round facies, epicanthal folds, strabismus, low-set ears

Neurology—severe *mental deficiency, cat-like cry* (attributed to abnormal laryngeal development), *microcephaly, hypotonia*

Other—low birth weight, *failure to thrive*

2. Deletion 13 q

Clinical

Cardiac—increased risk congenital heart disease

Extremities—*thumb hypoplasia,* 5th finger clinodactyly, short big toe, talipes equinovarus

Eyes—*colobomas,* increased risk of *retinoblastoma* (usually bilateral), small eyes

Facial—*microcephaly,* micrognathia, large malformed and low-set ears, *high nasal bridge,* hypertelorism, ptosis, epicanthal folds

Genitourinary—hypospadias, cryptorchidism

Neurology—mental deficiency, microcephaly

Other—intrauterine growth restriction, focal lumbar agenesis

C. MICRODELETIONS

1. Angelman syndrome

Etiology

~70% due to 15q11-13 deletion; <5% due to paternal uniparental disomy; 20–30% due to point mutations or other abnormality of maternal 15q11–13 region

Deleted piece is always of *maternal origin*

Clinical

Facial—inappropriate bursts of laughter, widely spaced teeth, large mouth, protruding tongue, 65% with blond hair color, decreased iris pigment, deep-set eyes, maxillary hypoplasia, microbrachycephaly

Neurology—severe mental deficiency, delayed motor skills, absent speech or < 6 word vocabulary, ataxia and jerky movements similar to a puppet, seizures (EEG with high-amplitude spikes, 2–3 hz slow waves), hypotonia
Skeletal—*"puppet-like" gait*

2. DiGeorge syndrome
Etiology
Majority with 22q11.2 deletion
= velocardiofacial syndrome = CATCH 22 (**C**ardiac, **A**bnormal facies, **T**hymic hypoplasia, **C**left palate, **H**ypocalcemia)
Due to a defect in 4th brachial arch and derivatives of the 3rd and 4th pharyngeal pouches
Clinical
Cardiac—aortic arch abnormalities (right-sided aortic arch, interrupted aorta, truncus arteriosus), ventricular septal defect, patent ductus arteriosus, tetralogy of Fallot
Facial—cleft palate, hypertelorism, misshapen ears, micrognathia, short philtrum, short palpebral fissures
Thymus—*hypoplastic to aplastic thymus*
Other—hypoplastic parathyroid glands leading to *hypocalcemia* and possible seizures, *deficient cellular immunity*, may have diaphragmatic hernia, imperforate anus, choanal atresia, or esophageal atresia,

3. Prader-Willi syndrome
Etiology
1 in 15,000
~70% with deletion of 15q 11-13; ~25% due to maternal uniparental disomy; ~5% due to maternal methylation at several loci within 15q11–13 region
Deleted piece is always of *paternal origin*
Clinical
Variability of features based on age
Extremities—*small hands and feet*
Facial—almond-shaped palpebral fissures, thin upper lip, light-colored hair and eye color
Genitourinary—*hypogenitalia, undescended testes*
Neurology—*hypotonia* (profound, generalized, greatest during infancy), mild-severe mental deficiency
Other—failure to thrive during infancy followed by *obesity* (associated with excessive appetite and decreased activity) presenting between 6 months to 6 years of age, scoliosis, typically in *breech* position at time of delivery

4. Rubenstein-Taybi syndrome
Etiology
Majority are sporadic
Locus at 16p13.3, which encodes the cAMP-regulated enhancer-binding protein
1/4 due to submicroscopic deletions, some may be due to point mutations
Clinical
Cardiac (25%)—patent ductus arteriosus, ventricular septal defect, atrial septal defect
Extremities—*broad thumbs, broad toes,* 5th finger clinodactyly, flat feet
Facial—*downward slanting of palpebral fissures, hypoplastic maxilla,* narrow palate, prominent and/or beaked nose, deviated nasal septum, low-set ears, long eyelashes, heavy eyebrows, strabismus
Other—speech difficulties, stiff and unsteady gait, hypotonia, cryptorchidism, developmental delay, postnatal growth deficiency, hirsutism

5. WAGR syndrome
Etiology
11p13 deletion, usually de novo
Phenotype variability due to different sized deletions
Clinical
Wilms tumor (50%), **A**niridia, **G**enitourinary abnormalities, mental deficiency (or **R**etardation – moderate to severe)

Facial—prominent lips, micrognathia, malformed ears, congenital cataracts, nystagmus, ptosis, blindness

Genitourinary—males may have cryptorchidism, hypospadius

Other—may develop gonadoblastomas, short stature, microcephaly

6. Williams syndrome

Etiology

7q11.23 deletion leading to deletion of an elastin gene

Majority sporadic

Clinical

Cardiac (50-70%)—*supravalvular subaortic stenosis* > *peripheral pulmonic stenosis,* ventricular septal defect, atrial septal defect, coarctation of the aorta

Extremities—*hypoplastic nails*

Facial—*prominent lips* with open mouth, *hoarse voice,* blue eyes, *stellate iris pattern,* periorbital fullness, enamel hypoplasia, depressed nasal bridge, short palpebral fissures, epicanthal folds, long philtrum

Neurology—*mental deficiency* (IQ 41-80), mild microcephaly

Renal—anomalies include renal asymmetry, pelvic kidney

Other—hypercalcemia (usually transient), mild perinatal growth restriction

D. AUTOSOMAL DOMINANT DISORDERS

1. Achondroplasia AD

Etiology

Autosomal dominant, *80-90% are due to new mutations;* 1 in 15,000

Increased risk with increased paternal age

Due to a mutation in the transmembrane domain of the fibroblast growth factor receptor 3 gene (at 4p16.3 locus)

Clinical

Endocrine—relative glucose intolerance

Extremities—*"trident hands"* (separation between middle and ring fingers), *short limbs*

Facial—*depressed nasal bridge,* prominent mandible, frontal bossing

Neurology—*megalocephaly,* mild hypotonia, small foramen magnum (may lead to hydrocephalus), *caudal narrowing of spinal cord, normal intelligence*

Skeletal—abnormal vertebrae, short stature, spinal complications, narrow chest

2. Apert and Crouzon syndromes AD

	Apert Syndrome = Acrocephalosyndactyly	Crouzon Syndrome = Craniofacial Dysostosis
Etiology	Autosomal dominant Majority sporadic Increased risk with increased paternal age Due to mutation in fibroblast growth factor receptor 2 gene	Autosomal dominant with variable expression Due to different mutation in fibroblast growth factor receptor 2 gene
Clinical	*Hypertelorism, midfacial hypoplasia,* shallow orbits, abnormally shaped skull, large fontanels, flat facies, down-slanting palpebral fissures, small nose, maxillary hypoplasia, narrow palate, dental anomalies, strabismus *Broad distal phalanx of thumb and big toe, syndactyly* of hands and feet *Irregular craniosynostosis* (especially coronal) VSD, PS, overriding aorta Greater risk of mental deficiency, neurological defects Other—increased risk of acne, fusion of cervical vertebrae	Hypertelorism, *maxillary hypoplasia, shallow orbits,* ocular proptosis, frontal bossing, may have curved parrot-beak nose, strabismus *Premature craniosynostosis* (especially coronal, lamboid, sagittal sutures) Mental deficiency less common Other—decreased visual acuity, conductive hearing loss

3. Beckwith-Wiedemann syndrome AD

Etiology

Autosomal dominant with variable expression and incomplete penetrance with gene located at 11p15.5

Usually sporadic

Different genetic mechanisms

Clinical

Typically with history of *polyhydramnios* and prematurity

Facial—*large tongue,* linear *earlobe fissures,* relative infraorbital hypoplasia, capillary nevus flammeus, large fontanel, *exophthalmos,* metopic ridge, prominent occiput

Gastrointestinal—*omphalocele,* diastasis recti

Growth—*macrosomia,* accelerated ossification, *organ hyperplasia*—particularly with renal, pancreatic, and pituitary hyperplasia, *fetal adrenocortical cytomegaly*

Neurology—usually without mental deficiency, large tongue may lead to speech difficulties, microcephaly

Other—neonatal polycythemia, cryptorchidism, congenital heart disease, *increased incidence (5–10%) of intraabdominal malignancies (especially Wilms tumor and hepatoblastoma),* limb hypertrophy, *hypoglycemia* (1/3–1/2, during early infancy, responsive to hydrocortisone)

4. Holt-Oram syndrome

Etiology

Autosomal dominant with variable expression

Some cases associated with 12q2 locus

Clinical

Cardiac (>50%)—*atrial septal defect* most common, ventricular septal defect, coarctation of aorta

Extremities—*upper limb defects* (may include ulna, humerus, clavicle), *absent, hypoplastic or abnormally-shaped thumbs, narrow shoulders,* decreased range of motion of upper extremities

Facial—may have hypertelorism

Other—no correlation between severity of limb defect and cardiac defect

5. Marfan syndrome AD

Etiology

Autosomal dominant with variable expression

Connective tissue disorder that is due to abnormal fibrillin gene located at 15q21.1

Clinical

Cardiac—*dilated aorta,* aortic aneurysm, aortic regurgitation, mitral valve prolapse

Extremities—*arachnodactyly, hyperextensibility,* joint laxity, *scoliosis,* kyphosis, disproportionate with arms and legs relatively longer than expected

Facial—*lens subluxation* (usually upward), myopia, increased risk of retinal detachment

Genitourinary—inguinal hernia

Other—there is a *severe neonatal form* that can occur [diagnosis typically within first 3 months of life, may present with cardiac defects (especially mitral valve abnormalities), contractures at birth, dolichocephaly, high-arched palate, micrognathia, hyperextensibility, arachnodactyly, chest deformity, lens dislocation; this neonatal disease is due to a different mutation in the fibrillin gene]

Management

Treatment with β-blocker recommended as soon as possible to decrease rate of aortic dilatation

6. Noonan syndrome AD

Etiology

Sporadic

Autosomal dominant with wide variable expression

Abnormality mapped to 12q22 region

Clinical

   Turner-like syndrome

   Cardiac (>50%)—*dysplastic pulmonary valve*, atrial septal defect, cardiomyopathy

   Chest—*pectus excavatum*

   Extremities—increased carrying angle

   Facial—*short or webbed neck*, low posterior hairline, epicanthal folds, hypertelorism, ptosis, low-set or abnormal ears, low nasal bridge, downslanting palpebral fissures

   Genitourinary—*cryptorchidism,* small penis

   Neurology—mental deficiency

   Other—*short stature* (50%), *abnormalities in coagulation pathway,* increased incidence of von Willebrand disease, 1/3 with thrombocytopenia, in utero cystic hygroma

Differential diagnosis

   45, X/XY mosaic, fetal hydantoin exposure, fetal alcohol syndrome

7. Osteogenesis imperfecta syndrome AD

Etiology

   Majority are autosomal dominant

   Defect in type I collagen

Clinical

   Type I—*blue sclera, increased risk of fractures* (~8% noted at birth, ~25% in first year of life), deafness, postnatal growth deficiency, abnormal dentition, *easy bruisability,* hyperextensible joints, Wormian bones in cranial sutures

   Type II—*blue sclera, increased risk of fractures, short and broad long bones, patients are usually stillborn or die in early infancy* due to respiratory failure, intrauterine growth restriction, Wormian bones, shallow orbits, small nose, low nasal bridge

   Type III—*blue sclera* during infancy that normalizes in adults, *increased risk of fractures* (usually present *at birth*), intrauterine growth restriction, macrocephaly, abnormal dentition, deafness, severe kyphoscoliosis, short stature

   Type IV—*normal sclera,* increased risk of bone deformities, may have abnormal dentition

   Note: there is significant overlap between all types, especially type II and type III

8. Stickler syndrome

Etiology

   Autosomal dominant with variable expression

   Due to mutation of type II collagen gene located at 12q13.11–q13.2 locus

   = hereditary arthro-ophthalmopathy

Clinical

   Facial—*flat facies,* depressed nasal bridge, prominent ears, epicanthal folds, short anteverted nose, midfacial or mandibular hypoplasia (can be associated with Pierre Robin sequence), palate, enamel anomalies, myopia, chorioretinal degeneration, cataracts, retinal detachment

   Neurology—deafness, hypotonia, hyperextensible joints

   Other—*myopia, spondyloepiphyseal dysplasia* (flat vertebrae with anterior wedging, poorly developed distal tibial epiphyses, flat femoral epiphyses), mitral valve prolapse

9. Thanatophoric dysplasia   AD

Etiology

   Autosomal dominant, all cases due to new mutations

   Due to a mutation in the extracellular domain or intracellular tyrosine kinase domain of the fibroblast growth factor receptor 3 gene (at 4p16.3 locus)

   Type I—more common, curved long bones, flat vertebral bodies

   Type 2—straight femoral bones, taller vertebral bodies, cloverleaf skull

Clinical

Extremities—*short limbs,* bowed long bones

Facial—*large cranium, low nasal bridge,* may have cloverleaf skull, bulging eyes, small facies

Neurology—temporal lobe dysplasia, hydrocephalus, brain stem hypoplasia, hypotonia, severe developmental delay if survive

Skeletal—*flat vertebrae*

Other—intrauterine growth restriction, narrow thorax, decreased activity and polyhydramnios in utero, high mortality shortly after birth partly due to small thorax and respiratory insufficiency

10. Treacher Collins syndrome AD

Etiology

Autosomal dominant with variable expression; 60% due to new mutations

= mandibulofacial dysostosis

Clinical

Facial—*defect of lower lid,* eyelid coloboma, *down-slanting of palpebral fissures, mandibular hypoplasia, malformed ears*

Neurology—conductive hearing loss (40%), visual loss (40%), normal intelligence

Other—may develop respiratory difficulties due to narrow airway

11. Waardenburg syndrome AD

Etiology

Autosomal dominant

Type I—due to mutation of PAX3 gene located at 2q35

Type II—due to mutation of microphthalmia gene at 3p12.3–p14.1

Clinical

Dermatology—white forelock, partial albinism

Facial—*lateral displacement of medial canthi* (in type I only), short palpebral fissures, broad nasal bridge, may have synophrys, broad mandible

Neurology—*deafness* (usually bilateral and severe, in 25% patients with type I and 50% patients with type II)

Other—premature graying, CT scan often demonstrates aplasia of posterior semicircular canal

E. AUTOSOMAL RECESSIVE DISORDERS

1. Carpenter syndrome

Etiology

Autosomal recessive

Clinical

Cardiac (50%)—patent ductus arteriosus, ventricular septal defect, atrial septal defect, pulmonary stenosis, tetralogy of Fallot, transposition of the great arteries

Extremities—*polydactyly, syndactyly* (feet), clinodactyly

Facial—*lateral displacement of inner canthus,* shallow supraorbital ridges, flat nasal bridge, corneal opacity, optic atrophy, low-set and malformed ears, hypoplastic mandible and/or maxilla, high-arched palate

Neurology—*brachycephaly,* mental deficiency

Other—failure to thrive, hypogenitalia, umbilical hernia, omphalocele

2. Ellis-van Creveld syndrome

Etiology

Autosomal recessive, chondroectodermal dysplasia

Clinical

Cardiac—(50%) single atrium and atrial septal defect

Extremities—*short distal extremities, polydactyly* (fingers more common than toes), *nail hypoplasia,* short stature

Facial—delayed teeth eruption, short upper lip

Other—intrauterine growth restriction, *narrow thorax,* typically with normal intelligence

Prognosis

50% mortality during infancy due to cardiorespiratory difficulties

3. Fanconi pancytopenia syndrome

Etiology

Autosomal recessive

Increased number of chromosomal breaks in lymphocytes and amniotic fluid cells (requires a breakage study to assess)

Clinical

Dermatology—*hyperpigmentation* (increases with age, especially involving groin, axilla, and trunk)

Extremities—*radial hypoplasia, thumb hypoplasia, short stature*

Facial—ptosis, nystagmus, microphthalmus, strabismus

Genitourinary—renal and urinary tract abnormalities (35%) (including malformed kidneys, double ureters), hypospadias, small genitalia

Hematology—*pancytopenia* (presents at ~ 7 years of age but may occur during infancy)

Neurology—microcephaly, mental deficiency (25%)

Other—intrauterine growth restriction, increased risk of respiratory infections, may have cardiac defect

Prognosis

~35% mortality due to hematological abnormalities, increased risk of acute myelogenous leukemia

4. Meckel-Gruber syndrome

Etiology

Autosomal recessive

Locus mapped to 17q21-q24

Clinical (large degree of phenotypic variability)

Cardiac—atrial septal defect, ventricular septal defect, patent ductus arteriosus, coarctation of the aorta, pulmonary stenosis

Extremities—*polydactyly* (usually postaxial)

Facial—microphthalmia, cleft palate, micrognathia, ear anomalies

Genitourinary—cryptorchidism, incomplete genitalia

Neurology—*occipital encephalocele,* microcephaly, cerebral and cerebellar hypoplasia, hydrocephaly, absence of corpus callosum, septum pellucidum, or olfactory lobes/tract

Renal—*cystic dysplastic kidneys*

Other—bile duct proliferation, hepatic cysts

Prenatal diagnosis with elevated alpha fetoprotein if encephalocele is present

Prognosis

Dependent on severity of illness

5. Smith-Lemli-Opitz syndrome

Etiology

Autosomal recessive, 1 in 20,000

Defect in cholesterol synthesis leading to low cholesterol levels and elevated precursor (7-dehydrocholesterol) levels

Clinical

Extremities—*2nd and 3rd toe syndactyly* (95%), transverse palmar crease

Facial—*ptosis,* cataracts, inner epicanthal folds, micrognathia, cleft palate, low-set or slanted ears, *anteverted nostrils*

Genitourinary—genital abnormalities (70%) due to failure of masculinization of male genitalia including *hypogenitalia, hypospadias,* cryptorchidism

Neurology—microcephaly, moderate-severe mental deficiency, tone may be hypotonic in early infancy and later becomes hypertonic

Renal—many types of anomalies

Other—intrauterine growth restriction, often with breech presentation in utero, failure to thrive

High mortality during first year of life if severely affected

Prenatal diagnosis possible (reduced amniotic fluid cholesterol and increased 7-dehydrocholesterol)

6. TAR (thrombocytopenia–radial aplasia) syndrome

Etiology

Autosomal recessive

Clinical

Cardiac (30%)—tetralogy of Fallot, atrial septal defect

Hematology (severest during infancy)—*thrombocytopenia* (may be precipitated by viral illness, especially gastrointestinal), granulocytosis, eosinophilia, anemia

Extremities—*absent bilateral radii* (100%), thumbs are always present, *ulnar abnormalities* (100%), hip dysplasia

Other—40% mortality due to hemorrhage early in infancy, abnormal humerus

F. X-LINKED DOMINANT DISORDERS

1. Fragile X syndrome

Incidence

Most common inherited cause of mental deficiency

1 in 1250–4000 males, 1 in 2000–8000 females

X-linked dominant with 80% penetrance in males and 30% penetrance in females

Etiology: name attributable to finding of X chromosomes cultured in a low folic acid medium that may break near the tip of the long arm

Due to expansion of premutation (with increased number of CGG repeats) leading to full mutation (with extremely high number of CGG repeats); the number of methylated repeats corresponds to the severity of expression

Clinical

Facial—*long facies, prominent forehead, large ears,* thick nasal bridge, epicanthal folds

Genitourinary—*large testes* post-puberty

Neurology—*mental deficiency* (mild to severe in males; 50% of females with mental deficiency and of remaining, large number with learning disabilities), speech pattern described as "cluttered," behavioral problems, *autism* (poor eye contact), macrocephaly

Other—*hyperextensible fingers/ joints, mild connective tissue dysplasia*

G. X-LINKED RECESSIVE DISORDERS

1. Menkes syndrome

Etiology

X-linked recessive, gene located at Xq13

= kinky hair syndrome

Due to abnormality of copper transport leading to *copper deficiency*

The phenotype is due to inability of copper to act as cofactor for multiple enzymes (e.g., tyrosinase, lysyl oxidase)

Clinical

Facial—*twisted, fractured, lightly pigmented hair* (hair color normal at birth but ~ 6 weeks of age, loses pigmentation), lack of expression, pudgy face

Neurology—*progressive cerebral deterioration* (typically presents at 1 to 2 months of age with hypertonia, irritability, *seizures,* feeding difficulties)

Skeletal—Wormian bones, increased risk of fractures due to lateral spur formation of bones

Other—gastric polyps (may lead to gastrointestinal bleeding), arterial tortuousity, growth deficiency

Prenatal diagnosis by abnormal copper uptake in cultured amniotic fluid cells
Prognosis
  Majority with death in early infancy

H. OTHER CHROMOSOMAL DISORDERS

1. Klinefelter syndrome
Incidence
  47,XXY; 1 in 500-1000 male births, equally derived from maternal or paternal errors; if maternally derived, increased risk with advancing maternal age
Clinical
  Cardiac (15%)—mitral valve prolapse, tetralogy of Fallot, atrial septal defect, patent ductus arteriosus
  Extremities—disproportionately long arms and legs, elbow dysplasia, 5th finger clinodactyly
  Genitourinary—*hypogonadism, hypogenitalia,* gynecomastia (~1/3), infertile due to atrophy of seminiferous tubules
  Neurology—*behavioral difficulty* (immaturity, shyness), learning disabilities
Management: testosterone at 11-12 years of age to increase secondary sexual traits, consider mastectomy if gynecomastia due to increased risk of breast cancer

2. Turner syndrome
Etiology
  1 in 2000 to 5000 live-born females
  ~50% 45, X; ~30-40% mosaics (45, X/ 46,XX is more common than 45, X/ 46,XY) and 10-20% due to deletions of X chromosome
  The chromosome that is deleted is usually *paternal* and thus, no increased risk with advanced maternal age
Clinical
  In utero—majority of fetuses undergo spontaneous abortion (only ~2% actually born and are thought to be mosaic)
  Cardiac (35%)—coarctation of aorta, bicuspid aortic valve, aortic stenosis, mitral valve prolapse, aortic dissection later in life, hypertension
  Extremities—*cubitus valgus,* knee anomalies
  Facial /neck—*cystic hygroma* in utero, *webbed posterior neck,* prominent ears, low posterior hairline, narrow maxilla
  Genitourinary—*gonadal dysgenesis* (cortical), don't usually develop secondary sexual traits and majority are infertile
  Renal—horseshoe kidney or other structural abnormality
  Other—*congenital lymphedema, short stature, broad chest with wide-spaced nipples,* poor coordination, visual-spatial deficits, bone dysplasia, increased risk of malignancy in gonadal streaks if mosaic with Y chromosome
    If survive, excellent prognosis
Management
  Growth hormone, estrogen to induce secondary sexual traits, anabolic steroids (controversial)
  + amoxicillin

3. Cat-eye syndrome
Etiology
  Extra part of chromosome 22 usually in quadruplicate or triplicate at 22q11 region (vs DiGeorge syndrome—deletion of 22q11)
Clinical
  Cardiac (>33%)—total anomalous pulmonary venous return, persistent left superior vena cava
  Facial—mild hypertelorism, *down-slanting palpebral fissure,* micrognathia
  Gastrointestinal—*anal atresia* with rectovestibular fistula
  Neurology—mild mental deficiency
  Ophthalmology—*coloboma of iris*
  Renal—renal agenesis

I. OTHER GENETIC DISORDERS

1. Mobius sequence

Etiology

Majority sporadic

6th and 7th nerve palsy (usually bilateral)

Nonspecific sign

4 types of abnormal development

1. Destruction of central brain nuclei
2. Hypoplasia or absence of central brain nuclei
3. Peripheral nerve involvement
4. Myopathy

Associated with limb reduction defects, Poland sequence, and Klippel-Feil anomaly

Clinical

Facial—*expressionless facies, micrognathia* (probably due to decreased movement of mandible in utero), may also have 3rd, 4th, 5th, 9th, 10th, or 12th nerve involvement, may have ocular ptosis or protruding ears

Extremities—talipes *equinovarus* (1/3)

Neurology—mental deficiency (15%)

Other—failure to thrive (attributable to feeding difficulties)

2. Pierre Robin sequence

Etiology

Due to mandibular hypoplasia prior to 9 weeks gestation

May be associated with genetic disorders (including trisomy 18 and Stickler syndrome)

Clinical

Facial—*micrognathia, glossoptosis, cleft palate* (U-shaped)

Other—may lead to posterior airway obstruction

J. DISORDERS OF UNKNOWN ETIOLOGY

1. CHARGE association

Etiology

Unknown

May be due to heterogeneous effects leading to arrested development between the 35th and 45th days following conception

Clinical

Coloboma (80%—usually retina)

Heart disease (50-70%) (tetralogy of Fallot, double outlet right ventricle, ventricular septal defect, atrial septal defect, patent ductus arteriosus, right-sided aortic arch)

Atresia of choanae (60%)

Retarded growth (90%, usually postnatal)

Genital hypoplasia (in males, 75%)

Ear anomalies and/or deafness (90%)

Other—mild to severe *mental deficiency* (94%), micrognathia, cleft lip and/or palate, cranial nerve abnormalities, feeding difficulties, renal anomalies, tracheoesophageal fistula, rib anomalies, hypertelorism, microcephaly, anal atresia, DiGeorge sequence, hypocalcemia

2. Cornelia de Lange syndrome

Etiology

Unknown etiology, majority are sporadic

Clinical

Cardiac—ventricular septal defect > tetralogy of Fallot

Extremities—*micromelia* (small hands and feet), 5th finger clinodactyly, syndactyly of 2nd and 3rd toes, ulnar abnormalities

Facial—*synophrys* (eyebrows joined in middle), *thin down-turning upper lip, long eyelashes,* depressed nasal bridge, anteverted nares, long philtrum, high-arched palate, micrognathia

Genitourinary—undescended testes

Neurology—mental deficiency (note: some patients with mild syndrome may not have mental deficiency), *initial hypertonicity,* microbrachycephaly

Other—intrauterine growth restriction, failure to thrive, *hirsutism, low posterior hairline,* cutis marmorata, hearing loss, may have gastroesophageal reflux

3. Goldenhar syndrome

Etiology

Unknown etiology, usually sporadic

1 in 3000 to 5000

Due to *1st and 2nd brachial arch abnormalities*

= oculo-auriculo-vertebral spectrum or facio-auriculo-vertebral spectrum

Clinical

Cardiac—ventricular septal defect > patent ductus arteriosus > tetralogy of Fallot > coarctation of aorta

Facial—malar, maxillary or mandibular hypoplasia, lateral extension of corner of mouth, malformed ears, ear tags and/or pits, tongue abnormalities

Neurology—deafness, mental deficiency (~13% with IQ < 85)

Skeletal—hemivertebrae or hypoplasia of vertebrae (cervical most common)

Other—70% unilateral (right > left), renal abnormalities

4. Klippel-Feil sequence

Etiology

Unknown etiology, majority sporadic

Leads to early developmental defect of cervical vertebrae

Clinical

Cardiac—ventricular septal defect

Facial—*short neck, low posterior hairline, limited movement of head* (may lead to webbed neck, torticollis, and/or facial asymmetry), deafness (conductive or neural)

Neurology—may have neurologic deficits, mental deficiency

Skeletal—*abnormal cervical vertebrae* (typically fused), can be associated with Sprengel deformity (failure of scapula to descend to normal location leading to elevation and medial rotation of inferior portion of scapula)

5. Klippel-Trenaunay Weber syndrome

Etiology

Unknown etiology, may be sporadic

Clinical

Extremities—*asymmetric limb hypertrophy* (congenital or early childhood, may involve one or more limbs, may lead to disproportionate growth)

Skin—*vascular lesions* (including capillary and cavernous hemangiomas, phlebectasia; typically located on legs, buttocks, abdomen or lower trunk)

6. Poland sequence

Etiology

Unknown etiology, majority sporadic

Possibly due to proximal subclavian arterial disruption in utero leading to poorly developed distal limb and pectoral region on that side

Male > female (3:1)

75% right-sided

Clinical

Cardiac—dextrocardia if left-sided Poland abnormality

Extremities—*syndactyly of hand, unilateral hypoplasia or absence of pectoralis muscle*

Renal—various anomalies

Skeletal—rib anomalies, may have hemivertebrae

7. Russell-Silver syndrome

Etiology

Majority are sporadic; some with uniparental disomy

Clinical

Facial—frontal bossing, *small triangular facies* (this may lead to appearance of large head, but head circumference is actually normal), down-turning corners of mouth, micrognathia

Skeletal—*short stature, congenital asymmetry of skeleton*

Other—café au lait spots, *small incurved 5th finger,* tendency for excess sweating, fontanels may be large, late closure of anterior fontanel

8. VACTERL association

Etiology

Unknown etiology, sporadic

Increased risk in infants of diabetic mothers

Clinical

Diagnosis requires 3 of following (note: of those who meet criteria, 1/2 will have isolated VACTERL association and other 1/2 will have another genetic abnormality):

Vertebral anomalies (70%, e.g., hemivertebrae)

Anal atresia (80%, may have fistula)

Cardiac (50%, ventricular septal defect > tetralogy of Fallot, coarctation of the aorta)

Tracheo**e**sophageal fistula (70%, with esophageal atresia)

Renal anomaly (53%), 35% with single umbilical artery

Limb dysplasia (65%, typically radial, may also have preaxial polydactyly or syndactyly)

Other less frequent associations—intrauterine growth restriction, ear anomalies, laryngeal stenosis, large fontanels, rib anomalies, spinal abnormalities

Majority with normal intelligence

K. TRAITS ASSOCIATED WITH SPECIFIC ANOMALIES

Trait	Associated Genetic Disorder
Arachnodactyly (long, spider-like fingers)	Homocystinuria, Marfan syndrome
Camptodactyly (flexed digits, usually 5th finger)	Isolated, trisomy 8
Cleft lip and/or palate	CHARGE association, DiGeorge syndrome (palate), Meckel-Gruber syndrome (palate), Pierre Robin sequence (palate), Smith-Lemli-Opitz syndrome (palate), trisomy 13 May also be seen in Goldenhar syndrome, Treacher Collins syndrome
Clinodactyly (curving or medial deviation of finger, 5th finger most commonly involved)	Carpenter syndrome, Cornelia de Lange syndrome, deletion 13q, Klinefelter syndrome, isolated, Rubenstein-Taybi syndrome, Russell-Silver syndrome, trisomy 21 (usually bilateral and 5th finger) Also observed in Holt-Oram syndrome, Prader-Willi syndrome
Coloboma	Cat-eye syndrome (iris), CHARGE association (usually retina), deletion 13q, Treacher Collins syndrome (eyelid), trisomy 13 (iris)

(continued on following page)

Trait	Associated Genetic Disorder
Cystic hygroma	Noonan syndrome and Turner syndrome May also be observed in deletion 13q, trisomy 13, 18 and 21
Hypertelorism	Apert syndrome, cat-eye syndrome, Cri du chat syndrome, Crouzon syndrome, deletion 13q, DiGeorge syndrome, Noonan syndrome, trisomy 8, Turner syndrome
Hypotelorism	High association with holoprosencephaly May also be observed in Meckel-Gruber syndrome, Williams syndrome, trisomy 13
Limb hypertrophy	Beckwith-Wiedemann syndrome, Klippel-Trenauney-Weber syndrome
Lips, thick and/or prominent	Trisomy 8, WAGR syndrome, Williams syndrome
Hypogenitalia	Carpenter syndrome, Klinefelter syndrome, Prader-Willi syndrome, Smith-Lemli-Opitz syndrome
Macroglossia	Beckwith-Wiedemann syndrome, congenital hypothyroidism, trisomy 21
Micrognathia	Cat-eye syndrome, CHARGE association, Cornelia de Lange syndrome, deletion 13q, DiGeorge syndrome, Marfan syndrome, Meckel-Gruber syndrome, Mobius sequence, Pierre Robin sequence, Russell-Silver syndrome, Smith-Lemli-Opitz syndrome, trisomy 8 and 18, WAGR syndrome
Polydactyly	Carpenter syndrome, Ellis-van Creveld syndrome, isolated, Meckel-Gruber syndrome, trisomy 13, VACTERL association May also be observed in DiGeorge syndrome, Holt-Oram syndrome, Smith-Lemli-Opitz syndrome
Radial hypoplasia	Fanconi pancytopenia syndrome, TAR syndrome, VACTERL association Also may be observed in Cornelia de Lange syndrome, Holt-Oram syndrome, Poland sequence, trisomy 13 and 18
Syndactyly (fusion of digits, bones may or may not be involved)	Apert syndrome, Carpenter syndrome, Cornelia de Lange syndrome, isolated, Poland sequence, Smith-Lemli-Opitz syndrome, VACTERL association

L. TERATOGENS (see Maternal-Fetal Medicine chapter)

References

Bianchi DW, Crombleholme TM and D'Alton ME: Fetology. New York, McGraw-Hill, 2000.

Gelehrter TD, Collins FS and Ginsburg D: Principles of Medical Genetics (2nd edition). Baltimore, Williams & Wilkins, 1998.

Jones KL: Smith's Recognizable Patterns of Human Malformations (5th edition). Philadelphia, WB Saunders Co, 1997.

Jorde LB, Carey JC, Bamshad MJ and White RL: Medical Genetics (2nd edition). St. Louis, Mosby, 2000.

CHAPTER 6

Infectious Diseases and Immunology

TOPICS COVERED IN THIS CHAPTER

I. Infection of Organ Systems
   A. Sepsis
   B. Pneumonia
   C. Osteomyelitis and septic arthritis
   D. Omphalitis
   E. Meningitis
   F. Urinary tract infection (UTI)
   G. Conjunctivitis
   H. Gastroenteritis
   I. Necrotizing enterocolitis

II. Etiologic Agents
   A. Bacteria
      1. *Streptococcus agalactiae* group B (group B Strep) and *Listeria monocytogenes*
      2. *Treponema pallidum*
      3. *Neisseria gonorrhoeae*
      4. *Chlamydia trachomatis*
      5. *Mycobacterium tuberculosis*
      6. *Clostridium botulinum*
      7. *Staphylococcus (Staph) epidermidis* and *aureus*
      8. Gram-negative bacilli
   B. Viral
      1. Herpes simplex virus (HSV)
      2. Respiratory syncytial virus (RSV)
      3. Hepatitis B
      4. Hepatitis D
      5. Hepatitis C
      6. Hepatitis A and E
      7. Parvovirus B19
      8. Varicella-zoster virus
      9. Rubella
     10. Cytomegalovirus (CMV)
     11. Toxoplasmosis (toxo)—protozoal not viral
     12. Comparison of rubella, CMV and toxo

     13. Human immunodeficiency virus (HIV)
     14. Enteroviruses
     15. Rotavirus
   C. Fungal
      1. *Candida*

III. Maternal Infections
   A. Urinary tract infection
   B. Bacterial vaginosis
   C. Mastitis
   D. Chorioamnionitis

IV. Immunizations
   A. Immunization schedule
   B. Immunization of pregnant women
   C. Immunization of premature infants
   D. *Bordetella pertussis*
   E. *Clostridium tetani*
   F. Mumps and measles

V. Transmission of Infections

VI. Breast Feeding and Infections

VII. Diagnosis

VIII. Therapeutics in Infectious Diseases
   A. Antibiotics
   B. Action of antibiotics
   C. Immune globulin

IX. Development of the Immune System

X. Natural Immune System Components, Neonatal Ability, and Disorders
   A. Components of natural immune system

XI. Acquired Immune System Components, Neonatal Ability, and Disorders
   A. Components of acquired immune system
   B. Immunoglobulin levels with age

XII. Blood Cells and Infection

XIII. Screening Tests

XIV. Splenic Function

I. Infections of Organ Systems

A. SEPSIS

Incidence
  1–8/1000 live births

Transmission
  Transplacental (viral infections, less common for bacterial infections except syphilis and *Listeria*)
  Ascending infection
  Amniotic fluid exposure
  Postnatal (breast milk, mastitis)

Risk factors
  Maternal risk factors: chorioamnionitis, premature rupture of membranes (ROM), Group B *Streptococcus* (GBS) colonization, untreated maternal urinary tract infection (UTI), maternal fever, malnutrition, sexually transmitted diseases, lower socioeconomic status
  Neonatal risk factors: prematurity, low birth weight, indwelling catheter, endotracheal tube

Types

	Early-Onset Sepsis	Late-Onset Sepsis
Timing	Presents less than 4–7 days of life	Presents greater than 4–7 days of life
Acquisition	Organism from maternal genital tract	Either maternal genital tract or environment
Organisms	GBS, *Escherichia coli* (*E. coli*), *Listeria*, non-typeable *Haemophilus influenzae* (*H. flu*) and enterococcus	*Staphylococcus* (*Staph*) coagulase (coag)-negative, *Staph. aureus*, *Pseudomonas*, GBS, *E. coli*, and *Listeria*
Clinical	Multisystem involvement (greater risk of pneumonia)	Usually focal involvement (greater risk of meningitis)
Mortality	Greater mortality (15–45%)	Lower mortality (10–20%)

  Of note: also late-late onset sepsis—majority due to candida or coagulase-negative *Staph;* associated with prematurity, central lines, and/or endotracheal intubation

Clinical
  Respiratory distress, lethargy, decreased peripheral perfusion, possible shock, fever or hypothermia, apnea, vomiting, diarrhea, abdominal distention, focality (e.g, cellulitis, osteomyelitis, meningitis), cyanosis, hypotonia, feeding intolerance, seizures, persistent unexplained jaundice, hypoglycemia, petechiae

Evaluation of Sepsis
  CBC (complete blood count with differential), glucose
  Blood, urine (if > 72 hours old, via catheterization or suprapubic aspiration), cerebrospinal (CSF) gram stain and culture, consider tracheal culture if intubated
  CSF protein/glucose, CSF white blood count (WBC) and CSF red blood count (RBC)
  CXR, abdominal Xray to assess for necrotizing enterocolitis
  CSF GBS latex agglutination test
  Immature: total neutrophil ratio helpful (especially if > 0.2)—can also be increased if prolonged oxytocin in mother, stressful labor, prolonged crying, isolated maternal fever
  CRP (C-reactive protein)—nonspecific acute phase reactant (hepatic protein that is increased during inflammation); no change with gestational age (GA); increased in 50-90% of patients with sepsis
  Other nonspecific markers of sepsis: erythrocyte sedimentation rate (ESR), fibrinogen, fibronectin, haptoglobulin and cytokines

Management
   Broad-empiric antibiotic treatment before culture results
   Monitor respiratory and hemodynamic status, monitor glucose, monitor platelets
   Always consider viral infection (e.g., herpes simplex virus, enterovirus), fungal infection and metabolic disease in
      differential diagnosis

B. PNEUMONIA (see Respiratory chapter)

C. OSTEOMYELITIS AND SEPTIC ARTHRITIS

	Osteomyelitis (osteo)	Septic Arthritis
Etiology	1. Hematogenous spread s/p bacteremia (#1 in neonates) 2. Directly from puncture wound 3. Spread from adjacent infection	1. Hematogenous spread following bacteremia 2. Local infection s/p puncture wound 3. Spread from adjacent infection
Pathology	Most common site of origin is metaphysis Femur > humerus > tibia > radius > maxilla Neonatal infection can spread to epiphysis since blood supply between metaphysis and epiphysis connected until 8–18 mos of life Can lead to septic arthritis Neonates often with multiple bone involvement	Leads to synovial inflammation, increased vascular permeability, and increased fluid production Fluid accumulates in joint Increased pressure due to pus-filled joint may lead to compression and/or vascular necrosis Often multiple joint involvement Often associated with osteomyelitis
Organisms	*Staph. aureus*, group B *Strep*, *E. coli*, *Candida*, *Neisseria gonorrhoeae*	*Staph. aureus*, group B *Strep*, *Staph. epi*, *Neisseria gonorrhoeae* (more commonly found with septic arthritis than osteo), *Candida*, *E. coli*, *Pseudomonas*
Clinical Diagnosis	Typically subtle, without systemic illness (in contrast to older children) Decreased movement, tenderness, erythema, swelling, pain with motion GBS osteo usually presents at 3–4 weeks of age, humerus is the most common site	Similar to osteo—decreased movement, tenderness, erythema, and joint effusion
Laboratory Diagnosis	Needle aspiration at point of greatest tenderness and fluctuance Positive blood culture in 60% Neonate with xray findings after 7–10 days X-ray—soft tissue swelling followed by periosteal thickening and cortical destruction and then new bone formation If one xray abnormality, should do complete skeletal survey to assess for other bone involvement (10–40%) Bone scan—controversial if this test is helpful in neonates due to high false-negative rates, often positive following aspiration Consider lumbar puncture (LP)	Needle aspiration—culture positive in ~70–80% Positive blood culture in 30–40% Imaging—same as for osteo except aspiration of joints affects bone scan results less than compared to osteo
Management	Initiate treatment with penicillinase-resistant penicillin and aminoglycoside or cephalosporin × 21–42 days After organism is identified, continue with appropriate antibiotics Surgical drainage if significant soft tissue collection Immobilize involved extremity Consider orthopedic consult	Penicillinase-resistant penicillin and aminoglycoside initially Surgical drainage necessary if hip/shoulder involved; aspiration for knee, ankle and elbow Immobilize involved joints Treat 2–6 weeks depending on organism (e.g., treat *Staph. aureus* 4–6 weeks while group B Strep can be treated for 2–3 weeks) Consider orthopedic consult
Prognosis	Decreased growth if epiphyseal plate damage, may lead to joint deformities	Greater risk of permanent abnormality

[handwritten note: treat Staph longer than GBS]

D. OMPHALITIS

Organisms
   Staph. aureus, group A *Strep,* also gram-negative bacilli, and anaerobes

Transmission

Acquisition by direct invasion from skin

Clinical

Purulent drainage from umbilical site or periumbilical erythema, edema or tenderness; diagnose by culturing drainage and blood culture

May be complicated by necrotizing fasciitis, peritonitis, and umbilical peritonitis

Management

Methicillin/nafcillin/oxacillin to treat penicillin (PCN)-ase resistant organisms

Consider empiric treatment with vancomycin if high local incidence of methicillin-resistant *Staph. aureus* (MRSA)

Gentamicin or 3rd generation cephalosporin for gram-negative coverage

Requires anaerobic coverage if black periumbilical region

E. MENINGITIS

Incidence

1 in 2500 infants, majority occurring during first month of life   *early signs*
= nonspecific
– lethargy, resp distress, temp instability

Premature infants 10× risk of meningitis

Organisms

GBS > *E. coli* (especially K1 antigen) > *Listeria* > *Klebsiella* and Enterobacter > *H. flu*; also *Neisseria meningitidis*

Transmission

Hematogenous (most common), focal infection leading to bacteremia and direct extension, following neurosurgery, open neurological defect

Clinical

40% with seizures, 30% bulging fontanel, 15% nuchal rigidity, increased risk of syndrome of inappropriate anti-diuretic hormone

Management

Ampicillin (coverage for GBS and *Listeria*) and cephalosporin

Aminoglycosides do not have adequate CSF penetration but can be useful for synergy

Vancomycin does penetrate CSF well and will also treat coagulase-negative *Staph*

Duration 10–14 days for GBS, 14–21 days for *Listeria* and at least 21 days for gram-negative organisms

Prognosis

1/3–1/2 with significant neurological sequelae (e.g., mental deficiency, motor delay, seizures, hydrocephalus, hearing/speech abnormalities)

Worse outcome if gram-negative meningitis, CSF WBC > 500, persistent CSF positive culture

E. coli with K1 antigen more likely to lead to meningitis

GBS meningitis: worse outcome if comatose, shock, WBC < 5000, absolute neutrophil count (ANC) < 1000, CSF protein > 300

Seizures are not predictive of outcome

F. URINARY TRACT INFECTION (UTI)

Incidence

Occurs in 0.1–1% of neonates; high association with reflux

Greater if very low birth weight infant

Neonatal UTI greater in males
Uncommon in first few days of life

Organisms
Gram-negative rods (*E. coli* #1, *Klebsiella*, Enterobacter), *Enterococcus*, coagulase-negative *Staph*, *Candida*

Transmission
Neonates develop UTI via hematogenous or ascending routes; neonates often with anatomic or physiologic
abnormalities of renal system
In contrast, older children mostly due to ascending route

Clinical
Nonspecific findings (poor feeding, weight loss, fever)

Diagnosis
Urine culture by catheterization or suprapubic bladder aspiration

Management
Intravenous ampicillin and aminoglycoside until organism identified
Voiding cystourethrography to rule out reflux and renal ultrasound to assess for underlying renal abnormality

G. CONJUNCTIVITIS

Organisms
Neisseria gonorrhoeae (abrupt onset, day of life #2-5, *purulent* discharge)
Chlamydia (most common cause in 1ˢᵗ month of life, presents 5-14 days of life, bilateral) watery → purulent
Other—*Staph. aureus* (golden crust around eyelids), GBS, *Pseudomonas*, *Strep. pneumoniae* (dacrocystitis),
Haemophilus influenzae (dacrocystitis) and herpes simplex virus
Note: also due to chemical irritation (usually soon after birth)

Clinical
Discharge (may be purulent), lid erythema and edema, conjunctival injection
Complications are rare, can include visual loss, corneal epithelial erosions

Management
Irrigation, intravenous (*N. gonorrhoeae* or *Pseudomonas*) or local antibiotics
Gonorrhea conjunctivitis is a medical emergency since can progress to involve cornea and ulceration/perforation if
untreated

H. GASTROENTERITIS

Organisms
Campylobacter, E. coli, Salmonella, Yersinia, rotavirus, adenovirus, *Clostridium difficile*
Less common—*Pseudomonas, Klebsiella*, Enterobacter, group A *Strep*, *Shigella*

Clinical
Typically self-limited, can be asymptomatic or present with diarrhea, fever, vomiting, abdominal distention, bloody stool
(e.g., *Shigella, Yersinia, Campylobacter* and some strains of *E. coli*)

Diagnosis

Stool culture, fecal leukocytes (*E. coli, Yersinia, Campylobacter, Salmonella* or *Shigella*), blood culture if *Salmonella, Shigella, Campylobacter,* or *Yersinia*

Management

Supportive, manage fluid/electrolyte status, possible oral or intravenous antibiotics (*Salmonella*—cefotaxime; *Shigella*—ampicillin; *Campylobacter* or *Yersinia*—-erythromycin)

I. Necrotizing enterocolitis (see Gastroenterology chapter)

II. Etiologic Agents

A. BACTERIA

1. Streptococcus agalactiae group B (group B Strep) and Listeria monocytogenes

[handwritten: MORe fatal → Early - first 24hr. (premature) pneumonia, meningitis   Late (Term) 7d-12wks, meningitis]

Group B Strep (GBS)	Listeria monocytogenes *[handwritten: common]*
Gram-positive diplococci in chains	Gram-positive *rod*
GI tract > vaginal > cervical; present in unpasteurized milk	Granulomatous rash in severe cases
Vaginal colonization increases with age	Associated with placental microabscesses
Note: vaginal colonization may be transient and thus cultures are not 100% predictive of status at delivery	Present in unpasteurized milk and soft cheeses, uncooked meat and unwashed raw vegetables
Greater risk of neonatal infection if prematurity, prolonged ROM, intrapartum fever, chorioamnionitis, maternal GBS bacteriuria	Increased risk stillbirth and premature delivery
NOT acquired by transplacental route	Early-onset disease acquired by:
Acquired through colonization during passage through vaginal canal or ascending after ROM	A. Transplacental route (more common) or
	B. Ingestion or aspiration of infected amniotic fluid
8-28% of all mothers are GBS positive, 1/2 of infants with GBS positive mothers are colonized and 1% of these infants are infected	Late-onset disease acquired:
	A. From colonized mother
Neonate may become colonized postnatally	B. By nosocomial infection (majority)
Early-onset disease (< 7 DOL): sepsis (25-40%), pneumonia (35-55%), and meningitis (5-10%); many serotypes since often from vaginal flora (serotype III most likely), increased in premature infants	Early-onset disease (< 7DOL): sepsis and pneumonia, serotypes Ia and Ib, often with chocolate colored amniotic fluid, increased in premature infants, mother often with symptoms (65% of mothers with prodrome flu-like illness—headache, gastrointestinal symptoms, malaise, fever)
Late-onset disease (>7 DOL): meningitis (30-40%), 1/2 with neurological sequelae, may have osteo, septic arthritis, cellulitis	Late-onset disease (> 7DOL): meningitis (may have increased CSF mononuclear cells), most common serotype is IV B, typically milder symptoms
Serotype III majority, presents typically 24 DOL, no increase in premature infants	
Lower mortality compared with early disease	
To prevent neonatal colonization, treat GBS-positive mothers with antibiotics > 4 hours PTD if:	Treatment with ampicillin and aminoglycoside 10-14 days, longer if meningitis
1. Previous infant with GBS disease	No isolation needed
2. Premature delivery	
3. Maternal temperature ≥100.4	
4. ROM > 18 hours	
5. GBS bacteriuria during pregnancy	
Treat neonate if inadequate maternal GBS prophylaxis, neonatal symptoms, premature	
Penicillin ideal treatment	
No isolation needed	
Mortality: early disease, 5-10%; late, 2-6%	Mortality: early disease, 25%; late, 15%

2. Treponema pallidum *[handwritten: * snuffles]*

Transmission

[handwritten: Ⓧ] Transplacental route in majority (risk to fetus 70-100% if untreated primary syphilis, 40% if early latent infection)

The greater the gestational age, greater risk of fetal infection

Can be acquired by contact with active lesion at delivery; however, lesion not always detected since it may be present within vagina or cervix or female can be in the latent asymptomatic stage

Clinical

30–40% infected fetuses are stillborn

Most symptomatic have hepatosplenomegaly & bone Δ's

The majority of fetuses acquire the infection hematogenously, and thus no chancre in neonate; increased risk of nonimmune hydrops fetalis and in utero growth restriction (IUGR)

Early congenital syphilis: before 2 years of age

⊗ 2/3 asymptomatic at birth; 1/3 symptomatic at birth

May have unexplained *large placenta*

Hepatosplenomegaly (HSM) and/or generalized lymphadenopathy and/or desquamating *maculopapular rash* (often involving palms and soles)

System review:

Respiratory: pneumonitis, persistent rhinitis (typically 1 week to 3 months of age)

Dermatologic: cutaneous bullous eruptions, pigmented macules

Hematologic: hyperbilirubinemia, hemolytic anemia, thrombocytopenia, leukopenia or leukocytosis

Renal: nephrotic syndrome; Ophthalmologic: chorioretinitis, uveitis

Orthopedic: osteochondritis (Wimberger sign = bilateral destruction of proximal medial metaphysis — tibia > humerus), periostitis

Neurologic: Erb palsy, leptomeningitis

⊗ *Late congenital syphilis:* after 2 years of age, will develop if congenital infection is not treated

Frontal bossing, saddle nose, high-arched palate, short maxilla, perioral fissures, saber shins (anterior bowing of tibia), hydrocephalus, seizures, deafness, Hutchinson teeth (peg-shaped upper central incisors), mental deficiency   *Hutchinson triad*

Diagnosis

Test all pregnant women for syphilis

Evaluation of following neonates

Infant born to seropositive mother with untreated syphilis

Mother treated for syphilis during pregnancy with a non-penicillin (PCN) antibiotic

Mother treated less than 30 days prior to delivery (since treatment failures can occur)

Mother treated appropriately during pregnancy without an appropriate serologic response ($\geq$ 4-fold decrease in titers)

Mother treated appropriately before pregnancy but had insufficient serological follow-up

Symptomatic neonate

Evaluation

Physical exam, VDRL (Venereal Disease Research Lab) or RPR (Rapid Plasma Reagin), FTA (fluorescent treponemal antibody absorption test), LP (increased CSF cell count, elevated CSF protein, positive VDRL), anti-treponemal IgM (if available, can be difficult to perform)

Long bone films (especially femur and humerus)

CBC, liver function tests (LFTs), direct bilirubin, urine analysis, CXR, strongly consider HIV test if positive for syphilis

Ophthalmologic exam, placenta and umbilical cord examination by darkfield microscopy

Non-treponemal test & *treponemal antibody test*

Detects a cell membrane cardiolipin nonspecific IgG Ab, which is a sign of response to host tissue damage = VDRL or RPR (RPR not appropriate for CSF)

Both are reported as titers; titers correlate with disease activity

Reactive in 75% adults with primary syphilis within 1–2 months of infection and reactive in all with secondary infection

Becomes negative 2 years following treatment

Neonate has a positive test if titer 4-fold higher than maternal titer

False-positive if autoimmune disorder, tuberculosis, Ebstein-Barr virus, endocarditis, passively transferred maternal IgG antibody to neonate

Prozone phenomenon = false-negative VDRL or RPR secondary to excess antibody in test sera which prevents antibody-antigen complex necessary for reactive test, occurs in 1–2% of secondary syphilis; avoid by diluting sera

Treponemal test–FTA

Detects a specific Ab (IgG or IgM) to *Treponema pallidum*–reactive for life; false-positive if antinuclear antibody present (e.g., lupus)

Does not correlate with disease activity (as does non-treponemal test)

Is not quantified

Guide for Interpretation of the Syphilis Serology of Mothers and Their Infants*				
Nontreponemal Test (eg, VDRL, RPR, ART)		**Treponemal Test (eg, MHA-TP, FTA-ABS)**		
Mother	**Infant**	**Mother**	**Infant**	**Intreparation†**
−	−	−	−	No syphilis or incubating syphilis in the mother and infant or prozone phenomenon
+	+	−	−	No syphilis in mother (false-positive nontreponemal test with passive transfer to infant)
+	+ or −	+	+	Maternal syphilis with possible infant infection; or mother treated for syphilis during pregnancy; or mother with latent syphilis and possible infection of infant:‡
+	+	+	+	Recent or previous syphilis in the mother; possible infection in infant
−	−	+	+	Mother successfully treated for syphilis before or early in pregnancy; or mother with Lyme disease, yaws, or pinta (ie, false-positive serology)

*RPR indicates rapid plasma reagin; ART, automated reagin test; MHA-TP, microhemagglutination test for *Treponema pallidum*; FTA-ABS, fluorescent treponemal antibody absorption; plus sign, reactive; and minus sign, nonreactive.

†Table presents a guide and not the definitive interpretation of serologic tests for syphilis in mothers and their newborn infants. Maternal history is the most important aspect for interpretation of test results. Factors that should be considered include the timing of maternal infection, the nature and timing of maternal treatment, quantitative maternal and infant titers, and serial determination of nontreponemal test titers in both mother and infant.

‡Mothers with latent syphilis may have nonreactive nontreponemal tests.

Printed with permission from Pickering LK (ed): 2000 Red Book: Report of the Committee on Infectious Diseases (25th edition), Elk Grove Village, IL. American Academy of Pediatrics, 2000, p. 552.

Management

Treatment of mother with syphilis: aqueous PCN G; if PCN allergic – desensitization to PCN is required followed by treatment with PCN; after treatment, monitor monthly titers during pregnancy (retreat if 4-fold increase in titers)

Treat neonate who meet any of following criteria:

1. Physical, laboratory, or radiographic evidence of syphilis
2. Visualization of spirochetes by dark-field microscopy or fluorescent antibody staining (including placental tissue, umbilical cord, skin lesions)
3. Reactive CSF VDRL and/or abnormal CSF
4. Non-treponemal test is 4-fold higher than mother's
5. Inadequately treated mother (no treatment, treatment with a non-penicillin antibiotic, treatment < 30 days prior to delivery, mother without documented response to therapy represented by 4-fold decrease in non-treponemal titers)

Medications

Aqueous PCN G (intravenous) × 10–14 days

Procaine = IM single-dose PCN G; CSF entry not as good as aqueous form, and thus not recommended in neonates

Benzathine PCN G, single-dose IM: long-acting, poor entry into CSF; can administer if asymptomatic neonate with normal laboratory and radiographic findings and mother inadequately treated; not recommended if active syphilis

Follow-up

If untreated neonate: follow VDRL and FTA 1, 2, 3–4, 6 and 12 months of age; if negative at 12 months, uninfected neonate

If VDRL is not decreasing by 3–4 months and/or remains detectable > 6 months, re-evaluate and need to treat

If treated neonate: follow VDRL 1, 2, 3–4, 6 and 12 months; check CSF every 6 months

If VDRL decreasing by 3–4 months, negative VDRL by 6 months, negative CSF VDRL by 6 months, decreasing CSF cell count, and normal CSF cell count by 2 years of age, adequate therapy

If not → retreat

3. *Neisseria gonorrhoeae*

"GC" George Clooney → Gonorrhoeae Cephalosporin

early discharge in eye

untrt mom → 1x IM ceftri-axone → baby

Characteristics
Gram-negative intracellular diplococci in pairs that can lead to gonorrhea (GC) infection

Transmission
Horizontal transmission: intercourse (cervical secretions most commonly infected)

Vertical transmission: vaginal secretions of infected pregnant woman at delivery, breast milk

Clinical
Neonatal conjunctivitis (typically 2–5 days of life, profuse bilateral purulent discharge, may lead to corneal ulcerations if untreated)

Scalp abscess from fetal monitoring

Systemic: pneumonia, sepsis, arthritis, osteomyelitis, meningitis, scalp infection

Concurrent infection with chlamydia is common

Gonorrhea in pregnant women usually asymptomatic —may have vaginal discharge, dysuria

Diagnosis
Conjunctival, blood, skin lesion, oropharyngeal, rectal Gram stain, and culture using Thayer-Martin growth medium

Note: need to plate *rapidly* for adequate growth

Management
GC conjunctivitis requires emergent intravenous treatment since can rapidly progress to corneal ulceration and/or perforation; frequent ophthalmic irrigation

Due to high chance of penicillin-resistance, treat with 3rd generation cephalosporin

Due to high co-infection rate with chlamydia, evaluate for chlamydia and consider adding erythromycin

If disseminated disease and CSF negative, treat for 7 days; if positive CSF, requires 14 days of therapy

Prevention
Eye ointment (0.5% erythromycin — most common > 1% tetracycline >>1% silver nitrate); ideal if applied < 1 hour of age; does decrease incidence of GC conjunctivitis from 10 to 0.5%; however, doesn't completely prevent chlamydia infection

If asymptomatic infant born to mother with untreated GC, one dose ceftriaxone IM

4. *Chlamydia trachomatis*

Eosinophilia, common newborn complication= pneumonia watery discharge, progresses to purulent

late discharge in eye

"CE" Chlamydia erythromycin (chris emily)

Incidence
25–60% of infants born to chlamydia-infected mother will become infected

Characteristics
Obligate intracellular bacteria, 18 serotypes

Transmission
Neonatal infection acquired during vaginal delivery

Clinical
Conjunctivitis: most common cause of conjunctivitis in 1st month of life

Most common neonatal manifestation of chlamydia (25–50%)

Typically bilateral, occurs 5 – 14 days post-delivery (can be earlier if premature rupture of membranes)

Initially watery discharge that becomes purulent; swollen eyelids and red, thickened conjunctivae

Pneumonia: 5–20% of patients with chlamydia

Presents at 4 – 12 weeks with *staccato cough,* URI, increased respiratory distress, hyperinflated lungs with bilateral infiltrates, *eosinophilia* in 70%

1/2 with history of chlamydia conjunctivitis

Diagnosis
Culture (Giemsa stain) of conjunctiva scrapings, nasopharynx

Neonates with pneumonia may have increased chlamydia-specific IgM levels

Note: not detectable by Gram stain

Management

Chlamydia conjunctivitis or pneumonia – oral erythromycin $\times$ 14 days (20% require second course)

5. *Mycobacterium tuberculosis*

Characteristics

Slow-growing, acid-fast bacillus that can lead to tuberculosis (TB)

Transmission

Congenital TB (extremely rare) acquired by:

1. Hematogenous spread from an infected placenta
2. Aspiration or ingestion of infected amniotic fluid

Postnatal acquisition by

1. Inhalation of infected respiratory secretions
2. Contamination of traumatized mucous membranes or skin

Clinical

Majority of symptoms in neonates with congenital infection present in 2nd or 3rd week of life

Nonspecific: HSM, respiratory distress, fever, lymphadenopathy, abdominal distention, lethargy, irritability, ear discharge, skin papules

Greater risk of dissemination in neonates compared with older children and adults

Diagnosis

PPD (infected neonate develops positive PPD defined as $\geq$ 10 mm only after infection present for 4–6 months and thus if negative PPD, requires repeat testing every 2–3 months)

CXR, acid-fast bacilli staining and culture of blood, urine, three early gastric aspirates, tracheal aspirates and spinal fluid

Liver function tests typically abnormal if disseminated disease

Examine placenta, lymph nodes, liver, lung, bone marrow, skin lesions for pathology

Evaluate all household members for TB

Management

Drug sensitivities should be done on any isolated organisms (especially maternal samples)

Pregnant mother

1. *Asymptomatic, positive PPD, negative sputum, and negative CXR:*

   Administer isoniazid (INH) to mother postpartum

   However, if recent known TB exposure, immunosuppressed (HIV seropositive), or converted to positive PPD within past 2 years, treat mother with INH and pyridoxine x 9 months starting in 2nd trimester

2. *Active disease:* INH, rifampin (RIF), and ethambutol (EMB); add pyridoxine to prevent vitamin B6 deficiency

   Therapy dependent on sensitivities:

   If sensitive to INH and RIF, treat for 9 months and discontinue EMB

   If sensitive to only INH or RIF, continue EMB and treat for 12–18 months

   Isolate mother, notify local health department

Asymptomatic neonate, mother with positive PPD, and no evidence of active infection

If mother with abnormal CXR $\longrightarrow$ separate infant and mother and determine if mother with active disease; if inactive disease, infant with minimal risk of infection; monitor infant with PPD (every 3 months for 1 year and yearly thereafter) and frequent clinical evaluations

If mother with normal CXR $\longrightarrow$ no need to separate infant and mother; no therapy required for infant; monitor infant with PPD and clinical evaluations

Asymptomatic neonate, active infection in mother

Administer INH to neonate until mother is culture negative for 2–3 months (RIF if INH-resistant)

If neonate with positive PPD at 2- 3 months of age $\longrightarrow$ continue INH x 9 months (12 months if HIV seropositive neonate); monitor neonate clinically

If neonate with negative PPD at 2–3 months of age→ can discontinue INH if mother is responding to therapy; repeat PPD every 2–3 months for 1 year and yearly thereafter, and monitor neonate clinically

Isolate infant from mother if mother is noncompliant, has respiratory symptoms, or has multidrug-resistant TB

Neonate with congenital TB

Initially treat with INH + RIF + pyrazinamide + streptomycin or EMB (4-drug regimen = broad therapy)

Consult with local TB and infectious disease specialist; isolate neonate

If extrapulmonary TB: treat with broad therapy x 2 months followed by 7–10 months of INH and RIF; add corticosteroids if TB meningitis

If multidrug-resistant TB: treat with broad therapy × 12–18 months

If breast-feeding and receiving INH: administer pyridoxine to neonate

Anti-tuberculosis medications and side effects

INH: hepatotoxicity, peripheral neuropathy, allergic reactivity

RIF: hepatotoxicity, vomiting, low platelets, orange color to body fluids

Pyrazinamide: hepatotoxicity, hyperuricemia

Streptomycin: ototoxicity, nephrotoxicity

EMB: optic neuritis, gastrointestinal symptoms

6. *Clostridium botulinum*

Characteristics

Anaerobe, gram-positive bacillus that may lead to botulism

Airborne spores from soil, dust, or honey

Emits a toxin that inhibits release of acetylcholine from nerves

Clinical

Disease most commonly presents at 2–4 months of age, usually < 6 months

Can be mild or severe

Lethargy, constipation, poor feeding, typically afebrile, weak cry

Can develop progressive hypotonia, progressive weakness, ocular nerve palsies

Respiratory muscle weakness

Diagnosis

Identify toxin in stool, identify organism by stool culture

Electromyograph (EMG): incremental response at high-frequency, abnormal spontaneous activity; abundant, brief, small-amplitude action potentials

Management

Supportive respiratory and nutritional care

Gavage feeding, close monitoring, +/− intubation

Administer human-derived botulinum antitoxin

Antibiotics not helpful (aminoglycosides can actually increase neuromuscular blockade)

Prognosis

Since toxin binds irreversibly, need to regenerate nerve endings that typically requires several weeks; ~5% recurrence rate

7. *Staphylococcus (Staph) epidermidis and aureus*

Staph epidermidis (epi) (−) Vancomysin	Staph aureus (+) Oxacillin Nafcillin
Coagulase-negative	Coagulase-positive
Increased risk if immunocompromised, indwelling catheter, often nosocomial	Leads to bullous impetigo, abscesses, sepsis
Leads to sepsis	Also associated with *Staph* scalded skin syndrome, toxic shock syndrome
Vancomycin ideal therapy since many methicillin-resistant strains	Oxacillin or nafcillin preferred
Consider synergy with gentamicin or rifampin	Consider empiric treatment with vancomycin (until sensitivity results) if high local incidence of methicillin-resistant Staph aureus (MRSA)
Contact precautions, no isolation required	If MRSA confirmed, treat with vancomycin +/− rifampin or gentamicin
	Contact precautions, no isolation required

8. Gram-negative bacilli

Organisms

Include *Escherichia coli (E. coli), Klebsiella, Serratia, Enterobacter, Proteus, Citrobacter, Pseudomonas, Haemophilus influenzae (H. flu)*

Transmission

Neonatal infection usually acquired from maternal genital tract; also can acquire nosocomially (person-to-person transmission and environment)

Seeding from colonized gastrointestinal tract

Clinical

Neutropenia, sepsis, meningitis (increased risk if *E. coli* with K1 capsular polysaccharide antigen), urinary tract infection, pneumonia, brain abscesses (*Citrobacter or Enterobacter*)

Diarrhea — *E. coli* associated with 5 types:

Enterohemorrhagic (hemorrhagic colitis and hemolytic uremic syndrome)

Enteropathogenic (watery diarrhea)

Enterotoxigenic (watery diarrhea)

Enteroinvasive (febrile)

Enteroaggregative (watery diarrhea)

Predisposing factors

Maternal infection, low birth weight, prolonged ROM, traumatic delivery, galactosemia (increased risk of *E. coli*), fetal hypoxia

Diagnosis

Blood, urine, CSF cultures

Management

Initial empiric treatment with double-coverage (e.g., ampicillin/cephalosporin and aminoglycoside)

Narrow coverage further after organism and sensitivities identified

Enterobacter, Citrobacter, Serratia and *Pseudomonas* require continued double-coverage

Consider consultation with infectious disease specialist

B. VIRAL

1. Herpes simplex virus (HSV)

Incidence

1 in 2000 to 5000 deliveries per year

Less common than CMV or toxo, similar incidence as syphilis

Mother with primary genital lesion during delivery → 40–50% of neonates will become infected due to high viral titer and neonate without protective antibodies

Mother with secondary genital lesion during delivery → < 5% of exposed neonates will become infected (low % probably due to maternally transmitted antibodies)

However, since secondary lesions are more common, ~50% of neonates with HSV are born to mothers with secondary HSV

60–80% of women with neonates who develop HSV are asymptomatic or without a history of HSV

~75% of neonatal disease due to HSV type 2

Characteristics

HSV type 1 (typically oral) or HSV type 2 (typically genital)

Belongs to a group of double-stranded herpes DNA viruses (cytomegalovirus, Ebstein-Barr virus, varicella-zoster virus, and human herpes virus 6)

Multinucleated giant cells

Transmission

At delivery (~95%): majority due to virus in birth canal

In utero (~5%): ascending or transplacental

Postnatal (rare): can be transmitted from breast milk or contact with infected skin lesion

Neonatal risks

Primary maternal genital infection during pregnancy: greatest risk factor, 10–20x risk compared with secondary/recurrent lesions due to high viral replication, longer excretion of virus from primary lesion (3 weeks if primary infection vs. 2–5 days shedding if recurrent HSV), and lack of maternal antibodies to infant

Prematurity: probably due to low transplacental IgG antibodies in premature infants

Fetal scalp monitoring: may break infant's skin barrier and thus contraindication if known HSV infection

Prolonged rupture of membranes: > 4–6 hours; increases risk of ascending infection

Screening

Previously screened all mothers with HSV weekly after 36 weeks to determine whether to deliver by C/S or not; this has been found to have poor predictive value and is no longer done since:

1. Most infants with HSV have mothers without any clinical history of HSV
2. Lower risk to neonate if maternal recurrent HSV exposure
3. Vaginal shedding of HSV difficult to test at appropriate time

Current recommendations: assess for visible lesions at time of delivery and if present, consider delivery by C/S

Clinical

Perinatal HSV (acquired at time of delivery or postnatally):

✓ liver, adrenal, lungs

	Disseminated (systemic)	SEM (skin, eye, mucous membranes)	Encephalitis (CNS)
Timing	4–10 day of life (DOL)	6–9 DOL	10–18 DOL
Clinical	Fever, lethargy, irritability, poor oral intake	Most common	Initially with fever, lethargy, and seizures
	Respiratory distress may be presenting sign in ~20% secondary to pneumonitis	Eyes: conjunctivitis, keratitis, chorioretinitis, retinal dysplasia	Irritability, apnea
	Hepatomegaly, adrenal gland involvement	Skin: papulovesicular lesions, often pustular	Bulging fontanel
	Coagulopathy, shock	and with erythematous base, often occurs at	Pyramidal tract signs
	May also have central nervous system (CNS, 60–75%, due to hematogenous spread) or SEM (80%)	sites of trauma, risk of scar formation	SEM disease in 40–60%
			CNS involvement (probably due to retrograde axonal transmission to brain)
Morbidity	~30–50% normal development if treated	Treatment minimizes risk of progression to disseminated or CNS disease	30% with normal development
		Normal development in >90% if treated	Increased risk microcephaly, spasticity, blindness, chorioretinitis, developmental delay
		Greatest risk of neurological sequelae if ≥ 3 skin recurrences	
Mortality	~55% (despite treatment)	Minimal	~15% (despite treatment)

Congenital HSV (acquired in utero): rare

Triad: 1. Brain — microcephaly, hydranencephaly, intracranial calcifications, hypertonicity, seizures

2. Eyes — microphthalmia, chorioretinitis, cataracts, blindness

3. Skin — vesicles (often present at birth, unlike perinatal HSV), scar, hypopigmented lesions

Also with in utero growth restriction

Elevated cord IgM levels

Diagnosis

CBC/differential, CSF (elevated protein, pleocytosis — especially mononuclear cells, increased RBCs, herpes PCR)

If low suspicion and not treating with acyclovir, obtain surface cultures of conjunctivae, nasopharynx and rectum 24–48 hours post-delivery (note: keep rectal sample separate from others due to meconium's ability to eradicate virus from culture media)

If high suspicion (i.e., ill infant, vesicles present) and treating with acyclovir, obtain surface cultures as well as CSF, urine and vesicular base cultures

May have abnormal LFTs, elevated direct bilirubin, thrombocytopenia, coagulopathy; CXR consistent with pneumonitis

Diffusely abnormal EEG (typically spike and slow-wave activity in temporal region)

Head imaging if high suspicion

Diagnosis in a timely manner requires high index of suspicion

Management

If mother with active lesion at delivery → C/S (ideal if ROM < 4 hours)

If mother with ROM and fetus is premature→ management controversial, some recommend acyclovir IV to mother if delay labor

If infant exposed to HSV→ obtain surface cultures at 24–48 hours of age and monitor infant closely

Treat if positive HSV culture, neonate with clinical symptoms consistent with HSV, or neonate with nonspecific symptoms and exposure to primary HSV

Acyclovir: inhibits viral DNA transcription; specifically is activated by thymidine kinase; monitor urine output and creatinine to assess for renal toxicity

Ophthalmic antiviral (e.g., trifluridine) in addition to acyclovir if SEM disease

Supportive care

Isolate infant with HSV; isolate infant born vaginally or by C/S to mother with ROM > 6 hours and active lesions

Delay circumcision until culture negative

2. RSV (respiratory syncytial virus)

Incidence

Most common respiratory infection in infants, very contagious

Most common in winter months

Almost all children infected by 2–3 years of age

Characteristics

Strain A (more common) and B, RNA paramyxovirus

Transmission

Direct contact with secretions, highly contagious

Virus can survive for hours in droplets on countertops, survives 1/2 hour on skin

Not transmitted to fetus since no viremia

Risk factors

< 1–2 years of age, premature infant (10× greater chance of hospitalization even without history of chronic lung disease or CLD), CLD, congenital heart disease, exposure to smoke

Clinical

URI, pneumonia, bronchiolitis, apnea (initial phase), otitis media, low-grade fever, cough, hypoxemia

Most improve in 3–4 days, but hypoxemia may persist for weeks

CXR with bilateral interstitial pneumonitis, hyperinflation, 20% with lobar consolidation

Long-term: recurrent wheezing, some with abnormal pulmonary function tests later in life

Management

Prevention:

Synagis = palivizumab (IM, monoclonal antibody)

Administer monthly to infants < 2 years of age with CLD who required medical treatment < 6 months prior to RSV season, premature birth at < 32 weeks gestation (note: check recent recommendations)

Has been shown to decrease risk of hospitalization by 55% and decrease number of hospital days

Previously used monthly RSV-IVIG (polyclonal antibody)

Good hand washing

Treatment: ribavarin (aerosol), effectiveness is controversial

Supportive care (hydration, supplemental oxygen)

Bronchodilators are controversial, systemic steroids not proven to be beneficial

3. Hepatitis (Hep) B

Incidence

0.8% of pregnant women in US are HepBsAg positive

Characteristic

Double-stranded DNA

Transmission

From infected blood or body secretions

Groups with greatest risk include intravenous drug users, person with multiple sexual partners, health-care workers and Alaskan Eskimos; increased prevalence in delivery population in Japan, China, and Taiwan

HepBsAg positive asymptomatic mother carrier greater risk of transmission from 10 to 85% if mother also HepBeAg positive (due to high degree of replication)

Greatest risk of transmission is at birth (due to exposure to contaminated genital tract secretions and/or blood) > postpartum > transplacental (3rd trimester) > transplacental (1st or 2nd trimester, rare)

Does cross into breast milk, but little risk of transmission

Diagnosis (adults)

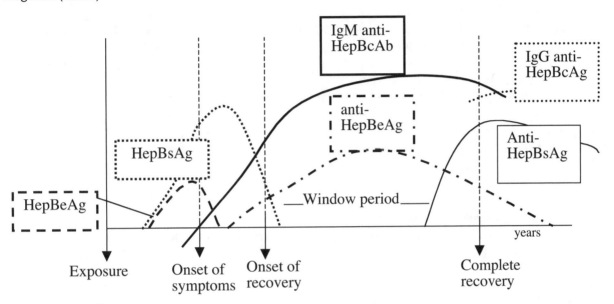

NOTE: chart representative of adult infection; c= core; s=surface; Ag=antigen; Ab=antibody; note that Ab to c then e then s while Ag to s then e. Modified from Braunwald E, Fauci AS, Kasper DL, et al (eds): Harrison's Principles of Internal Medicine (15th edition). McGraw-Hill, New York, 2001, p 1724.

HepBcAg: not present in high amounts to be clinically useful

HepBsAg: first marker to appear in acute infection

Present 1–3 months after exposure, typically before onset of symptoms and cleared 1–2 weeks after jaundice occurs

HepBeAg: detectable when HepB virus is rapidly replicating

Antigen initially present prior to clinical symptoms and disappears before clinical symptoms resolve; always detected with HepBsAg

Anti-HepBeAg: infected but low risk of transmission

Anti-HepBcAg: IgM initally (specific for acute infection) and followed by IgG; detected during "window period" between HepBsAg and anti-HepBsAg; can be detected in acute, resolved, or chronic infection

Anti-HepBsAg: antibody that protects against future re-infection

Indicates immunity (not present if person is a chronic carrier)

Clinical

Incubation period is 50–180 days (compared with Hep A, 28 days)

Elevated LFTs 2 weeks to 2 months after positive HepBsAg

Maternal infection: often self-limited, < 1% with severe liver failure, greater risk of prematurity and low birth weight

Most infants infected with hepatitis B are asymptomatic

80–90% of neonates will become chronic HepBsAg carriers if mother HepBeAg-positive

Neonate at higher risk of chronicity compared with older children

Management

    If mother with unknown HepBsAg status

        Test mother

        Administer HepB vaccine to neonate within 12 hours of age

        If mother is positive and full-term infant, administer hepatitis immune globulin (HBIG) to neonate within 7 days

        If mother is positive and premature infant, administer hepatitis immune globulin to neonate within 12 hours of age; if premature infant had 1st dose < 2 kg, administer vaccine for 4 doses

    If mother is HepBsAg positive

        Administer HepB vaccine to neonate within 12 hours (2nd dose at 1–2 mo, 3rd dose at 6 months of age); premature infants must receive total of 4 vaccines

        Administer HBIG concurrently at a different IM site

        Follow anti-HepBsAg and HepBsAg 1–3 months after vaccination series complete to identify chronic carriers and possible need for repeat vaccinations

    HBIG — decreases infection rate from 94 to 75% and decreases chronic carrier rate from 91 to 22%; if also give vaccine, chronic carrier rate is reduced to 0 –14%

    Universal neonatal hepatitis B vaccination — 90% efficacy in preventing HBV infection

4. Hepatitis D

A defective RNA virus that utilizes HepBsAg for its surface coat and thus necessitates co-infection with hepatitis B virus

Transmitted via blood, sexual contact; rare to have perinatal transmission

5. Hepatitis C

Characteristics: single-stranded RNA virus, 30–60 day incubation

Transmission: infected blood, contaminated needle sticks, rare to transmit via sexual intercourse

    From mother to infant (~5%; especially if high maternal titer, maternal co-infection with HIV or maternal chronic liver disease)

Clinical: neonatal effects uncertain

    Adults can have acute hepatitis (1/2 develop chronic hepatitis with 1/4 developing cirrhosis and liver failure), increased risk of hepatocellular cancer; high rate of relapse

Management: supportive, some adults treated with α-interferon and ribavirin (no trials in neonates)

6. Hepatitis A and E

Hepatitis A

    Characteristics: single-stranded RNA virus; spread by fecal/oral route

        Highly contagious, low risk of perinatal transmission

        No chronic carrier state, incubation for 4 weeks

    Clinical: majority asymptomatic, low mortality, no increased risk of congenital malformations, mild hepatitis with jaundice, mild abdominal pain, fever, malaise

    Diagnosis: anti-hepatitis IgM at onset of disease and may be present up to 3 months

    Management: IVIG soon after birth if maternal hepatitis A infection ≤ 2 weeks prior to delivery; enteric precautions

Hepatitis E

    Rare in US; RNA virus transmitted by fecal-oral route

    If maternal infection during pregnancy, high maternal mortality (~20%) and increased risk stillbirth and premature delivery; not associated with chronic hepatitis

7. Parvovirus B19

Characteristics

    Single-stranded DNA, B19 infects only humans

Incubation period 4–14 days, increased seropositivity with age

Replicates within RBC precursors

Transmission

Direct contact with respiratory secretions

Maternal to fetal transmission

From infected blood or fomites

Clinical

Asymptomatic in majority

Fifth disease = erythema infectiosum—occurs in older children; malaise, low-grade fever and "slapped-cheek" rash (low infection risk after rash develops)

Adults may have self-limited arthralgia or arthritis, transient RBC aplasia, myocarditis, peripheral nerve abnormalities, vasculitis

Fetal infection: majority normal, not teratogenic, increased risk of fetal loss

Anemia and congestive heart failure may lead to hydrops

Fetus may develop myocarditis, thrombocytopenia, neutropenia, liver disease

Diagnosis

Diagnose by parvovirus maternal IgM levels

PCR of amniotic fluid or fetal blood

Management

If pregnant infected mother — monitor fetus for development of anemia, congestive heart failure and possible hydrops and treat accordingly (e.g., in utero blood transfusion)

Postnatally, supportive care

8. Varicella-zoster virus

Characteristics

DNA herpes virus

Contagious 1–2 days before onset of rash to 6 days after rash

Incubation 10–21 days unless varicella-zoster immune globulin (VZIG), which lengthens incubation period to 28 days

Neonates often with shorter incubation (9–15 days)

Transmission

Respiratory droplets

Contact with rash

Transplacental

Varicella infection in pregnant mother

Uncommon

No increased risk of spontaneous abortion

Previously thought greater chance of pneumonia if pregnant, now controversial

If asymptomatic, exposed and not immune, administer VZIG to pregnant mother within 72 hours of exposure; no evidence of this protecting fetus

If symptomatic, exposed and not immune, treat pregnant mother with acyclovir if pneumonia

If uncomplicated maternal varicella, prefer not to treat pregnant mother since unknown risk of acyclovir to fetus

Congenital varicella syndrome

Low incidence

Could occur even if mild maternal infection

Time of Maternal Infection	Risk of Congenital Varicella
During first 20 weeks gestation	High risk
During 2nd 1/2 of pregnancy up to 21 days prior to delivery	Low risk
Between 20 days prior to delivery to 6 days before delivery	Mild symptoms, little risk of severe disease
Between 5 days before delivery until 2 days after delivery	Greatest risk since insufficient time for protective antibodies to cross to fetus (17% chance of acute infection; if untreated, 30% mortality)

*give VZIG

Mild to severe disease (usually < 10 days of life) including: cutaneous lesions (= cicatricial lesions, along dermatomes, scarred or segmental), limb abnormalities (including limb atrophy, typically distal to cutaneous lesions), eye abnormalities (cataracts, chorioretinitis), severe mental deficiency, seizures, intracranial calcifications, pneumonia, encephalopathy, hepatitis, possible early death

Management

Vaccine: = Varivax, live, attenuated; given prior to pregnancy, protects about 85%

VZIG: if administered within 3–5 days of maternal exposure (ideal if < 3 days), modifies infection; doesn't prevent infection

Indications for VZIG:

Infant with mother who develops varicella 5 days prior to delivery to 2 days after delivery

Premature infant ≥ 28 weeks gestation if significant exposure and mother without history of chickenpox and/or seronegative

Premature infant < 28 weeks gestation or ≤ 1000 g if significant exposure, regardless of maternal history since inadequate maternal antibody protection

Acyclovir: any infant with generalized disease, higher dose than HSV therapy

If mother develops varicella 5 days prior to delivery to 2 days after delivery, administer VZIG to infant; prefer not to induce labor since ideal if maternal antibodies have more time to cross to fetus; VZIG not recommended to mother prior to delivery; isolate mother from infant until lesions crusted

If infant exposed postnatally 2–7 days of life, low risk, consider VZIG (especially if premature infant)

Isolation:

Isolate mother from infant if active lesions at delivery

If mother with lesions < 5 days prior to delivery and > 2 days after → infant given VZIG and isolated until maternal lesions crusted

If mother s/p varicella and lesions healed → no isolation of mother from infant but isolate infant from other infants around time of delivery

Isolate infant with congenital varicella

9. Rubella

cong. rubella syndrome
Deafness, glaucoma, VSD

Women aquire in 1st 20 wks
20-25% chance
first 8 wks = 85% chance
of cong. rub. syndrome
P 20 wk - seldom causes defect

Characteristics

RNA virus, high frequency in late winter and early spring, humans are only host

Incubation period 14–21 days after contact

Transmission

Majority spread by respiratory secretions

Transplacental acquisition with risk to fetus dependent on gestational age at time of maternal infection:

Weeks Gestation	Risk Fetal Infection
1–12	~80% (greatest risk congenital anomalies)
	If < 10 weeks gestation, 100% fetuses with cardiac abnormalities and deafness
13–16	54% (deafness in 1/3 infected)
17–22	36%
23–30	30%
31–36	60%
Last month	100%

Congenital anomalies rare after 20 weeks gestation

Clinical

In utero — hydrops

Congenital rubella syndrome:

General — ~60% IUGR, poor growth postnatally

Neurologic – *sensorineural hearing loss* (65–75%, occurs if maternal infection < 20 weeks gestation), meningoencephalitis, mental deficiency, hypotonia, microcephaly (5%)

Ophthalmologic – cloudy cornea, *cataracts*, microphthalmia, *salt and pepper chorioretinitis*

Hematologic – thrombocytopenia, hemolytic anemia, petechiae/purpura, *blueberry muffin rash* (due to dermal extramedullary hematopoiesis, resolves)

Cardiac – if infection < 8 weeks gestation, there is a 50% chance of cardiac disease including *patent ductus arteriosus* > peripheral pulmonary stenosis > pulmonary valvar stenosis > aortic stenosis, tetralogy of Fallot, and myocarditis

Other – long bone striated radiolucencies (i.e. "celery stalking" of long bone metaphyses), interstitial pneumonia, myositis, hepatitis, HSM

20% with delayed symptoms including insulin-dependent diabetes and thyroid disease

Diagnosis

In utero: fetal rubella IgM levels by percutaneous umbilical blood sampling

Neonate: viral culture of nasopharynx, blood, CSF, and urine (need to notify laboratory in advance prior to sending cultures)

Rubella IgM serum levels and serial IgG levels, abnormal long bone films

Management

Rubella vaccination of nonimmune pregnant women is not recommended, yet no proven risk; no contraindication to breast-feeding if mother with rubella infection

Congenital rubella infection: isolate neonate from other newborns; may be contagious for 1 year unless repeat urine and blood cultures are negative; hearing screen, ophthalmologic exam, assess for heart disease

Postnatal rubella infection: isolate x 7 days after rash develops

10. Cytomegalovirus (CMV)

Ganciclovir — trt chionoretinitis — can cause thrombo- cytopenia

Incidence

The most common intrauterine infection worldwide

Greater chance of being CMV positive with advancing age

~2–2.5% seroconvert during pregnancy, and majority asymptomatic

If maternal primary CMV – transplacentally 30–40% fetuses infected with only 10% symptomatic at birth; if symptomatic, 20–30% mortality with sequelae ~90%; if asymptomatic at birth, ~5–15% sequelae

If maternal secondary CMV/recurrent CMV – 1% of fetuses infected, almost all asymptomatic at birth; less morbidity to neonate than if exposure to primary maternal CMV infection

If maternal infection is during first 1/2 of pregnancy, greater risk of neonatal disease and greater severity of neonatal illness

Characteristics

Double-stranded herpes DNA virus; intranuclear and cytoplasmic inclusions

Transmission

Secretions (requires close contact), sexual intercourse, blood products, transplacental (all trimesters) and intrapartum

CMV can also be transmitted via human milk (uncommon due to passively transferred maternal antibodies); decreased risk if pasteurization or freezing; increased risk if premature infant

Clinical

Can be asymptomatic at birth (90% of congenital CMV, minimal mortality):

Increased risk of hearing loss (sensorineural, often bilateral, moderate to profound) that correlates with presence of periventricular calcifications; hearing loss often progressive and may not be detected until > 1 year of age

Chorioretinitis

Increased risk of cavities due to abnormal tooth enamel

Possible neurological abnormalities

May reactivate later

Can be symptomatic at birth (10% of infected infants, 20–30% mortality):

    Usually due to primary maternal infection at time of conception

    IUGR, HSM, hyperbilirubinemia, petechiae

    Dermal hematopoiesis (blueberry muffin rash), thrombocytopenia

    Microcephaly, periventricular calcifications, chorioretinitis (~20%)

    Hearing loss, mental deficiency, seizures

    High likelihood long-term neurological sequelae (~45%)

    Inguinal hernias, dental cavities, disseminated intravascular coagulopathy, liver failure, sepsis, possible death

If acquired intrapartum, via infected breast milk, or infected blood products:

    Incubation 4–12 weeks; can lead to pneumonitis, possible sepsis, HSM, thrombocytopenia, microcephaly or hearing loss

Diagnosis

    Spin-enhanced culture or shell virus (results in 1–2 days), urine viral culture (results in 2–6 weeks)

    Less definitive tests include increase in IgG titers by 4-fold and positive IgM anti-CMV

    Prenatal evidence of fetal infection — US (microcephaly, ventricular dilatation, periventricular calcifications, IUGR, hepatic lesions, hydrops, echogenic abdominal foci); amniocentesis (amniotic fluid culture, PCR); and cordocentesis (IgM anti-CMV, PCR)

Management

    If congenital infection: head CT or MRI, ophthalmologic exam, hearing screen, platelet count, LFTs, CSF evaluation

    Ganciclovir — especially to treat chorioretinitis and neurological abnormalities, can lead to thrombocytopenia, neutropenia, anemia; increased relapse after discontinue ganciclovir

    Can't use acyclovir since CMV doesn't induce thymidine kinase required by acyclovir

    Consider consultation with infectious disease specialist

11. Toxoplasmosis (toxo)

[handwritten: Infected Neonate: pyrimethamine & sulfadiazine X 1 YR.]
[handwritten: ** Folinic acid prevent neutropenia]

Incidence

    1/2 pregnant women are susceptible to primary toxoplasmosis

Characteristics

    Although placed in the viral section, toxo is due to a *protozoal* organism

    Intracellular parasite (*Toxoplasma gondii*)

    Sources include meat that is poorly cooked and cat feces

Transmission

    Almost all congenital toxo due to primary maternal infection

    Transmission during pregnancy greater as increased gestational age; however, if fetus acquires infection early in pregnancy, there is a greater risk of severe disease

Clinical

[handwritten: * Hydro, chorioretinitis, brain calcif = triad]

    Mother typically asymptomatic or mild symptoms

    Greater then 75% neonates are asymptomatic in early infancy

    Common: lymphadenopathy, chorioretinitis, cortical brain calcifications, hydrocephalus, thrombocytopenia, HSM, jaundice

    Other: anemia, rash, pneumonitis, diarrhea

Presentations:

    Well infant, subclinical infection, symptoms later in childhood

    Well infant, symptoms during first few months of life

    Systemic illness in neonate — IUGR, prematurity, HSM, lymphadenopathy, cutaneous lesions (blueberry muffin lesions due to dermal erythropoiesis typically within first few days of life, also with CMV and rubella)

    Neurologic abnormalities at birth, may be associated with microcephaly

Diagnosis

    Prenatal — ultrasound (ventricular dilatation, ascites, hepatomegaly, intracranial calcifications); fetal toxo IgG and IgM; amniotic fluid PCR and culture

Toxo IgM ideal, can monitor for rising toxo IgG antibodies over several months

Management

If mother infected, treat with spiramycin during pregnancy to attempt to decrease transmission rate

If mother *and* fetus infected with toxo, treat with pyrimethamine and sulfadiazine to attempt to decrease fetal effects

If symptomatic or asymptomatic infected neonate, treat with pyrimethamine and sulfadiazine $\times$ 1 year

Monitor with ophthalmologic exams, head imaging, CSF evaluation

Monitor CBC and differential, UA, LFTs, creatinine, toxo IgG and IgM levels

Requires folinic acid supplementation to prevent neutropenia from pyrimethamine

Consider consultation with infectious disease specialist

Prognosis

Normal development in 70% of treated infants despite initial neurological symptoms

Poor outcome if delayed diagnosis and/or delayed treatment

12. Comparison of rubella, CMV and toxo

Clinical Findings	Incidence				
Low birth weight	CMV (~65%)	>	Rubella (~ 60%)	>	Toxo (~30%)
Hepatomegaly	CMV (70%)	>	Rubella (65%)	>	Toxo (35%)
Splenomegaly	CMV (70%)	>	Rubella (60%)	>	Toxo (40%)
Jaundice	CMV (70%)	>	Toxo (~40%)	>	Rubella (15%)
Petechiae/purpura	CMV (65%)	>	Rubella (55%)	>	Toxo (5%)
Congenital heart disease	Rubella (75%)	>	CMV (5%)		
Cataracts	Rubella (50%)	>	Toxo (5%)		
Retinopathy	Toxo (90%)	>	CMV (20%)	>	Rubella (5%)
Microcephaly	CMV (40%)	>	Toxo (10%)	>	Rubella (5%)
Cerebral calcifications	Toxo (cortical) (40%)	>	CMV (periventricular) (15%)		
Pneumonia	CMV (35%)	>	Rubella (15%)	>	Toxo (10%)

Modified from Fanaroff AA and Martin RJ (eds): Neonatal-Perinatal Medicine (6th edition). St Louis, Mosby-Year Book Inc, 1997, p 768.

13. Human immunodeficiency virus (HIV)

Characteristics

Retrovirus that has its own reverse transcriptase (RNA to DNA synthesis), DNA then incorporated into genomic host DNA

Infects cells (helper T lymphocytes and macrophages)

Affects both antibody and cell-mediated immunity

Transmission

Perinatal transmission rate without maternal medications is 25–30% with majority of transmission occurring immediately before or during delivery and if outside US, via breast milk

Increased risk for transmission:

1. Maternal CD4 count < 200, increased maternal viral RNA load
2. Newly acquired infection during pregnancy: increases risk vertical transmission since primary infection associated with greater viral load
3. ROM > 4 hours, regardless of delivery mode

HIV exposed
~ ZDV prophylaxis
first 6 wks
P. carinii pneum proph.
@ 4-6 wks & continue
for 1st year of life

Initial testing: viral cx, PCR, viral load
in first 48 hrs
Repeat 1, 2 and 3-6 mo.
IgG levels inacc. until 18 mo.
b/c reflects maternal antibody

4. Vaginal delivery (especially if prolonged ROM and in labor)
5. Maternal vitamin A deficiency
6. Fetal scalp monitoring
7. Twin: first twin more likely to be HIV positive compared with second twin
8. Breast feeding: in US, recommendations to avoid breast feeding if HIV positive mother since increases transmission rate by 14%

Clinical

Usually asymptomatic at birth and symptomatic by 1–2 years of age

Infants typically have shorter incubation periods compared with adults and more rapidly progressive course

FTT, HSM, lymphadenopathy, diarrhea, recurrent bacterial infections (due to early decrease in B cell function) including sepsis, pneumonia, meningitis, cardiac dysfunction

Developmental delay

Pneumocystis carinii pneumonia (PCP) — majority of children with HIV develop PCP between 2 and 8 months of age, often the presenting illness

Presents with fever, cough, congestion, respiratory distress

Severe hypoxemia, increased LDH levels

Radiographic findings of diffuse alveolar infiltrative pneumonia

Lymphocytic interstitial pneumonia (LIP) — respiratory distress, diffuse infiltrates

Diagnosis in neonate

HIV DNA PCR	Preferred test to diagnose HIV in infant
	Tests mononuclear blood cells
	~30% infants with HIV infection will have positive PCR by 48 hours of age, while ~93% will be positive by 2 weeks of age
	If positive at birth, suggests infant infected in utero
	If positive, confirm with HIV culture
HIV culture	Expensive
	Results may take up to 4 weeks
HIV p24 antigen	Specific yet less sensitive compared with DNA PCR or culture
	May have false-positive if < 1 month of age
HIV RNA PCR	Diagnostic if elevated but if negative test, may still be infected

Note: neonate with HIV infection if positive results on 2 separate specimens (excluding cord blood) using above techniques, Modified from Pickering LK (ed). 2000 Red Book: Report of the Committee on Infectious Diseases (25th edition), Elk Grove Village, IL, American Academy of Pediatrics, 2000, p 332.

If mother HIV-positive, test neonate with PCR at birth (don't use umbilical cord blood due to possible contamination with maternal blood), 1–2, and 3–6 months of age

If initial PCR is positive, confirm; culture neonate prior to therapy

ELISA and Western positive due to neonatal infection; if positive ELISA, must confirm by Western to be valid

Laboratory

Initial lymphocyte count low or normal; at several years of age, lymphocytopenia observed

Decrease in CD4/CD8 T lymphocyte ratio

B lymphocytes with normal amount yet dysfunctional; associated with increased immunoglobulins

Management

Maternal (US strategies):

Test prenatally; if positive, treat with anti-retroviral drug during pregnancy beginning at 14–34 weeks gestation to control maternal HIV viral load; C/S if high viral load

Intrapartum intravenous (IV) AZT

If mother did not receive prenatal anti-retroviral therapy: IV AZT, deliver by C/S, administer neonatal AZT, test neonate, consider maternal intrapartum and neonatal nevirapine

Breast feeding contraindicated

Class of Maternal Anti-retroviral Drugs	Medications	Comments
Nucleoside analogue reverse transcriptase inhibitors	Zidovudine (ZDV, AZT, Retrovir) Didanosine (DDI, Videx) Lamivudine (3TC, Epivir) Stavudine (D4T, Zerit) Zalcitabine (DDC, Hivid) Tenofovir (TNV)	Does cross placenta *Maternal AZT therapy:* Decreases risk from 25.5% to 8.3% The combination of DDI and D4T not recommended due to increased risk hepatitis, lactic acidosis, and nephrocalcinosis
Non-nucleoside reverse transcriptase inhibitors	Nevirapine (NVP, Viramune) Efavirenz (EFV, Sustiva) Delavirdine (DLV, Rescriptor)	EFV — teratogenic in animal models NVP — maternal (during labor) and neonatal therapy; long-acting; does cross placenta; reduces vertical HIV transmission; possible increased risk of hepatitis
Protease inhibitors	Ritonavir (RTV, Norvir) Nelfinavir (NFV, Viracept) Indinavir (IDV, Crixivan) Amprenavir (AMP, Agenerase) Saquinavir (FTV, Fortavase, Inverase) Lopinavir (LPV) Lopinavir and Ritonavir combination (Kaletra)	Large molecules with high amount of protein-binding and thus don't cross the placenta Not teratogenic Hyperglycemia Ritonavir and Nelfinavir approved in children > 2 years of age None are approved in children < 2 years

Note: long-term neonatal effects are UNKNOWN; if more than 2 anti-retroviral agents, transmission rate is less than ~2% (especially with controlled viral load). Modified from lecture by Sandra Burchett, MS, MD, "Neonatal Core Conference: HIV" Children's Hospital, Boston, 2001.

Neonatal (note: *evolving management*—please refer to CDC and/or infectious disease specialist for most recent recommendations):

Consult infectious disease specialist

Commonly used anti-retrovirals in neonates: AZT, DDI, 3TC, nevirapine, nelfinavir, and ritonavir (last 2 are still being evaluated, use in neonates not approved by FDA); limited data for premature infants

If controlled maternal viral load: AZT (2 mg/kg orally every 6 hours; different dose if IV or premature infant); monitor for anemia, abnormal LFTs; unknown long-term effects

Treat neonate with AZT by 8 – 12 hours of age for 6 weeks

Neonates who begin AZT < 72 hours of age still will have decreased risk of acquiring HIV even if mother not treated

If uncontrolled maternal viral load: AZT and consider neonatal nevirapine, lamivudine, or nelfinavir

If confirmed neonatal diagnosis of HIV: requires at least 3 anti-retroviral medications (usually 1 protease inhibitor and 2 reverse transcriptase inhibitors)

All HIV-exposed infants should receive PCP prophylaxis with trimethoprim-sulfamethaxole (Bactrim) at 1 month of age until determined to be uninfected

Polio vaccination with IPV to patient and all household members

Worse prognosis if clinical symptoms < 1 year of age

14. Enteroviruses

Characteristics

Single-stranded RNA virus

=echoviruses, coxsackievirus, poliovirus (polio), enterovirus

Typically greatest in summer and fall

Transmission

Transmitted fecal/oral, oral/oral route, swimming pools, contaminated hands

Transmitted transplacentally (usually 3rd trimester) through vaginal canal

Infection during pregnancy

Polio: increased risk of abortion (greatest if 1st trimester and increased severity of maternal illness); live attenuated vaccine not associated with increased risk of abortions, but vaccine should still be avoided during pregnancy

No increased risk of congenital malformations

Slight increased risk of premature delivery

Coxsackie and echoviruses: no increased risk of abortion

    Coxsackie possibly increases risk of congenital anomalies

    Slight increased risk of premature delivery

Neonatal infection

    Greater severity in neonates compared with older age groups

    Greater risk if low birth weight, antibiotic therapy, intubation, nasogastric feeding

    Polio: majority severe, 50% mortality, 1/2 survivors with paralysis

    Echoviruses: type 11 — sepsis-like illness and hepatic necrosis, coagulopathy, often fatal

    Rest of enteroviruses: mild to severe illness

        Symptoms can be similar to sepsis

        Apnea, fever, vomiting, diarrhea, decreased oral intake, maculopapular rash

        Can include hepatitis, myocarditis (especially coxsackie B), meningitis, encephalitis

Diagnosis

    Rectal, nasopharyngeal, blood, CSF and urine viral culture, PCR of CSF available

Management

    Supportive, IVIG (controversial, consider if life-threatening disease)

15. Rotavirus

Characteristics

    Double-stranded RNA

    Greatest cause of acute viral gastroenteritis in infants and children

    Localized to intestine, does not cross breast milk, greatest during winter months in temperate climates

    Intestinal lactase may be a receptor for rotavirus — possible explanation for the lower incidence in premature infants since their lactase activity is lower

    Possible that breast milk antibodies may prevent or decrease symptoms early in life

Transmission

    Majority fecal/oral route

    Can occur during delivery (probably due to exposure to maternal stool)

    Isolette does not protect infant from acquiring infection

    Hand washing critical to prevent transmission

Clinical

    Asymptomatic or gastroenteritis

    Can be associated with poor feeding, irritability, watery stools, dehydration

Diagnosis

    ELISA detection of viral antigen

Management

    Hydration, monitor electrolytes

C. FUNGAL

1. Candida

Amph B
c̄ Meningitis: add 5-Flurouracil (5-FU)

Incidence

    2-3% of very low birth weight (VLBW) infants who are infected develop systemic candidiasis (*Candida albicans* most common type)

Clinical

    Oral: = thrush most common, white patches over oral mucosa, can't scrape off, underneath there is an erythematous base, may become pustular, usually appears at 1 week of age

    Cutaneous: erythematous vesiculopapular rash with satellite lesions located typically in the groin/buttock regions but can also involve the neck and axilla

        Increased risk of systemic candida

Typically present 20-30 days

Congenital cutaneous candidiasis (rare): present at birth or within few hours of life due to ascending infection in utero

At birth may have an erythematous generalized maculopapular rash that can become pustular; usually benign

May have respiratory symptoms; if isolated skin lesions, can treat locally

Systemic candidiasis: increased risk if antibiotic treatment (due to candidal GI overgrowth), prematurity, VLBW, prolonged central venous catheter, prolonged intubation, corticosteroid usage

Respiratory symptoms, feeding intolerance, temperature instability, hypotension, hyperglycemia, typically ~5 weeks of age

Can lead to meningitis, brain abscesses, fungal renal masses, arthritis, otitis media, endophthalmitis, endocarditis

Diagnosis

Blood (multiple), CSF, and urine cultures

If candidemia, renal US and/or CT, head CT, echocardiogram, ophthalmologic exam

Management

Nystatin: oral suspension for thrush (can also use 1% gentian violet, nystatin ointment for skin infection)

Amphotericin B: first-line, can lead to nephrotoxicity (related to total dose), seizures, hypokalemia, low magnesium, hepatotoxicity, arrhythmia (especially if rapid injection), bone marrow suppression

Fluconazole: has been used successfully to treat candidiasis; can consider using in combination with amphotericin B

Liposomal amphotericin B: less nephrotoxicity compared with amphotericin B

Flucytosine: entry into CSF better than amphotericin

Use only in combination with amphotericin B for synergy

Toxicity includes bone marrow suppression, hepatotoxicity, GI disturbances

III. Maternal Infections

A. URINARY TRACT INFECTION (UTI)

Incidence

Increased risk during pregnancy of symptomatic UTI due to "physiologic hydronephrosis" during pregnancy attributable to decreased muscle tone around ureters, mechanical obstruction from increased uterine size, and decreased bladder tone with incomplete emptying

4–7% of pregnant women with asymptomatic bacteriuria (1/4 of these women can develop symptomatic UTI)

~2% of pregnant women with acute pyelonephritis

Increased risk with increased parity, lower socioeconomic status, sickle cell trait

Organisms

E. coli (80–90%), *Klebsiella pneumoniae, Proteus, Enterobacter,* GBS

Clinical

Cystitis (infection that involves lower urinary tract) — dysuria, urgency and frequency; often with microscopic hematuria

Pyelonephritis (infection that involves renal calyces, pelvis and/or parenchyma) — abrupt onset of fever, chills, costovertebral angle tenderness, nausea, vomiting, dysuria, may develop respiratory distress

Management

Asymptomatic bacteriuria: oral antibiotics to decrease associated preterm labor and prevent progression to symptomatic infection

Cystitis: oral antibiotics (ampicillin, sulfonamides, nitrofurantoin or cephalosporins)

Acute pyelonephritis: hospitalize until afebrile for at least 24 hours, intravenous hydration, intravenous antibiotics (ampicillin and aminoglycoside, cefazolin, ceftriaxone) and change to oral antibiotics when afebrile; administer antibiotics × 7–10 days; repeat urine culture 1–2 weeks

Monitor with monthly urine cultures since ~30% recurrence rate

B. BACTERIAL VAGINOSIS

Incidence
  10–30% of pregnant women, majority are symptomatic

Organisms
  Gardnerella vaginalis, anaerobes, Mycoplasma hominis

Characteristics
  Homogeneous gray-white vaginal discharge, pH > 4.5, fishy odor when mixed with 10% KOH, clue cells on wet prep
    (i.e., vaginal epithelial cells coated with bacilli)
  Possibly associated with premature rupture of membranes and chorioamnionitis

Management
  Intravaginal metronidazole
  Ampicillin (only 40–50% effective)

C. MASTITIS

Organisms
  Staph. aureus (most common), coag-negative Staph., Strep. viridans

Clinical
  Symptoms usually after 3rd–4th week postpartum
  Usually unilateral
  Breast engorgement followed by inflammation with chills, fever, tachycardia
  Erythematous, firm, tender breast
  10% develop an abscess (especially if due to Staph. aureus)

Management
  Culture expressed milk
  Empiric antibiotics with dicloxacillin, erythromycin if PCN-resistant, vancomycin if resistant to dicloxacillin or
    erythromycin
  Recommend continued lactation (if too tender to breast feed, use breast pump)

D. CHORIOAMNIONITIS (see Maternal-Fetal Medicine chapter)

IV. Immunizations

A. IMMUNIZATION SCHEDULE

Vaccine	Birth	2 mos	4 mos	6 mos	12 mos	Other
DPT Diphtheria Pertussis Tetanus		#1	#2	#3		Defer pertussis if recent seizure, febrile, shock or progressive neurological disorder #4 at 15–18 mos, #5 at 4–6 yrs Td booster 11–18 yrs and then every 10 yrs *(continued on following page)*

Vaccine	Birth	2 mos	4 mos	6 mos	12 mos	Other
IPV Inactivated poliovirus		#1	#2		#3 (6-18 mos)	#4 at 4–6 yrs
Hib *Haemophilus Influenzae* B		#1	#2	#3	#4 (12-15 mos)	
Hep B	#1 (birth to 2 mos)		#2 (1-4 mos)	#3 (6-18 mos)		4th dose if #1 given when premature infant < 2 kg Refer to Hepatitis section for dosing of neonate born to mother with positive or unknown HepBsAg
Pneumococcal conjugate		#1	#2	#3	#4 (12-15 mos)	
MMR Mumps, measles, rubella					#1 (12-15 mos)	#2 at 4–6 yrs Mumps and measles contraindicated if egg-allergy
Varicella					#1 (12-18 mos)	If first dose ≥ 13 yrs, requires 2 doses with ≥ 1 month between each dose

Notes: (1) vaccination schedules change frequently, so confirm above with most recent available information; (2) minimal age of first dose of DPT, IPV, Hib and pneumococcal conjugate is 6 weeks; and (3) avoid all live vaccines for immunodeficient patients. Modified from "Childhood Immunization Guidelines February 2001." Massachusetts, Department of Public Health.

B. IMMUNIZATION OF PREGNANT WOMEN

Vaccinate only if high risk for disease exposure, if infection would lead to high risk to fetus/neonate, and vaccine not known to be harmful

If vaccination is necessary, delay until 2nd or 3rd trimester to decrease risk of teratogenicity

Vaccines routinely recommended during pregnancy: tetanus, diphtheria, influenza (if >14 weeks gestation)

Vaccines not contraindicated during pregnancy: pneumococcal, hepatitis B

Vaccines that are contraindicated during pregnancy: live-virus vaccines – MMR, varicella

C. IMMUNIZATION OF NEONATES WITH HIV OR SUSPECTED HIV

Contraindications: OPV (oral poliovirus), bacille Calmette-Guérin vaccine (in US)

Relative contraindications: MMR (can administer if neonate is not severely immunocompromised); varicella (can administer if CD4 count is high)

D. IMMUNIZATION OF PREMATURE INFANTS

Premature infants should be vaccinated based on their chronological age

If first dose of hepatitis B vaccine given to a premature infant who weighs < 2 kg, a 4th dose is need

E. BORDETELLA PERTUSSIS

Characteristics
Gram-negative pleomorphic bacillus that may lead to pertussis; humans only host

Clinical
Infants develop mild upper respiratory infection (catarrhal stage) that progresses to paroxysmal cough (paroxysmal stage); may have respiratory whoop, posttussive emesis, mild fever, apnea

May be complicated by pneumonia, seizures, or encephalopathy

Diagnosis
Mucous culture using Bordet-Gengou medium; lymphocytosis often present

Management
Oral erythromycin (estolate preparation) often decreases infectivity and may decrease spread

F. CLOSTRIDIUM TETANI

Characteristics
Gram-positive bacillus that may lead to tetanus
Anaerobe, spore-forming, present in soil and feces, rare in US

Clinical
Neonatal disease usually due to improper umbilical cord handling
Presents with difficulty swallowing, rigidity, muscle spasms, fever, continuous crying, seizure activity, hyperreflexia, lockjaw (less common in neonates compared with adults)
Symptoms due to toxin leading to decreased acetylcholine release
Infection can spread through umbilical vessels

Management
Supportive care
PCN G and tetanus immune globulin to neutralize circulating unbound toxin
Diazepam to decrease spasms
Still need to vaccinate since disease does not lead to immunity

G. MUMPS AND MEASLES

	Mumps	Measles
Organism	Paramyxovirus	Paramyxovirus
Transmission	Respiratory droplets Fomites Saliva	Respiratory droplets Fomites Transplacental – hematogenous
Incubation	12–25 days	8–12 days, infectious with onset of symptoms until 3 days after rash
Clinical	Fever, malaise, myalgia Bilateral parotitis Orchitis (greatest after puberty) Aseptic meningitis and pancreatitis are less common Reports of aqueductal stenosis and mumps infection Congenital/postnatal—very rare, majority with mild symptoms	Fever, cough, coryza and conjunctivitis Koplik spots – white spots on buccal mucosa with surrounding erythema Rash from head to trunk that fades 7–10 days Pneumonia (mortality 0.1%) Encephalitis (mortality 11%) Myocarditis, pneumonia, otitis media, panencephalitis Diagnose with hemagglutination test and IgM titers Congenital—if symptoms occur < 10 days of life, increased mortality
Pregnancy	No evidence of more severe symptoms Increased risk of first-trimester abortions	No evidence of more severe symptoms No increased risk of abortions Not teratogenic Increased incidence of prematurity Pregnant, nonimmunized women exposed to measles: Immune globulin within 72 hours after exposure; vaccine is contraindicated during pregnancy; administer vaccine to infant at 15 months

V. Transmission of Infections

Intrauterine: transplacental — rubella (greatest risk during 1st and 3rd trimester), CMV, syphilis, toxo (greatest risk during 3rd trimester), varicella-zoster, coxsackie (greatest risk during 3rd trimester), parvovirus, *Listeria,* HIV
Ascending chorioamnionitis

Intrapartum: exposure during delivery — gonorrhea, chlamydia, herpes simplex, GBS, hepatitis B, HIV, *Listeria,* CMV

Blood transfusion: CMV, HIV, hepatitis B, hepatitis C (thus, blood is filtered to avoid these pathogens)

VI. Breast Feeding and Infections

If HSV lesion lower abd. cover-ok to feed

Lactoferrin: present in high amounts in breast milk; bacteriostatic against numerous bacteria

Lactoperoxidase: present in low amounts in breast milk; requires hydrogen peroxide and thiocyanate for antibacterial effect

CMV, HIV, Hep B, Rub, HSV

Infections that can cross breast milk: CMV, HIV, hepatitis B, rubella, HSV
Note: if mother with hepatitis B, does cross into breast milk but little risk of transmission (especially if infant received IVIG and vaccine) and thus can still breast feed

Contraindications to breast feeding (in US): maternal HIV, mother with HSV lesions on breast, symptomatic mother with positive PPD and CXR (i.e., presumed active TB), active breast abscess

Relative contraindications to breast feeding: consider not breast feeding if premature infant and CMV-seropositive mother (due to low amount transplacentally acquired maternal antibodies), oral HSV lesions (mother to use mask)

VII. Diagnosis

Chlamydia	Giemsa stain
Neisseria gonorrhoeae	Thayer-Martin growth medium
Pertussis	Bordet-Gengou medium
Pseudomonas aeruginosa	Oxidase-positive, catalase-positive
Rubella	Hemagglutination inhibition

VIII. Therapeutics in Infectious Diseases

A. ANTIBIOTICS

Medication	Organism Coverage	Comments
Ampicillin (beta-lactam) A PCN with greater gram-negative coverage	GBS, *Listeria* Gram-positive organisms except *Staph* Some susceptible gram-negative organisms (*Salmonella, Shigella, Haemophilus, E. coli*)	Renal excretion Unasyn= ampicillin + sulbactam; broader coverage
Anti-*Pseudomonas* antibiotics (beta-lactam) Pipercillin (with tazobactam = Zosyn) Ticarcillin (with clavulanate = Timentin)	*Pseudomonas*	Ideal to use with aminoglycoside
		(continued on following page)

Medication	Organism Coverage	Comments
Aztreonam Ceftazidime **Cephalosporin (beta-lactam)** (1st generation)	Most gram-positive cocci, *E. coli*, *Klebsiella* and *Proteus* *None* of the cephalosporins cover enterococcus or Listeria	e.g., cephalexin, cefazolin Treatment of cellulitis Poor CSF penetration
Cephalosporin (beta-lactam) (2nd generation)	More gram-negative coverage compared with 1st generation cephalosporin	e.g., cefoxitin, cefuroxime, cefaclor, cefotetan
Cephalosporin (beta-lactam) 3rd generation)	Excellent gram-negative coverage Cefotaxime and ceftriaxone: GBS, many gram-negative enteric bacilli; gonorrhea and *Salmonella;* some species of *Citrobacter;* no coverage for *Staph* Ceftazidime: ideal for *Pseudomonas* (in combination with aminoglycoside)	e.g., cefotaxime, ceftriaxone and ceftazidime Good CSF penetration Ceftriaxone: possible increased risk of bilirubin displacement from albumin Ceftazidime: may yield false-positive Coombs reaction
Chloramphenicol	Broad-spectrum	Contraindicated in pregnancy due to "gray-baby syndrome" (cyanosis, respiratory distress, vasomotor collapse, gray-ashen color)
Clindamycin	Anaerobic infections, *Staph. aureus* and *Strep*	Good for septic arthritis and osteomyelitis Poor CSF entry Can cause pseudomembranous colitis in older children (rare in neonates)
Erythromycin (macrolide)	*Chlamydia*, *Pertussis*, some minor *Staph* or *Strep* skin infections, *Mycoplasma*, *Ureaplasma*	Poor CSF entry Interferes with hepatic metabolism of aminophylline Increases effect of carbamazepine and digoxin Decreases midazolam clearance Increases gastrointestinal motor activity Association with oral erythromycin and infantile hypertrophic pyloric stenosis in infants < 6 weeks of age
Gentamicin (aminoglycoside)	Most gram-negative enteric bacilli Many *Staph* Provides synergy to *Listeria*, GBS and *Enterococcus* if used with cell wall synthesis inhibitors (e.g., β-lactam antibiotics and vancomycin)	Low CSF penetration Good penetration into synovial, peritoneal, ascitic, and pleural cavities Monitor levels since possible nephrotoxicity (greatest of all aminoglycosides) and ototoxicity At toxic levels, may lead to neuromuscular blockade (worse with hypermagnesemia)
Meropenem (carbapenem) (similar to Imipenem)	Broad-spectrum (except methicillin-resistant *Staph. aureus*, *Enterobacter*, *Pseudomonas*)	Good CSF penetration Imipenem with increased risk of seizures if underlying CNS disease; Meropenem with less neurotoxicity
Penicillin G (beta-lactam)	Majority of *Strep* (pneumococcus coverage is variable), *Treponema pallidum*, *Bacteroides* (except *Bacteroides fragilis*), *Neisseria meningitidis*, some *Staph* infections	Other penicillins include ureido PCN (piperacillin, mezlocillin; for anaerobe coverage, *Pseudomonas*) and carboxy PCN (ticarcillin and carbenicillin; for *Pseudomonas*)
Penicillinase-resistant PCN (methicillin, nafcillin, oxacillin)	*Staph. aureus, Strep* infections, some coag-negative *Staph*	Interstitial nephritis sometimes with methicillin and oxacillin Bone marrow suppression Oral form is dicloxacillin
Sulfonamide (trimethoprim-sulfamethoxazole, sulfadiazine)	Gram-positive organisms and gram-negative organisms (including *H. flu*, *E. coli*), PCP, toxoplasmosis, *Shigella*	NOT recommended in neonates Increased risk of Stevens-Johnson syndrome Displaces bilirubin from albumin Exacerbation of glucose-6 phosphate dehydrogenase deficiency Ideal for urinary tract infections in older children
Tetracycline	Broad-spectrum (gram-negative and gram-positive organisms)	Contraindicated in neonates due to teeth discoloration Blocks skeletal growth Not used in children < 9 years of age
Tobramycin (aminoglycoside)	Broad gram-negative organisms, *Staph. aureus* Usually used with β-lactam antibiotic	Possible nephrotoxicity (< gent) and ototoxicity
Vancomycin	Coagulase-negative *Staph*, methicillin-resistant *Staph aureus*, most gram-positive aerobic organisms, *Clostridium difficile* No activity against gram-negative organisms	Poor CSF penetration Monitor levels since possible nephrotoxicity and ototoxicity If rapid infusion, may lead to flushing and/or hypotension (=red-man syndrome)

Modified from Fanaroff AA and Martin RJ (eds): Neonatal-Perinatal Medicine (6th edition). St Louis, Mosby–Year Book Inc, 1997, p 729 and 730.

B. ACTION OF ANTIBIOTICS

Action	Antibiotics
Bactericidal Completely destroy bacteria (ideal for endocarditis, meningitis, severe *Staph* and gram-negative infections)	Penicillins — inhibit bacterial enzymes (penicillin-binding proteins) necessary for the synthesis of peptidoglycan (important component of cell wall) Cephalosporins—bind to penicillin-binding proteins and inhibit bacterial cell wall synthesis Aminoglycosides — bind to 30S subunit of bacterial ribosomes and inhibit protein synthesis Vancomycin — inhibit peptidoglycan synthesis in bacteria cell wall Quinolones — inhibit DNA gyrase
Bacteriostatic Inhibit growth and reproduction of bacteria	Erythromycin — bind reversibly to the 50S subunit of bacterial ribosomes and inhibit protein synthesis Clindamycin Chloramphenicol Tetracycline (at therapeutic concentrations)—bind reversibly to 30S subunit of bacterial ribosome Sulfonamides — inhibit folate synthesis Vancomycin

C. IMMUNE GLOBULIN (IG)

Characteristics
   From pooled adult plasma
   95% IgG, trace IgA, and IgM
   Concentrated protein solution with specific antibodies present in population

Clinical
   Intramuscular IG for hepatitis A and measles prophylaxis (causes pain at site)
   Specific IG for hepatitis B, rabies, tetanus, varicella-zoster, CMV, RSV
   Intravenous IG for primary immunodeficiency, Kawasaki disease, HIV, premature infants (controversial use to prevent late-onset infection)

Contraindication
   IgA deficiency with antibodies to IgA

IX. Development of the immune system

Hematopoiesis in yolk sac during 3rd week of development, in fetal liver at ~8 weeks gestation, and in bone marrow at ~5 months gestation

T- cell lymphopoiesis:
8.5 weeks gestation	Precursors in fetal lever
10 weeks gestation	Thymus becomes lymphoid
11–12 weeks gestation	T cells emigrate from thymus to spleen, nodes
16–18 weeks gestation	Hassall's bodies in thymus

B-cell lymphopoiesis:
~8 weeks gestation	Pre-B cells in fetal liver
8-10 weeks gestation	In fetal bone marrow
18–22 weeks gestation	Also in liver, lung, and kidney
>30 weeks gestation	B cell production solely in bone marrow

X. Natural Immune System Components, Neonatal Ability, and Disorders

A. COMPONENTS OF NATURAL IMMUNE SYSTEM

Natural immune system: first-line defense, non-specific, rapid availability, does not rely on T or B cells, does not require prior exposure to organism or antigen for function

Component	Function	Neonate	Examples of Abnormalities
Neutrophils	Chemotaxis Phagocytosis Bacterial killing	Decreased migration Normal bacterial killing if healthy, decreased ability if ill Limited neutrophil pool and thus decreased ability to increase # of neutrophils	Chédiak-Higashi (partial oculocutaneous albinism, nystagmus, peripheral neuropathy, recurrent infections) Hyper IgE syndrome (= Job's syndrome, abnormal neutrophil chemotaxis, recurrent infections — especially involving skin, coarse facial features, broad nasal bridge, eczema) Leukocyte adhesion defects (increased neutrophils but they are defective, recurrent bacterial infections with poor wound healing, necrotic skin lesions, delayed separation of umbilical cord at birth) Chronic granulomatous disease (X-linked in majority, dysfunctional NADPH oxidase and abnormal phagocytic microbial ability, normal B and T cell function, increased risk abscesses, poor wound healing, granuloma formation) Myeloperoxidase deficiency (increased risk fungal infections)
Monocyte	Chemotaxis Phagocytosis Bacterial killing Wound repair	Decreased migration	Leukocyte adhesion defects Histiocytosis Chédiak-Higashi syndrome (defective monocyte chemotaxis) Wiskott-Aldrich syndrome Chronic granulomatous disease
Complement	Important for opsonization of foreign particles Chemoattraction Inflammation Classical complement pathway (requires antigen-antibody reaction) and alternative complement pathway (can be antibody-independent)	Decreased complement (premature infants lower amounts compared with full-term infants) Most neonates reach adult levels at 3–6 mos of age	Deficiency of early components (C1-C4; C2 is most common), increased risk of infections (especially pneumococcal) and collagen vascular disease Deficiency of late components (C5-C9), increased risk of *Neisseria* infection Hereditary angioedema (autosomal dominant, absence of esterase inhibitor, recurrent swelling) Leiner syndrome (generalized erythematous desquamative dermatitis, failure to thrive, diarrhea, and recurrent infections; associated with functional complement 5 abnormality)

Modified from Fanaroff AA and Martin RJ (eds): Neonatal-Perinatal Medicine (6th edition), St Louis, Mosby-Year Book Inc, 1997, p 719.

Basophils/mast cells
Release inflammatory mediators, important in atopic allergies

Eosinophils
Release inflammatory mediators (such as leukotrienes, prostaglandins, and cytokines), modulate immediate hypersensitivity reactions, and antiparasitic activity
Leukotrienes: important in leukocyte motility and metabolism, platelet aggregation
Prostaglandins: important in leukocyte motility and metabolism, platelet aggregation, contribute to fever production

Cytokines

Regulate cellular activity, important in intercellular signaling, mediators of host's response to infection

Interferon-alpha: majority from lymphocytes and macrophages, inhibits viral replication, blocks cellular proliferation, activates natural killer cells

Tumor necrosis factor alpha: secreted by macrophages, T and B cells, mast cells, and eosinophils; promotes inflammation

Interleukins (IL)-1: secreted by macrophages, activates T-cells and macrophages, promotes inflammation, contributes to septic shock, and induces fever by increasing prostaglandin production

Acute phase reactants

Promote phagocytosis, stimulate cytokines, promote tissue repair

e.g., C-reactive protein, proteinase inhibitors, protein C and protein S, fibrinogen and haptoglobin

Innate system also includes

Physical barrier (skin and mucous membranes), normal flora, natural antibodies, hormones, and natural killer cells

XI. Acquired Immune System Components, Neonatal Ability, and Disorders

A. COMPONENTS OF ACQUIRED IMMUNE SYSTEM

Acquired immune system: a specific response that relies on T and B cells, requires memory

Component	Function	Neonate	Disorder
T lymphocytes: CD4 T cells (cytokine secreting helper cells) and CD8 T cells (cytotoxic killer cells)	Must travel to thymus to complete development Activate macrophages Cell-mediated T-helper cells (with macrophages) present antigen to B-lymphocytes	Decreased T-cell function including cytotoxicity, participation in delayed-type hypersensitivity and assistance in B-cell differentiation	Severe combined immunodeficiency Adenosine deaminase deficiency Ataxia-telangiectasia DiGeorge syndrome Wiskott-Aldrich syndrome (X-linked, thrombocytopenia, eczema, recurrent infections) Chronic mucocutaneous candidiasis

B lymphocytes	Mature within bone marrow
	Humoral-mediated
	Produce immunoglobulins (Ig = antibodies)
	  IgA (secretory, in saliva, colostrum, respiratory secretions, and gastrointestinal secretions)
	  IgG (binds and activates complement, binds to Fc receptor to facilitate action)
	  IgM (binds and activates complement, first antibody expressed after infectivity)
	  IgE (allergic reaction – binds to basophils and mast cells leading to histamine and leukotriene release)
	  IgD (seems to function as an antigen receptor, important in regulation of B-cell development)
		Premature infants with poor antibody response to infection
		IgG is only antibody that crosses the placenta to provide passive protection to neonate
			X-linked agammaglobulinemia: severe deficiency of B cells leading to hypogammaglobulinemia, recurrent infections 4–12 months of age including pneumonia, otitis, sepsis, meningitis, septic arthritis, diarrhea, and sinusitis
			X-linked hyper IgM syndrome (low IgG, IgA and IgE but normal or increased IgM, increased risk of infections 6 mos-2 years of age)
			Selective IgA and subclass IgG deficiency
			Job's syndrome (increased IgE levels)
			Common variable immunodeficiency

B. IMMUNOGLOBULIN LEVELS WITH AGE

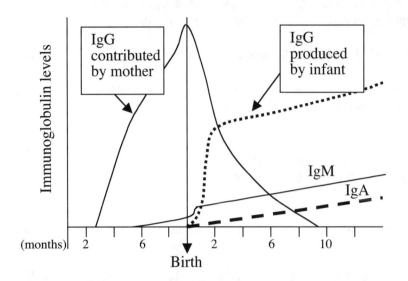

IgG contributed by mother

IgG produced by infant

IgM

IgA

IgG: during fetal period, all IgG from mother following active placental transport, maternal IgG disappears by 9 months of age

IgM: 75% of adult levels are reached by 1 year of age, some fetal IgM production

IgA: no fetal IgA production, levels at 1 year of age about 20% adult amount

Modified from Stiehm ER (ed): Immunologic Disorders in Infants and Children (4th edition), WB Saunders Company, Philadelphia, 1996, p 67.

XII. Blood Cells and Infection

Anemia	Chronic infection (increased risk with fungi, TB, osteo)
	May also be due to hemolysis (e.g., syphilis, rubella) or direct infection of progenitor cells (parvovirus B19, HIV)
Disseminated intravascular Coagulation	= low platelets, increased D-dimers, prolonged PT and PTT, prolonged thrombin time, decreased fibrinogen
	Often initiated by endotoxin
Eosinophilia	Due to increased bone marrow proliferation
	Parasitic and fungal infections
	Often observed in *chlamydia* pneumonia
Lymphocytopenia	HIV, some viral infectious (due to direct destruction or trapping in spleen or lymph nodes)
Lymphocytosis	Infection — CMV, toxo, viral hepatitis, HIV
Neutropenia	Infection (direct damage of precursors, demand > supply, bone marrow suppression, splenic sequestration), especially with gram-negative sepsis
	Also observed in :
	Maternal autoimmune disease (e.g., lupus)
	Congenital disorders (Schwachman-Diamond syndrome, Chédiak-Higashi)
	Drug-induced (phenothiazines, non-steroidal anti-inflammatory medications, sulfonamides)
	Metabolic diseases (e.g., glycogen storage type Ib)
	Following in utero growth restriction
Neutrophilia	Infection (mobilization from bone marrow, increased proliferation)
Thrombocytopenia	Consumptive coagulopathy, sequestration in spleen, disseminated infection (e.g., rubella, CMV, toxo)
	Also observed following in utero growth restriction
Thrombocytosis	Acute phase reaction during infection
	Also can be observed in growing premature infants

XIII. Screening Tests

Ab-mediated immunity	Quantitative immunoglobulin levels
	Isohemagglutinin titers
	Antibody response to vaccines
Cell-mediated immunity	Total T cells and subset CD4/ CD8
	Delayed-type hypersensitivity skin tests (mumps, candida, tetanus)
Phagocytosis	Quantitative nitroblue tetrazolium (NBT) test
Complement	Total hemolytic complement (CH50)
	Quantitative complement levels
Chronic granulomatous disease (CGD)	NBT test—neutrophils in patients with CGD cannot produce superoxide and thus NBT test is negative

XIV. Splenic Function

Splenic role
  Synthesis of antibodies against carbohydrate antigens
  Clears microorganisms from bloodstream

Effect of splenectomy
  Increased susceptibility to infection
  Usually rapid onset to infection, greater likelihood of infection being fatal
  Majority of infections are pneumococcal but can also involve meningococci, *E. coli,* H. flu, Staph infections, *Strep. pyogenes,* malaria and viruses

References

Cloherty JC and Stark AR (eds): Manual of Neonatal Care (4th edition), Infectious Disease Section. Philadelphia, Lippincott–Raven Publishers, 1998.

Cunningham FG, Gant NF, Leveno KJ, et al (eds): Williams Obstetrics (21st edition). New York, McGraw-Hill, 2001.

Fanaroff AA and Martin RJ (eds): Neonatal-Perinatal Medicine (6th edition). St Louis, Mosby–Year Book Inc, 1997.

Gerdes, JS: Clinicopathologic approach to the diagnosis of neonatal sepsis. *Clinics Perinatol* 1991; 18(2):361–381.

Hall CB: RSV *Contemporary Pediatrics,* November 1993: 92–110.

Jenkins M. and Kohl S: New aspects of neonatal herpes. *Infect Dis Clin No Amer* 1992; 6(2):57-74.

Mandell GL, Bennett JE and Dolin R (eds): Principles and Practice of Infectious Diseases (5th edition). Philadelphia, Churchill Livingstone, 2000.

Pickering LK (ed): 2000 Red Book: Report of the Committee on Infectious Diseases (25th edition), Elk Grove Village, IL, American Academy of Pediatrics, 2000.

Remington JS and Klein JO (eds): Infectious Diseases of the Fetus and Newborn Infant (5th edition), Philadelphia, WB Saunders Company, 2001.

Stoll B: Congenital syphilis. *Pediatr Infect Dis J* 1994; 13:845-53.

References for Immunology

Delves PJ and Roitt IM. The immune system: First of two parts. *N Engl J Med* 2000; 343(1):37-49.

Delves PJ and Roitt IM. The immune system: Second of two parts. *N Engl J Med* 2000; 343(2):108–117

Mandell GL, Bennett JE and Dolin R (eds): Principles and Practice of Infectious Diseases (5th edition). Philadelphia, Churchill Livingstone, 2000.

Remington JS and Klein JO (eds): Infectious Diseases of the Fetus and Newborn Infant (5th edition), Philadelphia, WB Saunders Company, 2001.

Stiehm ER (ed): Immunologic Disorders in Infants and Children (4th edition). Philadelphia, WB Saunders Company, 1996.

CHAPTER 7

Fluids, Electrolytes, and Renal System

TOPICS COVERED IN THIS CHAPTER

I. Water Metabolism

A. BODY WATER COMPARTMENTS

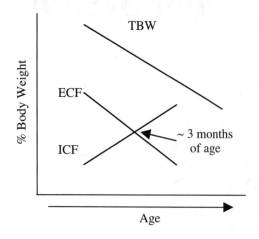

	24 Weeks GA	32 Weeks GA	Birth	3 Months of Age	1 Year of Age
TBW (% body weight)	90	83	80	70	65
ECF (% body weight)	65	53	45	35	20
ICF (% body weight)	25	30	35	35	45

TBW = total body water; ECF = extracellular fluid; and ICF = intracellular fluid; Modified from Fanaroff, AA and Martin RJ (eds): Neonatal and Perinatal Medicine: Diseases of the Fetus and Newborn (6th Edition). St. Louis, Mosby, 1997, p 623.

TBW and ECF decreases with increasing gestational age, while ICF increases with age

Early weight loss in newborns primarily due to water loss from the extracellular fluid compartment

B. MONITORING WATER BALANCE

Monitoring water balance can be accomplished by close monitoring of:
  Serial weight change—weight loss of 5–15% can be observed with fluid loss
  Fluid balance with input and output measurements; normal urine output is 1–3 cc/kg/day, stool may contain 5–10 cc/kg/day of water
  Electrolytes
  Physiologic and environmental states that can increase or decrease water losses

To correct free H_2O deficit, administer 4 cc/kg of free H_2O for every 1 mEq/L increase in Na^+ over 145; if $Na^+ > 170$ mEq/L, replace with 3 cc/kg of free H_2O

C. MECHANISM OF INSENSIBLE WATER LOSS

Neonatal evaporative water loss
  1/3 via respiratory tract, 2/3 through skin

Factors leading to increased insensible losses
  Decreasing gestational age
  Increased environmental and body temperatures
  Skin breakdown
  Congenital skin defects
  Radiant warmer
  Phototherapy

Factors leading to decreased insensible losses
  Humidity
  Plastic heat shield

D. ENDOCRINE CONTROL OF WATER METABOLISM

1. Arginine vasopressin (AVP)/antidiuretic hormone (ADH)
Physiology: present in fetus at 11 weeks
  This octapeptide is produced in cell bodies of neurons located in supraoptic and paraventricular nuclei of the hypothalamus
  It is stored in secretory granules in posterior pituitary gland and released when small increases in plasma osmolality occur (as small as 3 milliosm);

$$\text{Plasma osmolality} = 2 \times (\text{plasma Na}^+) + \frac{\text{glucose mg/dL}}{18} + \frac{\text{BUN mg/dL}}{2.8}$$

  The hormone then acts directly on late distal tubule as well as cortical and medullary collecting ducts
Actions:
  Primary determinant of water excretion in kidney
  Increases permeability of the cortical and medullary collecting tubules to water
  Secondary increase in urine osmolality
  Extrarenal effect of arterial vasoconstriction
  Note that the response of fetus and premature infant to vasopressin is blunted (indicating end-organ insensitivity)

2. Syndrome of inappropriate ADH secretion (SIADH)
Etiology: pain, opiates, intraventricular hemorrhage, perinatal depression, pneumothorax, positive pressure ventilation
Clinical: water retention (weight gain), dilution and expansion of body fluids, hyponatremia (note that Na$^+$ is still excreted in urine despite hyponatremia), higher than appropriate urine osmolality in setting of low plasma osmolality, decreased urine output
Management: free water restriction; if Na $<$ 120 mEq/L, replace with NaCl; consider furosemide

3. Nephrogenic diabetes insipidus (NDI)
Etiology: insensitivity of renal tubule to ADH
  Congenital—X-linked recessive [V2 (vasopressin) receptor defect]; autosomal (aquaporin defect)
  Secondary—hypokalemia, hypercalcemia, renal failure
Clinical: increased urine output, dehydration, failure to thrive
Labs: increased Na$^+$, hypotonic urine in presence of serum hypertonicity, increased calcium, decreased K$^+$
Management: hydrate, monitor electrolytes, thiazides to increase urine concentrating ability (K$^+$ supplementation as needed)
Prognosis: good outcome if diagnosed early

E. MANAGEMENT OF WATER BALANCE

1. Fluid changes in disease states
Perinatal depression
  Decreased urine output secondary to SIADH and/or renal parenchymal injury (acute tubular necrosis or ATN)
  Restrict fluid intake to avoid fluid overload
  Replace insensible losses ($\sim$30–40 cc/kg/day, this replacement is higher in premature infants)
  Avoid hyperkalemia by limiting K$^+$ supplementation
  During recovery of ATN, some patients may have large losses of Na$^+$, so need to quantify and replace
Respiratory distress syndrome (RDS)
  Although it was previously thought that the diuretic phase led to improvement of RDS, it now seems more likely that these two events are not directly related; rather,
    Diuresis probably coincides with contraction of body fluid, which occurs at the same time as RDS naturally improves; and
    Artificial surfactant improves respiratory status and does not depend on diuresis

Patent ductus arteriosus (PDA)
  Increased risk for PDA with fluid overload
  During treatment of PDA, indomethacin may decrease urine output and lead to fluid overload
Chronic lung disease (CLD)
  During treatment of CLD, ideal to achieve a balance of high-caloric intake and basic fluid requirements without leading to fluid overload
  Management of CLD with diuretics increases risk for electrolyte abnormalities and osteopenia of prematurity

II. Electrolyte Metabolism

A. ELECTROLYTE CONTENT IN BODY FLUIDS (mmol/L)

Fluid source	Na^+	K^+	Cl^-
Stomach	20–80	5–20	100–150
Small intestine	100–140	5–15	90–120
Bile	120–140	5–15	90–120
Ileostomy	45–135	3–15	20–120
Diarrheal stool	10–90	10–80	10–110

Printed with permission from Fanaroff, AA and Martin RJ (eds): Neonatal and Perinatal Medicine: Diseases of the Fetus and Newborn (6th Edition). St. Louis, Mosby, 1997, p 625.

Electrolyte replacement can be calculated by multiplying the total volume of body fluid loss by the corresponding electrolyte composition

B. HYPONATREMIA

Factitious values can result from:
  Hyperlipidemia—Na^+ decreased by 0.002 × lipid concentration in mg/dL
  Hyperproteinemia—Na^+ decreased by 0.25 × protein concentration in gm/dL
  Hyperglycemia—Na^+ decreased by 1.6 mEq/L for each 100 increase in glucose (mg/dL)

Differential diagnosis of nonfactitious hyponatremia

HYPONATREMIA*		
Decreased Weight		
Renal Losses	**Extrarenal Losses**	**Increased or Normal Weight**
CAUSE		
Na^+-losing nephropathy	GI losses	Nephrotic syndrome
Diuretics	Skin losses	Congestive heart failure
Adrenal insufficiency	Third spacing	SIADH
	Cystic fibrosis	Acute/chronic renal failure
		Water intoxication
		Cirrhosis
		Excess salt-free infusions
LABORATORY DATA		
↑ Urine Na^+	↓ Urine Na^+	↓ Urine Na^+
↑ Urine volume	↓ Urine volume	↓ Urine volume
↓ Specific gravity	↑ Specific gravity	↑ Specific gravity
↓ Urine osmolality	↑ Urine osmolality	↑ Urine osmolality

(continued on following page)

Renal Losses	Extrarenal Losses	Increased or Normal Weight
MANAGEMENT		
Replace losses Treat cause	Replace losses Treat cause	Restrict fluids Treat cause

GI, gastrointestinal; *SIADH*, syndrome of inappropriate antidiuretic hormone secretion.

  *Hyperglycemia and hyperlipidemia cause spurious hyponatremia.

  †Urine Na^+ may be appropriate for level of Na^+ intake in patients with SIADH (or increased) and water intoxication.

  Printed with permission from Gunn VL and Nechyba C (eds): The Harriet Lane Handbook (16th Edition). Philadelphia, Mosby, 2002, p 244.

Na^+ deficit (mEq) = [Na^+ desired (mEq/L) − Na^+ current (mEq/L)] × 0.6 × weight (kg); 0.6 represents volume of distribution (L/kg)

C. HYPERNATREMIA

HYPERNATREMIA

	Decreased Weight		Increased Weight
Renal Losses	**Extrarenal Losses**		**Increased Weight**
CAUSE			
Nephropathy Diuretic use Diabetes insipidus Postobstructive diuresis Diuretic phase of ATN	GI losses Respiratory losses* Skin losses		Exogenous $Na^{+†}$ Mineralocorticoid excess Hyperaldosteronism
LABORATORY DATA			
↑ Urine volume ↑ Urine Na^+ ↓ Specific gravity	↓ Urine volume ↓ Urine Na^+ ↑ Specific gravity		Relative ↓ urine volume Relative ↓ urine Na^+ Relative ↑ specific gravity
MANAGEMENT			
Replace FW losses based on calculations in text and treat cause. Consider a natriuretic agent if there is increased weight.			

ATN, Acute tubular necrosis; *FW*, free water; *GI*, gastrointestinal.

  *This cause of hypernatremia is usually secondary to free water loss, so that the fractional excretion of sodium may be decreased or normal.

  †Exogenous Na^+ administration will cause an increase in the fractional excretion of sodium.

  Printed with permission from Gunn VL and Nechyba C (eds): The Harriet Lane Handbook (16th Edition). Philadelphia, Mosby, 2002, p 245.

D. HYPOKALEMIA

HYPOKALEMIA

	Decreased Stores		Normal Stores
		Normal BP	
Hypertension	**Renal**	**Extrarenal**	**Normal Stores**
Renovascular disease Excess renin Excess mineralocorticoid Cushing syndrome	RTA Fanconi syndrome Bartter syndrome DKA Antibiotics Diuretics Amphotericin B	Skin losses GI losses High CHO diet Enema abuse Laxative abuse Malnutrition	Metabolic alkalosis ↑ Insulin Leukemia β_2 catecholamines Familial hypokalemic periodic alkalosis

(continued on following page)

Hypertension	Renal	Extrarenal	Normal Stores
LABORATORY DATA			
↑ Urine K^+	↑ Urine K^+	↓ Urine K^+	↑ Urine K^+

CHO, Carbohydrate; *DKA*, diabetic ketoacidosis; *GI*, gastrointestinal; *RTA*, renal tubular acidosis.
Printed with permission from Gunn VL and Nechyba C (eds): The Harriet Lane Handbook (16th Edition). Philadelphia, Mosby, 2002, p 242.

EKG changes
  Atrioventricular conduction defect, U wave, ventricular arrhythmias, depressed ST segment

Mechanisms
  Alkalosis—H^+ exits cell to compensate, K^+ enters the cell
  Insulin—increased intracellular uptake of K^+ by direct stimulation via Na/K ATPase
  Volume contraction and hypokalemia (as occurs with diuretic use)
    Reduction in ECF volume → increased Na^+ reabsorption (although competing with losses induced by diuretic) → increased renal K^+ and H^+ secretion → HCO_3^- reabsorption increases to maintain neutrality
    Volume depletion → stimulates renin → increases aldosterone → promotes further Na^+ reabsorption and K^+/H^+ secretion
    Management of volume contraction and hypokalemia:
      Potassium chloride repletion—this will restore K^+ and Cl^- levels; in addition, the increased K^+ levels will limit net H^+ excretion and therefore, reduce HCO_3^- reabsorption and normalize plasma levels of HCO_3^-
      Volume repletion with saline bolus to replete volume status and replace Na^+ losses

E. HYPERKALEMIA

HYPERKALEMIA		
Increased Stores		
Increased Urine K^+	**Decreased Urine K^+**	**Normal Stores**
Transfusion with aged blood	Renal failure	Cell lysis syndromes
Exogenous K^+ (e.g., salt substitutes)	Hypoaldosteronism	Leukocytosis (>100 K/mm²)
	Aldosterone insensitivity	Thrombocytosis (>750 K/mm²)
	↓ Insulin	Metabolic acidosis*
	K^+-sparing diuretics	Blood drawing (hemolyzed sample)
	Congenital adrenal hyperplasia	Type IV RTA
		Rhabdomyolysis/crush injury
		Malignant hyperthermia
		Theophylline intoxication

*For every 0.1-unit reduction in arterial pH, there is an approximately 0.2–0.4 mEq/L increase in plasma K^+.
  In addition to above, tissue destruction (e.g. necrotizing enterocolitis) may lead to hyperkalemia with normal stores; Printed with permission from Gunn VL and Nechyba C (eds): The Harriet Lane Handbook (16th Edition). Philadelphia, Mosby, 2002, p 243.

EKG changes (in order of increasing [K^+])
  Peaked T waves
  Loss of P waves, wide QRS
  ST segment depression, increasing width of QRS
  Bradycardia, first-degree atrioventricular block, ventricular arrhythmias, cardiac arrest

Management
  Remove all exogenous potassium sources
  10% Ca Gluconate—1–2 cc/kg
  Glucose—$D_{10}W$ 2 cc/kg + insulin 0.05 units/kg

Insulin increases intracellular uptake of K^+ by direct stimulation of Na/K ATPase

Lasix—1 mg/kg (effective only if renal function is normal)

$NaHCO_3^-$—1–2 mEq/kg (theoretical concern for acute hypocalcemia and may not be as effective as above)

Kayexalate—cation exchange resin, 1 g/kg rectally; use cautiously with premature infants who may have bowel ischemia

III. Acid-Base Balance

A. ACID-BASE REGULATION

Extracellular pH in newborn $\sim$ 7.35–7.43

1. Acute compensation

Acid-base balance maintained by the use of intracellular and extracellular buffers

a. *Intracellular buffers*

   Bone apatite (major buffer system)

   Hemoglobin

   Organic phosphates

b. *Extracellular buffers*

   HCO_3^-

   Phosphates

   Proteins

   Major buffer system is:

$$HCO_3^- + H^+ \leftrightarrow H_2CO_3 \xleftrightarrow{\text{carbonic anhydrase}} H_2O + CO_2$$

The CO_2 that is generated crosses into brain, decreases the pH, and stimulates chemoreceptors; this increases respiratory drive, thereby eliminating CO_2

$$pH = 6.1 + \log\left[\frac{[HCO_3^-]}{0.03 \times P_{co_2}}\right]$$

(6.1 is the pKa of the carbonic acid-bicarbonate buffer)

H^+ crosses the cell membrane to gain access to the intracellular or extracellular space and reaches these buffer systems by using *3 exchange mechanisms:* Na^+/H^+, K^+/H^+, and HCO_3^-/Cl^-

Therefore, acidosis can lead to hyperkalemia (for each 0.1 decrease in pH $\rightarrow$ increase K by 0.6 mEq/L) and alkalosis can lead to hypokalemia   *each 0.1 ↑ in ph – ↓ K+ by 0.6 meq/L*

2. Chronic compensation

Balance between intake/production and metabolism/excretion of acid

The intracellular buffer of bone apatite can also assist with chronic acidosis; may get increased bone resorption and decreased bone Na^+, K^+, and calcium carbonate

Acid production:

1. CO_2 production primarily excreted by respiratory system (volatile acid)

2. By-products of metabolism (nonvolatile acid):

   Sulfuric acid from methionine and cysteine

   Organic acids

Phosphoric acid
Hydrochloric acid
Kidney plays primary role in handling nonvolatile acid load by:
Excretion
Reabsorption of HCO_3^-
Maintenance of pH by regulation of HCO_3^- excretion/reabsorption (depending on pCO_2 concentration)
Kidney accomplishes above tasks by *urinary acidification*
60–80% of bicarbonate reabsorption occurs in the *proximal tubule*
Depends on Na^+/H^+ exchange (see figure below)

3. Mechanisms of acid-base balance in kidney

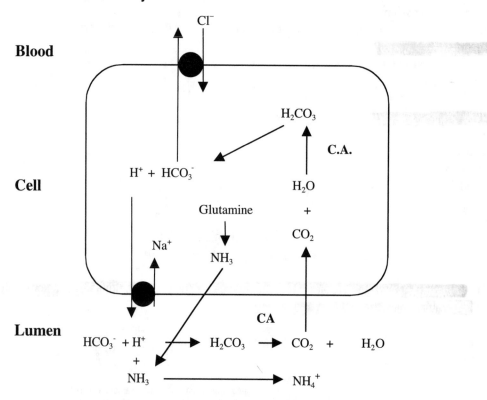

Mechanisms of acid-base balance in proximal tubule.
CA = carbonic anhydrase; Printed with permission from Fanaroff, AA and Martin RJ (eds): Neonatal and Perinatal Medicine:
Diseases of the Fetus and Newborn (6th Edition). St. Louis, Mosby, 1997, p 631.

CO_2 is formed and enters cell
Bicarbonate is produced and reabsorbed into blood stream in exchange for Cl^-
NH_4^+ is produced from glutamine

Loop of Henle and *distal tubule* do not play a significant role in urinary acidification

Cortical and medullary collecting tubule
Electrogenic H^+ secretion against a pH gradient; the H^+ that exits the cell can then bind to any available substrates
(see below figure)
Adsorption and secretion of NH_4^+ into urine, and this prevents loss of other cations (Na^+, K^+, Ca^{++})

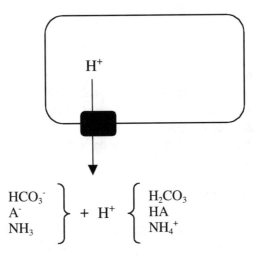

$$\left.\begin{array}{l} HCO_3^- \\ A^- \\ NH_3 \end{array}\right\} + H^+ \left\{\begin{array}{l} H_2CO_3 \\ HA \\ NH_4^+ \end{array}\right.$$

Modified from Fanaroff, AA and Martin RJ (eds): Neonatal and Perinatal Medicine: Diseases of the Fetus and Newborn (6th Edition). St. Louis, Mosby, 1997, p 632.

Newborn acid-base balance

Reduced HCO_3^- reabsorption in proximal tubule

Immature distal acidification

4. Laboratory analysis of acid-base disorders

	ΔP_{CO2} (mm Hg)	ΔHCO_3^- (mEq/L)	pH
Respiratory			
Acute acidosis	↑ 1	↑ 0.1	
Acute alkalosis	↓ 1	↓ 0.1-0.3	
Chronic acidosis	↑ 1	↑ 0.4-0.5	
Chronic alkalosis	↓ 1	↓ 0.2-0.5	
Pure respiratory	$\Delta +/- 10$		$\Delta +/- 0.08$

	ΔHCO_3^- (mEq/L)	ΔP_{CO2} (mm Hg)	pH
Metabolic			
Acidosis	↓ 1	↓ 1.0-1.5	
Alkalosis	↑ 1	↑ 0.2-1.0	
Pure metabolic	$\Delta +/- 10$		$\Delta +/- 0.15$

Note: pH never completely normalizes; Modified from Fanaroff, AA and Martin RJ (eds): Neonatal and Perinatal Medicine: Diseases of the Fetus and Newborn (6th Edition). St. Louis, Mosby, 1997, p 634; and Gunn VL and Nechyba C (eds): The Harriet Lane Handbook (16th Edition). Philadelphia, Mosby, 2002, p 519-520.

B. METABOLIC ACIDOSIS

Anion gap

$= [Na^+] - ([Cl^-] + [HCO_3^-])$

Metabolic acidosis with increased anion gap

Lactic acidosis (hypoxemia, shock, sepsis)

Acute renal failure

Inborn errors of metabolism

Organic acidemias—e.g., methylmalonic acidemia

Lactic acidosis—e.g., pyruvate dehydrogenase or carboxylase deficiency

Mitochondrial respiratory chain abnormalities

Glycogen storage disease type I

Galactosemia

Hereditary fructose intolerance

Toxins

Metabolic acidosis with normal anion gap

Renal—renal tubular acidosis, acetazolamide administration, renal dysplasia, obstructive uropathy, early uremia

Gastrointestinal—diarrhea, ileal drainage, cholestyramine administration, small bowel drainage

Decreased aldosterone—congenital adrenal hyperplasia

Hyperalimentation and administration of excess acid and amino acids

High-protein formula

Congenital hypothyroidism

Administration of $NaHCO_3^-$

HCO_3^- replacement $= 0.3 \times$ base excess $\times$ weight (in kg)

During administration:

1. Can worsen acidosis if poor pulmonary blood flow/ventilation ratio since cannot eliminate CO_2
2. Increased risk of hypernatremia
3. Calcium decreases since HCO_3^- causes Ca to bind to albumin and thus decreases ionized Ca concentration
4. K^+ may decrease
5. Increased risk of developing intraventricular hemorrhage secondary to hypertonicity

C. METABOLIC ALKALOSIS

Etiologies

Metabolic alkalosis with low urine chloride

Acid loss—vomiting, nasogastric suctioning

Diuretics (late)—secondary severe contraction alkalosis

Secretory diarrhea

Correction of chronic respiratory acidosis

Metabolic alkalosis with high urine chloride

Bartter syndrome with mineralocorticoid excess

Cl^- deficiency—e.g., Bartter syndrome, hypochloremic diet, chloride losses in diarrhea

Exogenous HCO_3^-, acetate, or citrate

Increased aldosterone—stimulates distal H^+ secretion

Diuretic therapy (early)

Hypochloremic, metabolic alkalosis

Pyloric stenosis

Cystic fibrosis

Bartter syndrome

Diuretic therapy

D. ACID-BASE DISORDERS

1. Renal tubular acidosis (RTA)

Normal anion gap metabolic acidosis

Secondary to decreased H^+ renal tubular secretion or decreased HCO_3^- reabsorption independent of glomerular filtration rate

Clinical presentation:

Polyuria, induced by:

Hypercalciuria (increased bone mobilization occurs to buffer evolving acidosis and this leads to increased excretion of excess Ca)

Increased risk for nephrocalcinosis, more common in Type I RTA (this type of nephrocalcinosis usually does not resolve in contrast to diuretic-induced nephrocalcinosis)

Chronic hypokalemia (volume contraction leads to increased aldosterone, which increases K^+ excretion)

Decreased K^+ also contributes to decreased ability to concentrate urine

Constipation—due to hypokalemia associated muscle weakness

Failure to thrive—metabolic acidosis blunts growth hormone axis and release; also decreased interest in feeding (anorexia) with acidosis

Evaluation:

Serum electrolytes

Urine pH and electrolytes including calcium, citrate, potassium, and oxalate

Renal ultrasound

Urine—blood partial pressure of CO_2 (normal values $>$ 20 mm Hg, type I RTA $<$ 20 mm Hg)

Tubular reabsorption of phosphate (TRP)

Type I = distal or "classic" RTA

Etiology:

Primary—majority autosomal dominant, can be autosomal recessive (particularly if associated with deafness)

Secondary—interstitial renal disease, genetic syndromes, autoimmune disease, hyponatriuric states, drug-induced

Pathology:

Cannot secrete H^+ in distal tubule, renal bicarbonate threshold is normal

Studies:

Urine pH $>$ 6.2—can't acidify urine

Decreased urine: blood pCO_2 gradient after HCO_3^- administration

Management and prognosis:

HCO_3^- or citrate

Minimize calcium excretion in urine to prevent stones

If effective treatment, expect adequate growth and normal renal function

Type II = proximal RTA

Etiology:

Primary—autosomal recessive, autosomal dominant, sporadic

Secondary—prematurity, Fanconi syndrome, cystinosis, tyrosinemia, Lowe syndrome

Pathology:

Decreased or absent proximal tubular HCO_3^- reabsorption, reduced renal bicarbonate reabsorption threshold

Normal distal acidification

Urinary findings:

Large urine losses HCO_3^-

Can have urine pH $<$ 5.3 when reach plasma HCO_3^- concentrations less than the renal threshold (or Tm—tubular maximum for reabsorption of HCO_3^-) with the aid of an intact distal acidification system

Normal urine concentrating ability

Lack of renal stones

Substantial K^+ losses ($>$ than type I) since K^+ excretion instead of H^+ excretion

Management:

HCO_3^- or citrate, $+/-$ phosphate, vitamin D

Prognosis:

Recovery usually expected in 2-3 years

Require more HCO_3^- to treat proximal RTA since constant HCO_3^- wasting compared with distal RTA; however, proximal RTA more likely to resolve

Type III RTA

Old nomenclature, no longer used since it is now known to be an infantile variant of type I

Type IV RTA
  Etiology:
    Aldosterone deficiency and aldosterone resistance
  Pathology:
    Abnormal aldosterone production or change in tubular sensitivity to aldosterone
  Clinical:
    Hyperkalemic RTA with hyperchloremic metabolic acidosis
    Subtypes (5 subtypes, 1, 4, 5 most common):
      1. Aldosterone deficiency—NaCl wasting, increased renin, decreased pH, increased K^+, decreased urine aldosterone; associated with Addison's disease and congenital adrenal hyperplasia; treat with aldosterone
      2. Pseudohypoaldosteronism (rare)—increased urine aldosterone but tubule insensitive to aldosterone leading to salt-wasting, decreased pH, and increased K^+; treat with HCO_3^-
      3. "Early childhood RTA" (most common)—tubule insensitive to aldosterone effect, salt reabsorption normal; typically matures with age; treat with HCO_3^-

2. Bartter syndrome

Definition:
  Hypertrophy and hyperplasia of renal juxtaglomerular apparatus
Pathophysiology:
  Increased renin, increased aldosterone, hypokalemic metabolic alkalosis, normal parathyroid hormone
Etiology:
  Defect of chloride transport in ascending loop preventing reabsorption
Clinical:
  Often diagnosed late in neonatal period; can present with dehydration and/or failure to thrive
  Blood pressure remains normal
  Nephrocalcinosis secondary to hypercalciuria
  Polyuria $\rightarrow$ dehydration
  Normal serum calcium
Management:
  Potassium supplementation
  $+/-$ thiazide diuretics
  $+/-$ indomethacin

IV. Renal Development and Function

A. RENAL MORPHOGENESIS

Embryology
  Develops from 3 successive *mesodermic structures:*
    Pronephros—transient, limited function in human
    Mesonephros—epididymis, vas deferens, seminal vesicles (unilateral dysgenesis of mesonephros = dysgenesis of unilateral kidney and gonad)
    Metanephros—pelvicalyceal system, 5th week gestation, first nephrons at 8 weeks

Nephrogenesis
  Deep nephrons are formed first
  Prenatally:
    Number of nephrons increase until 34–35 weeks gestation and then size of nephrons increases
    In second 1/2 gestation—kidney weight increases in proportion to gestational age, birth weight, and body surface area

Fetal growth restriction reduces number of nephrons
Kidney size cm = 16.19 + [0.61 × gestational age (weeks)]
At birth:
  Juxtaglomerular nephrons are more mature than superficial nephrons
Postnatal growth:
  Accelerated growth of proximal tubule volume

	Birth	Adult
Glomerular diameter	110 μm	250 μm
Proximal tubule length	2 mm	20 mm
Glomerular basement membrane	100 ηm	300 ηm—thinner, more permeable

B. RENAL FUNCTION

Urine production
Occurs at 10–12 weeks gestation
Urine is the major constituent of amniotic fluid production; increases with age:

GA (Weeks)	Urine Flow Rate (cc/Hour)
22	2-5
30	10-20
40	25-50

Renal concentrating ability
Fetal urine is hypotonic (osmolality increases with gestational age)
Newborn concentrating ability less efficient compared to older children and adults; premature infant even less efficient than full-term infant
Maximum osmolality for premature infants is 500 mOsm/L compared to 800 mOsm/L in full-term infants; concentrating capacity of kidney reaches the adult value ~1200 osm/kg @ age 6–12 months
This limited concentrating ability places the premature infant at risk for dehydration
Reduced ability of premature infant to concentrate urine due to:
  Tubule insensitivity to vasopressin
  Short loop of Henle
  Low osmolality of medullary interstitium (due to limited Na^+ reabsorption in thick ascending loop)
  Low serum urea

Dilutional capacity
Decreased in neonates due to low GFR, which limits ability to handle water load

Renal blood flow (RBF)
At 25 weeks gestation—20 cc/min; this low rate is associated with elevated renal vascular resistance; RBF accounts for only 2–3% of cardiac output in utero
Full-term—60 cc/min; RBF is higher than premature neonate due to decreased renovascular pressure and increased systemic blood pressure; RBF accounts for 5–18% of cardiac output postnatally

Glomerular filtration rate (GFR)
Increased with increasing number and size of nephrons
Doubles by 2 weeks of age
Adult levels at 1 year of age
Not altered by prematurity
If serum *creatinine* doubles, GFR falls by ~50%

Serum creatinine level (see Vc)

Creatinine is a reflection of GFR

In neonates, serum creatinine must be > 2.0 mg/dL to be considered abnormal

C. GLOMERULAR AND TUBULAR FUNCTION

Sodium

2/3 filtered Na^+ reabsorbed in proximal tubule, 20% reabsorbed in ascending loop of Henle, and 10% reabsorbed in distal tubule/collecting duct

Capacity to reabsorb Na^+ is developed by 24 weeks; this remains low until 34 weeks; at that time, 99% of filtered Na^+ is reabsorbed, yielding FeNa $< 1\%$

In severely ill infants, Na^+ losses can be high

FeNa $=$ urinary fractional excretion of Na^+

$$FeNa\ (\%) = \frac{(\text{urine } Na^+ \times \text{Plasma Cr})}{(\text{urine Cr} \times \text{Plasma } Na^+)} \times 100$$

Cr $=$ creatinine

Interpretation: $< 1\%$ normal

1–$2.5\% =$ pre-renal

$> 3\% =$ intrinsic renal failure

Neonates have difficulty holding onto Na (especially premature infants), and thus their fractional excretions may be elevated even though they are actually intravascularly depleted; in contrast, neonates also with limited ability to excrete Na^+ load secondary to lower GFR

Potassium

Reabsorbed in proximal tubule and ascending loop of Henle

Secreted in distal tubule and collecting ducts

Limited ability to excrete K^+ load secondary to decreased number and activity of apical membrane potassium channels

Bicarbonate

Low serum bicarbonate threshold in proximal tubule (14–16 mEq/L in premature infants, 18–21 mEq/L in full-term infants, and 22–24 mEq/L in older children and adults) and once threshold surpassed, bicarbonate is excreted in urine

Limited ability to excrete acid load (reduced distal urinary acidification) due to limited buffer availability for H^+ load

Calcium

Reabsorption in proximal tubule and loop of Henle (passive, limited by Na^+) as well as distal tubule and collecting ducts (active, independent of Na^+ transport)

Usually high reabsorption of Ca with low fractional excretion $(< 1\%)$

With immaturity may get increased excretion due to reduced reabsorption at loop of Henle

Phosphorus

80% of phosphorous reabsorbed in proximal tubule, 10% reabsorbed in distal tubule, and remaining phosphorous is excreted

Usually high level of reabsorption

Low serum phosphorus levels most likely due to inadequate intake rather than low tubular reabsorption of phosphorus (TRP)

$$TRP = 1 - \frac{(\text{urine phos} \times \text{Plasma Cr})}{(\text{urine Cr} \times \text{Plasma phos})} \times 100$$

Parathyroid hormone (in response to low calcium) has little effect on phosphate excretion

Magnesium
65% passive reabsorption in proximal tubule and thick ascending loop
This ability is established early and fractional excretion remains low

Glucose urine excretion
Renal glucose threshold increases with increasing gestational age
When plasma glucose concentration exceeds the renal transport maximum for glucose, glycosuria will occur

D. HORMONAL CONTROL OF RENAL FUNCTION

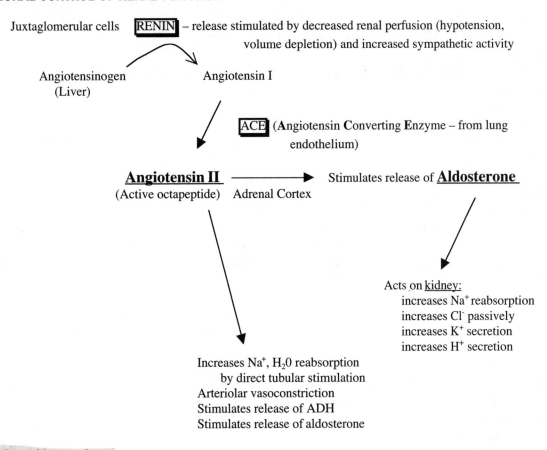

Juxtaglomerular cells RENIN – release stimulated by decreased renal perfusion (hypotension, volume depletion) and increased sympathetic activity

Angiotensinogen   Angiotensin I
(Liver)

ACE (**A**ngiotensin **C**onverting **E**nzyme – from lung endothelium)

Angiotensin II ⟶ Stimulates release of **Aldosterone**
(Active octapeptide)   Adrenal Cortex

Acts on kidney:
increases Na^+ reabsorption
increases Cl^- passively
increases K^+ secretion
increases H^+ secretion

Increases Na^+, H_2O reabsorption
by direct tubular stimulation
Arteriolar vasoconstriction
Stimulates release of ADH
Stimulates release of aldosterone

Pseudohypoaldosteronism
Etiology: X-linked recessive
Pathogenesis: unresponsiveness of renal tubule to aldosterone
Labs: decreased sodium, increased K^+, metabolic acidosis, increased aldosterone, increased renin
Clinical: prenatally, will have increased urine output and polyhydramnios; at 2–3 months of age, may have decreased feeding, vomiting, failure to thrive
Differential diagnosis: rule out congenital adrenal hyperplasia (decreased mineralocorticoids)
Management: administer increased amount of Na^+ and Cl^-
May need to give indomethacin to reduce urine output

V. Evaluation of Renal Function

A. HISTORY

Family history
Oligo/anhydramnios (suggests bilateral renal agenesis, severe renal dysplasia, obstructive uropathy)

Lg placenta, ↑AFP — Cong. Nephrotic Syndrome

Polyhydramnios (fetal nephrogenic diabetes insipidus, tubular dysfunction)
Increased abdominal girth (renal masses)
Large placenta (congenital nephrotic syndrome)
History of asphyxia, acute hemorrhage, infection, respiratory distress syndrome, indomethacin administration,
    hypernatremic dehydration (all increase risk for for acute tubular necrosis and acute renal failure)
Maternal drugs (e.g., captopril, indomethacin)
Increased α-fetoprotein (associated with congenital nephrotic syndrome)

B. PHYSICAL EXAM

Micturition
Majority of neonates (92–100%) with first void by 12–24 hours of age
Normal urine output 1–3 cc/kg/hour
If $>$ 24 hours of age without void or if oliguria ($<$ 1 cc/kg/hr), consider evaluation for:
    Hypovolemia
    Compensated shock
    Severe bilateral renal/urinary tract anomalies

Polyuria
Definition: urine output $>$ 4 cc/kg/hr
Etiologies:
1. Decreased antidiuretic hormone—central DI, hypervolemia
2. Decreased corticomedullary concentration gradiant
    Observed in medullary cystic disease, polycystic kidney disease, bilateral dysplastic kidneys, renal tract
    obstruction, medullary necrosis, interstitial nephritis, pyelonephritis, nephrocalcinosis, malnutrition, diuresis,
    polyuric phase post-acute tubular necrosis
3. Decreased ADH effect on tubules
    Observed in hypercalcemia, prostaglandin E2 administration, Bartter syndrome, proximal RTA
4. Transient diuretic phase in premature infant in first few days of life

Abdominal mass
2/3 secondary to renal origin including:
    Hydronephrosis
    Renal dysplasia
    Polycystic kidney disease
    Midline—posterior urethral valves (large bladder), hemorrhagic bladder, edema

Generalized edema—acute renal failure, nephrotic syndrome

Ascites

Abnormal external genitalia—ambiguous genitalia, hypospadias, epispadias, cryptorchidism

Hypertension—in newborns, hypertension is predominantly secondary

Other—physical exam findings associated with renal disease:
    Low-set malformed ears, anal atresia, abdominal wall defects, vertebral anomalies, aniridia, myelomeningocele,
    pneumothorax, hemihypertrophy and persistent urachus

C. LABS/STUDIES

Creatinine (Cr)
  At birth, levels reflect maternal renal function
  GFR decreased in premature infants and thus they are unable to efficiently eliminate excess Cr transferred in utero from mom

Age	Preterm Creatinine (mg/dL)	Full-Term Creatinine (mg/dL)
Day 1	0.8-1.8	1.2 +/− 0.5
7 days	<0.6	0.6 +/− 0.3
1-4 weeks	<0.7	< 0.7

Estimated GFR

$$\text{Estimated GFR (ml/min)} = \frac{0.45 \times \text{length (cm)}}{\text{plasma Cr (mg/dL)}}$$

  0.33 is the constant value for premature infants instead of 0.45

Blood urea nitrogen (BUN)
  Increased by dehydration, increased protein intake, hypercatabolic states/hypoxia, sequestered blood, and tissue breakdown

Renal tubular function (see FeNa, section IV.C)

Urinalysis
  Ideal to obtain urine by catheterization or suprapubic aspiration
  Specific gravity:
    1.001 to 1.021 (maximum specific gravity can be as high as 1.025)
    Premature newborns with a relatively impaired concentrating ability
  Proteinuria:
    > 95% of protein is reabsorbed in the proximal tubule
    Proteinuria may be present in up to 75% of healthy newborns with values of 5–10 mg/dL
    Transient proteinuria may be observed secondary to reduced renal blood flow, dehydration, asphyxia
    However, urine protein levels are difficult to interpret due to variability in urinary concentration
    If proteinuria persists, suggests glomerular/tubular injury
  Hematuria:
    > 5 red blood cells per high-power field
    Uncommon, always requires an evaluation
    Etiologies include moderate-severe perinatal depression (leading to ATN), glomerular disease, acute renal failure, renal vein or artery thrombosis [history of umbilical line access, coagulation abnormalities (e.g., Factor V Leiden)], congenital urinary malformation (autosomal recessive polycystic kidney disease, obstructive uropathies), coagulopathies, urinary tract infection (UTI), trauma (suprapubic or catheterization), tumors (Wilms, neuroblastoma, angiomas), and nephrocalcinosis
    Management:
      Microscopic analysis
      Urine culture
      Cr, BUN
      Renal ultrasound
      Assess for intrabdominal vascular clot by ultrasound
      Coagulation studies
  Hemoglobinuria: abnormal, due to hemolysis

Myoglobinuria: due to rhabdomyolysis
Sediment:
Leukocyturia—UTI, obstructive uropathy, glomerulonephritis
Red blood cell casts—glomerular injury
White blood cell casts—infection, renal interstitial/tubular injury
Epithelial, granular casts—dehydration, or renal interstitial/tubular injury
Hyaline casts—severe proteinuria, dehydration
Glycosuria—commonly present if < 34 weeks gestation

Radiographic studies
Plain film—may reveal an abdominal mass
Ultrasound
Length of kidneys in mm is approximately proportional to GA in weeks
Detection of bladder and bladder volume can be determined by 15 weeks gestation
Excellent tool to assess renal anatomy
Indications—fetal hydronephrosis or pelviectasis, UTI, detection of abdominal mass, oliguria of unknown etiology, unexplained tension pneumothorax, failure to void, poor urinary streams, perineal abnormalities, VACTERL association, decreased abdominal wall musculature, increased creatinine, hematuria (particularly with chronic diuretic therapy to rule out nephrocalcinosis), proteinuria, RTA, rule out renal arterial or venous thrombosis (assess with Doppler flow)
Voiding cystourethrogram
Detects anatomical and functional abnormalities in lower urinary tract (e.g., reflux)
Radionuclide renal imaging
Isotopes: DTPA, MAG-3, DMSA (binds to tubules, produces static images of renal cortex); while DMSA is static, DTPA and MAG-3 give dynamic images
Can assess position and size of kidneys
Determines renal blood flow distribution and function
Helpful to diagnose acute pyelonephritis and renal scarring

VI. Abnormal Renal Development

Renal anomalies 1/200

Most common: horseshoe kidney, unilateral renal agenesis (left $>$ right), pelvic kidney (left $>$ right)

A. CONGENITAL NEPHROTIC SYNDROME

Proteinuria, hypoproteinemia, hyperlipidemia, and edema

Presents in first 3 months

Most often in Finland (1/8000—secondary to increased consanguinity)

Two major types (both autosomal recessive):
1. Finnish (CNF)
Chromosome 19 (autosomal recessive, gene on 19q13.1, gene name *NPHS1*, gene product is called nephrin)
90% with symptoms by 1 month of age (can be symptomatic at birth): usually diagnosed at $\sim$3 months of age
Associated with large placenta and increased α-fetoprotein; may develop hydrops
$\sim$40% born prematurely
Typically small for gestational age

May develop edema, abdominal distention (~25%), and/or proteinuria (~20%)

Complications include infection and thromboemboli (secondary to urinary losses of IgG and coagulation proteins)

2. **Diffuse mesangial sclerosis (DMS)**

Later onset (up to 1 yr of life)

Normal placenta, AFP, and birthweight

Often rapidly develop renal insufficiency

Early-onset hypertension

B. RENAL AGENESIS AND DYSPLASIA

Agenesis

1/10,000

Recurrence risk 3–5%

Bilateral most common

40% stillborn or die shortly after birth

Associations: oligohydramnios sequence, pulmonary hypoplasia, Potter's syndrome, and single umbilical artery

Dysplasia

Incidence: 1/4300

Characteristics: unilateral or bilateral involvement; may be aplastic or multicystic; renal architecture is disorganized; may have ectopic cartilage and muscle tissue

Unilateral multicystic dysplasia is most common form

90% with other genitourinary anomalies

Clinical:

Unilateral (more common)

Sporadic, often found incidentally

More common in males

Greater on left

Moderate renal enlargement

Bilateral

Sporadic

Associated with oligohydramnios sequence/Potter's syndrome

Variable expression

C. POLYCYSTIC KIDNEY DISEASE (PKD)

Autosomal Recessive	Autosomal Dominant
= "infantile polycystic disease" since more common in newborns	Most common inherited kidney disease
1/40,000	1/1000
Chromosome 6p (6p21), variable expression	Chromosome 16, variable expression (the PKD1 gene is on 16p13.3 and codes for polycystin 1 while the PKD2 gene is on 4q and codes for polycystin 2; there are also patients with PKD who seem to have normal genes at these two sites, suggesting other loci can be involved)
Fetal ultrasound with large echogenic kidneys, oligohydramnios, and empty bladder	Rarely with findings at birth (however, if abnormalities at birth, ~50% die from respiratory failure or sepsis)
Cysts are large (>2 cm in diameter) with "snowstorm" appearance on ultrasound	Cysts are variable size
During neonatal period, kidney > liver involvement, while in older child, liver > kidney involvement	Cysts in kidneys and may also be observed in liver, pancreas, and spleen
Often with severe hypertension (may respond to angiotensin-converting enzyme inhibitors or loop diuretics)	Hypertension
	Renal insufficiency
Decreased renin and aldosterone levels as well as hepatic fibrosis and biliary dysgenesis	Many do well thoughout infancy

D. TUBULAR DYSFUNCTION

Fanconi syndrome
Genetics: inheritance: rare, autosomal dominant, generally sporadic
Pathologenesis: proximal tubule dysfunction leading to excess urinary losses of amino acids, glucose, phosphate, and bicarbonate
Etiology: can be primary or secondary (e.g., cystinosis, tyrosinemia, fructose intolerance, galactosemia, Lowe syndrome/oculocerebrorenal syndrome)
Clinical: polyuria with increased risk for dehydration; may develop rickets
Labs: decreased phosphate, decreased TRP
   Metabolic acidosis, hypokalemia
   Normal glomerular function
Management: supplement with sodium phosphate, sodium and potassium citrate, vitamin D

Cystinosis
Genetics: autosomal recessive
Pathogenesis: defective carrier-mediated transport of cystine leading to excess cystine in lysosomes of many cells
Clinical: infantile form (most severe) presents with vomiting, diarrhea, dehydration, failure to thrive
   Development of end-stage renal disease ~9 years of age
Labs: normal plasma cystine levels
Diagnosis: cornea-slit lamp exam—cystine crystals
Management: cysteamine, renal transplant

Lowe syndrome = oculocerebrorenal syndrome
Genetics: X-linked recessive (thus, males > females)
Pathogenesis: gene defect leads to an enzyme deficiency disrupting the Golgi apparatus, which plays a role in regulating specific cell lines (especially polarized epithelial cells)
Clinical and labs: time of onset ranges from early infancy to late childhood
   Oculo—cataracts, glaucoma, severe eye anomalies
   Cerebro—mental deficiency (severe), muscular hypotonia, areflexia
   Renal—tubular dysfunction, proteinuria, aminoaciduria, +/− congenital nephrotic syndrome
   Other—cryptorchidism
Diagnosis: prenatal—increased maternal AFP, increased amniotic fluid AFP
   Increased nucleotide pyro-phosphatase in skin fibroblasts
Management: symptom directed, no specific treatment will reverse the enzyme deficiency and disruption to the cellular Golgi apparatus

E. HYDRONEPHROSIS AND OBSTRUCTIVE UROPATHIES

Obstruction leads to:
   Dilation of the urinary tract above the level of lesion
   Risk for maldevelopment of kidney (both structural and functional)
   Possibility of associated oligohydramnios and pulmonary hypoplasia

1. Hydronephrosis (HN)
Etiologies:
   Uretopelvic junction obstruction (most common)
   Bladder outlet or urethral obstruction:
      1. Posterior urethral valves
      2. *Prune belly syndrome (Eagle-Barrett syndrome)*
         Renal dysplasia due to obstructive uropathy

Deficient abdominal muscles

After urinary decompression, "prune-belly" appearance becomes noticeable

Cryptorchidism

Patent urachus—allows for decompression of urinary obstruction and development of functioning kidney

Polycystic kidney disease, multicystic dysplastic kidney disease, renal agenesis, congenital megaureter

Prenatal management:

Mildly dilated 1–2 mm renal pelvis reported in 40% of routine prenatal ultrasounds; this is often normal and reflects functional dilation of urinary tract secondary to high fetal urine flow rates

If fetal ultrasound demonstrates HN, assess if upper tract involved, examine renal parenchyma, and measure bladder size and thickness

If oligohydramnios, there is increased chance of posterior urethral valves; if there is a normal amount of amniotic fluid, there is increased chance of reflux

Assess for other organ abnormalities

Monitor with repeat ultrasounds to determine if increasing severity, change in amniotic fluid volume, and/or bilateral involvement

Intrauterine intervention should be considered if severe HN and oligohydramnios to attempt to increase amniotic fluid volume and prevent pulmonary hypoplasia; in addition, shunting in utero may minimize renal injury

Postnatal management:

Postnatal studies should always confirm prenatal diagnosis—important to avoid studying within the first few days of life due to body fluid changes that may result in unreliable ultrasound results

Prophylactic antibiotics

Monitor with ultrasounds (do ultrasound immediately after birth if high suspicion of posterior urethral valves or severe bilateral HN that may require immediate intervention)

If moderate-severe → VCUG at 1–3 months, urology consultation, renal functional assessment tests later in life

Consider surgery if decreased renal function

Consider chromosome analysis (especially if bilateral and other anomalies on exam)

Prognosis: majority of mild HN resolve, while ~20% moderate-severe HN require surgery

Patients with evidence of vesicoureteral reflux by VCUG:

While males have reflux mostly during newborn period (due to short ureters), females present with reflux at later age (usually acquired)

30% associated with other genitourinary abnormalities (e.g., dysplasia, hypoplasia, or cortical scarring)

40% of neonates with urinary tract infection will have reflux

Expectant management since reflux often will spontaneously resolve

Higher grades of severity may require surgery but newer data suggest that this doesn't change the ultimate renal outcome

2. Ectopic ureterocele

Incidence: greater in females (5–7:1), 10% bilateral

Pathology:

Renal pelvis and ureter are duplicated

One of the ureters (usually the one that drains the upper pole of the duplex kidney) enters ectopically into the neck of the bladder

The portion of the obstructed kidney (upper pole) is abnormally developed

Diagnosis: voiding cystourethrogram shows filling defect in bladder (the ureterocele) and can evaluate for reflex

Management: excision of ureterocele, may need to remove upper pole of the kidney

3. Posterior urethral valves

Males

Diagnosis suggested by ultrasound findings of bilateral hydronephrosis, hydroureter, and thick-walled large bladder

Definitive diagnosis by VCUG with visualization of valve leaflets
Surgery for valve ablation

F. OTHER MISCELLANEOUS GENITOURINARY DEVELOPMENTAL ANOMALIES

Ectopic kidney, horseshoe kidney, crossed, and fused ectopia
Abnormalities in renal location
May be associated with reflux or obstruction
Horseshoe kidney—increased association with Turner syndrome

Urachal sinus
Isolated finding
Urine excreted from umbilicus

Hypospadias and epispadias (refer to Endocrinology chapter)

Exstrophy of cloaca sequence
Incidence: 1/400,000
Pathology:
    Primary defect of early mesoderm (role in formation of infraumbilical mesenchyme, cloacal septum, and lumbosacral vertebrae)
    Leads to failure of cloacal septation and the ureters, ileum and rudimentary hindgut are connected to a common cloaca
Clinical findings:
    Exstrophy of bladder
    Often associated with an omphalocele
    Incomplete development of lumbosacral vertebrae with herniation of a grossly dilated central canal of the spinal cord (hydromyelia)
    No anal opening
    Cryptorchidism
    Other genitourinary anomalies—pelvic kidneys, renal agenesis, multicystic kidneys, ureteral duplication
    Females may have bifid uterine horns, short, duplicated atretic vagina
    Other abnormalities include single umbilical artery, anomalies of lower limbs, congenital hip dislocation, talipes equinovarus, and agenesis of limbs
Management/prognosis:
    Excellent survival rates following surgical repair
    Gender assignment for 46, XY
    Urinary continence achieved in some patients
    Low chance of fecal continence
    Reconstruction to create vagina in teenage years

Exstrophy of bladder sequence
Incidence:
    1 in 30,000, male > female
    Recurrence risk:
        Unaffected parents with one affected child with bladder exstrophy <1%
        If affected parents—1/70 risk
Pathology:
    Primary defect of infraumbilical mesoderm
    At 6-7 weeks gestation, the infraumbilical mesenchyme migrates to give rise to lower abdominal wall, genital tubercles, pubic rami

Clinical:
    Exposed posterior wall of bladder
    Short, low abdominal wall
    May have inguinal hernia
    Epispadias
    Perforate anus
Management/outcome:
    Close defect in first few days of life
    Genital function usually satisfactory
    Good urinary control

G. DISORDERS ASSOCIATED WITH RENAL DISEASE

Disorders	Features	Renal Abnormalities
Oligohydramnios sequence (Potter syndrome)	Altered facies, pulmonary hypoplasia, abnormal limb and head position	Renal agenesis, severe bilateral obstruction, severe bilateral dysplasia, autosomal recessive polycystic kidney disease
VACTERL association	Vertebral anomalies, anal atresia, cardiac defects, tracheoesophageal fistula, radial dysplasia, limb defects	(~53%) renal agenesis, renal dysplasia, renal ectopia
"Prune belly" (Eagle-Barrett syndrome)	Hypoplasia of abdominal muscle, cryptorchidism	Megaureters, hydronephrosis, dysplastic kidneys, atonic bladder
Spina bifida	Meningomyelocele	Neurogenic bladder, vesicoureteral reflux, hydronephrosis, double ureter, horseshoe kidney
Caudal dysplasia sequence (caudal regression syndrome)	Sacral and lumbar hypoplasia, disruption of the distal spinal cord	Neurogenic bladder, vesicoureteral reflux, hydronephrosis, renal agenesis
Anal atresia (high imperforate anus)	Rectovaginal, rectovesical or rectourethral fistula tethered to the spinal cord	Renal agenesis, renal dysplasia

Autosomal Recessive disorder	Features	Renal Abnormality
Cerebrohepatorenal syndrome (Zellweger syndrome)	Hepatomegaly, glaucoma, brain anomalies, chrondrodystrophy	Cortical renal cysts
Jeune syndrome (thoracic asphyxiating dystrophy)	Small thoracic cage, short ribs, abnormal costochondro junctions, pulmonary hypoplasia	Cystic tubular dysplasia, glomerulosclerosis, hydronephrosis, horseshoe kidneys
Meckel-Gruber syndrome	Encephalocele, microcephaly, polydactyly, cryptorchidism, cardiac anomalies, liver disease	Polycystic/dysplastic kidneys

Autosomal Dominant	Features	Renal Abnormalities
Tuberous sclerosis	Fibrous-angiomatous lesions, hypopigmented macules, intracranial calcifications, seizures, bone lesions	Polycystic kidneys, renal angiomyolipomata
Nail-patella syndrome (hereditary osteoonychodysplasia)	Hypoplastic nails, hypoplastic or absent patella, other bone anomalies	Proteinuria, nephritic syndrome

Chromosomal Syndromes	Features	Renal Abnormalities
Trisomy 21	Abnormal facies, brachycephaly, congenital heart disease	May have cystic dysplastic kidney and other renal abnormalities
Turner syndrome	Small stature, congenital heart disease, amenorrhea	Horseshoe kidney, duplication and malrotations of the urinary collecting system
Trisomy 13 (Patau syndrome)	Abnormal facies, cleft lip and palate, congenital heart disease	May have cystic dysplastic kidneys and other renal anomalies
Trisomy 18 (Edwards syndrome)	Abnormal facies, cardiac defects, hypospadias and crytorchidism, syndactyly	Various renal anomalies
Partial trisomy 10q	Abnormal facies, microcephaly, limb and cardiac anomalies	Various renal anomalies

Modified Cloherty JP and Stark AR (ed): Manual of Neonatal Care (4th Edition). Philadelphia, Lippincott-Raven, 1998, p 594–596.

VII. Acquired Renal Disease

A. RENAL VASCULAR THROMBOSIS

Clinical triad
  Enlargement of kidney
  Hematuria
  Renal failure

Diagnosis
  Renal ultrasound with doppler flow

Management
  Controversial
  Conservative including:
    Anti-hypertensive medications (if unilateral—usually normotensive by 2 years of age with normal Cr clearance); remove indwelling vascular catheters
  Routine use of systemic antithrombolytic therapy not shown to improve outcomes (however, consider if massive thombosis)
  Surgical thrombectomy—shown to be no better than conservative management, mortality ~30%

1. Renal artery thrombosis
Risks:
  Indwelling umbilical arterial catheter
  Hyperviscosity
  Thrombophilia
Clinical: triad of renal vascular thromobosis, may also have hypertension

2. Renal vein thrombosis
Risks:
  Hyperosmolarity
  Polycythemia (small for gestational age, infant of diabetic mother)
  Hypovolumia (dehydration, hypotension)
  Hypercoagulable states (e.g., Factor V Leiden)
Clinical:
  Often unilateral
  Triad of renal vascular thrombosis
  Hypertension
  Thrombocytopenia and depletion of coagulation factors

B. CORTICAL OR MEDULLARY NECROSIS

Etiology: renal ischemia (shock, severe anemia, asphyxia)

Clinical: nonspecific, increased kidney size, oliguria, hematuria

Diagnosis: ultrasound shows bilateral increased echogenicity of kidneys

Management: nonspecific, treat renal failure

Outcome: increased mortality secondary to severity of underlying disease; increased risk for hypertension and tubular dysfunction

C. NEPHROCALCINOSIS

Incidence in neonates < 32 weeks gestation—25-60%

Associated with hypercalciuric states
  Loop diuretics (Lasix)
  Methylxanthines
  Glucocorticoids
  Vitamin D

Most spontaneously resolve over first year of life, some reports of tubular dysfunction

D. HYPERTENSION

Definition
  BP > 2 S.D. above normal values for age and weight

Differential diagnosis
  Vascular—renal artery thrombosis (common, often related to umbilical arterial line), renal vein thrombosis, coarctation
    of aorta, renal artery stenosis, idiopathic arterial calcifications
  Renal—obstructive uropathy, polycystic kidney disease, renal insufficiency, tumor (Wilms), glomerulonephritis,
    pyelonephritis
  Endocrine—congenital adrenal hypoplasia, primary hyperaldosteronism, hyperthyroidism
  Neurologic—increased intracranial pressure (intraventricular hemorrhage, hydrocephalus, meningitis, subdural
    hemorrhage), neural crest tumor (neuroblastoma, pheochromocytoma), cerebral angioma, drug withdrawal, seizures
  Pulmonary—chronic lung disease (etiology probably multifactorial)
  Drugs—corticosteroids, theophylline, adrenergic agents (dopamine, epinephrine), pancuronium
  Other—fluid/electrolyte overload, pain

Evaluation
  History:
    Determine how the BP was obtained
      Intra-arterial device versus cuff
      Which extremity—lower extremity blood pressure > upper
      Check cuff size—cuff bladder width should be 2/3 circumference of extremity
      BP should be taken when infant is comfortable
    If presence or history of umbilical arterial line, infant is at increased risk for renovascular HTN and thrombosis
    Pain or agitation
    History of chronic lung disease
    Medications
  Physical examination:
    Check 4 extremity BP
    Check femoral pulses
    Check for abdominal masses (to rule out tumor, polycystic kidneys, obstruction, renal vein thrombosis)
    Rule out ambiguous genitalia (CAH)
  Lab evaluation:
    Cr, BUN, Ca, urinalysis, urine culture, electrolytes (decreased K^+ and increased CO_2 suggests primary
      hyperaldosteronism), plasma renin levels (increased with renovascular disease, decreased with primary
      aldosteronism)
  Imaging:
    Renal ultrasound with Doppler flow

Cranial ultrasound (rule out intraventricular hemorrhage)
Echocardiogram to rule out cardiomyopathy
Renal scan to assess for segmental renal arterial infarctions

Management:
Treat underlying cause (e.g., pain, volume overload)
Antihypertensives agents
ACE inhibitors (captopril, enalapril)
Beta blockers (labetalol, propranolol)
Calcium channel blockers (amlodipine, isradipine, nicardipine); note that verapamil is contraindicated in neonates
Vasodilators (hydralazine, nitroprusside)

E. ACUTE RENAL FAILURE

Differential diagnosis
Prerenal (most common cause)—hypoperfusion of the kidneys
Intrinsic—due to direct injury or congenital anomaly
Postrenal—obstruction to urinary flow in both kidneys; in males, consider posterior urethral valves (renal function may be abnormal even after correction)

Diagnosis
Suspect renal failure if oliguria present with BUN > 20 mg/dL and Cr >1 mg/dL
Evaluate history
Urinalysis

Indices	Pre-renal	Intrinsic	SIADH
FeNa (%)	< 2.5	> 3.0	~ 1.0
Urine osmolality (osms)	> 400	< 400	> 500
U Na (mEq/L)	< 40	> 40	> 40
Urine specific gravity	> 1.015	< 1.015	> 1.020

Note: standard measurements used to evaluate renal function should be used with caution in newborns due to developmental renal immaturity; Modified from Gunn VL and Nechyba C (eds): The Harriet Lane Handbook (16th Edition). Philadelphia, Mosby, 2002, p 411.

Renal ultrasound
Bladder catheterization to rule out urinary tract obstruction
Fluid challenge (10–20 cc/kg) over 1 hour followed by Lasix 1 mg/kg
Consider low dose dopamine to improve renal blood flow and urine output

Management
Discontinue any potassium infusion
Fluid management minimized based on patient's fluid status, insensible losses, and urine output
Restrict Na^+ and monitor serum Na^+ concentration (hyponatremia usually secondary to excess free water)
Restrict phosphorus (calcium carbonate can be used as a phosphate-binding agent)
Ca supplementation if decreased Ca or if patient symptomatic
Correct metabolic acidosis with $NaHCO_3$
Nutrition—breast milk, low-phosphate formula (PM 60/40), high calories (due to fluid restriction), limit protein
Adjust dosing of nephrotoxic drugs
Dialysis may be required

F. CHRONIC RENAL FAILURE

Defined as a decrease in GFR to $< 25\%$ normal for a period $\geq$ 3 months

Complications
  End-stage renal disease:
      Rare in neonatal period
      Majority secondary to congenital urinary tract anomalies
      Majority require dialysis or transplant to survive
  Failure to thrive:
      Secondary to inadequate calories, abnormal electrolytes, renal osteodystrophy, hormonal abnormalities, anemia,
        infections, and use of steroids
      Normal growth hormone, normal insulin-like growth levels and decreased insulin-like growth factor binding proteins
      Increase caloric intake to 120–180% recommended daily allowance, limit amount of Na^+ and phosphate
      If severe, limit protein
      HCO_3^- as needed
  Renal osteodystrophy
      Secondary to decreased vitamin D hydroxylation due to loss of renal tissue, increased PTH, and excess aluminum
      Increased calcium/phosphorus ratio
      Provide 1,25 (OH) Vitamin D to prevent secondary hyperparathyroidism and hypocalcemia
  Possible neurologic complications:
      Encephalopathy, neuropathy, motor delay
      These neurologic manifestations due to excess aluminum, hypertension, electrolyte abnormalities, and underlying
        primary disease

Management
  Dialysis
  Renal transplant (still with increased mortality)

Prognosis
  Outcome depends on underlying etiology
      Congenital nephritic syndrome—15% mortality post-transplant
      Pyelonephritis and interstitial nephritis—11% mortality post-transplant
  Majority of patients improve post-transplant with increased growth and better long-term neurodevelopmental outcome
      compared with patients who receive long-term dialysis

REFERENCES

Chan JCM, Williams DM, and Roth HSR: Kidney failure in infants and children. *Pediatrics in Review.* 2002; 23(2): 47–59.

Chan JCM, Scheinman JI, and Roth HSR: Renal tubular acidosis. *Pediatrics in Review.* 2001; 22(8): 277–286.

Ettinger LM and Flynn JT: Hypertension in the neonate. *Neo Reviews.* 2002; 3(8): c151–c156.

Fanaroff, AA and Martin RJ (eds): Neonatal and Perinatal Medicine: Diseases of the Fetus and Newborn (7th Ed). St. Louis, Mosby, 2001.

Gunn VL and Nechyba C (eds): The Harriet Lane Handbook (16th Ed). Philadelphia, Mosby, 2002.

Jones KL: Smith's Recognizable Patterns of Human Malformation (5th Ed). Philadelphia, W.B. Saunders Company, 1997.

Peters C: Neonatal Core Conference: Hydronephrosis. Children's Hospital, Boston, MA, June 1999.

Rose BD: Clinical Physiology of Acid-Base and Electrolyte Disorders (5th Ed). New York, McGraw-Hill, 2001.

CHAPTER 8

Nutrition

TOPICS COVERED IN THIS CHAPTER

I. Fetal Growth

Fetal growth rate increases with advancing gestational age (GA):

Gestational age (weeks)	Growth rate (g/day)
16	5
21	10
29	20
37	35

II. Fetal Composition

Decreases with advancing GA and birth weight	Increases with advancing GA and birth weight
Total body water	Intracellular water
Extracellular water	Protein
Sodium content	Fat
Chloride content	Calcium
	Phosphorous
	Magnesium
	Iron

III. Fetal Energy Expenditure and Sources

Estimated fetal energy expenditure = 35 to 55 kcal/kg/day

Energy sources

1. Maternal glucose (2/3)

   Transferred across placenta by facilitated diffusion

   Acquired glucose has three major roles in fetal life:

   Glycolysis (major pathway for fetal glucose utilization)

   Carbon source (essential for fetal growth)

   Glycogen storage

2. Placental lactate (1/4)

3. Maternal amino acids (remaining)

   Transferred across placenta by active transport

   Acquired amino acids are important for fetus:

   Tissue growth

   Metabolic fuel

   Source of gluconeogenic substrates (alanine, glutamic acid, aspartic acid)

IV. Neonatal Energy Expenditure and Requirements

Estimated caloric expenditure and requirements:

Form of energy	Caloric expenditure in neonate
Resting metabolic rate	50 kcal/kg/day
Activity	15 kcal/kg/day
Cold stress	10 kcal/kg/day
Nutrition processing	Excretion: 12 kcal/kg/day
	Storage: 25 kcal/kg/day
	(continued on following page)

Form of energy	Caloric expenditure in neonate
Total	Synthesis: 8 kcal/kg/day 120 kcal/kg/day

Note: 1 kcal = 1 cal and is defined as the amount of heat required to raise the temperature of 1 kg of water from 14.5°C to 15.5°C
Modified from: Fanaroff AA, Martin RJ (eds): Neonatal-Perinatal Medicine (6th edition). St Louis, Mosby 1997, p. 564.

Resting metabolic rate is greater with increased prematurity, disease states, and low birth weight
Most sources recommend neonatal caloric requirement of 120 to 150 kcal/kg/day to balance energy expenditure and to allow for proper growth

V. Proteins *Nec. for cell growth; synthesis of enzymes; hormones*

Whey and casein
Whey and casein are major protein sources in neonates
Whey has greater cysteine and less methionine than casein

Milk source	Whey-to-casein ratio
Colostrum	80:20
Mature milk	55:45
Predominantly casein formulas	20:80
Predominantly whey formulas	60:40

Preterm formulas have greater protein content and whey-to-casein ratio is 60:40
Properties of selected amino acids:

Human milk
70% whey
30% casein

Preterm infants have limited ability to use excess AA → @ risk for hyperammonemia, azotemia, meth. acidosis (↑BUN)

Property	Amino acids
Glucose precursor	Salanine Glutamic acid Aspartic acid
Methylated in muscle protein	Homocysteine Methionine Creatinine Phosphatidylcholine

Essential	Lysine
	Phenylalanine*
	Threonine
	Tryptophan
	Methionine*
	Histidine
	Branched chain:
	  Valine
	  Leucine
	  Isoleucine

Considered essential amino acids in premature newborns	Cysteine Tyrosine Arginine Taurine

*There is decreased requirement for methionine and phenylalanine if enough cysteine and tyrosine in diet

Human milk 50% fat Formula 40-50%
L easier to digest d/t FA composition, presence
of bile salt-stimulated lipase (major)
1st energy source

combo of fat f/formula : human milk
↑fat absorption in LBW
and fat soluble vits (A,D,E,K)

VI. Fats

Placental transfer of both essential and nonessential fatty acids

Fats are a major source of energy (9 kcal/g)   (10 kcal/g parenteral)

Composition and types of fatty acids
Neutral fat
  = three long-chain fatty acids and one glycerol
Most common fatty acids
  Stearic acid: C18, fully saturated
  Oleic acid: C18, 1 double bond
  Palmitic acid: C16, fully saturated

source of fat
• Release of FFA stored
  in adipose tissue
• absorption f/milk
• IV lipids

Essential fatty acids imp. for brain: Retinal growth
  Linoleic
  Linolenic
Long-chain polyunsaturated (omega-6, omega-3) fatty acids—(LCPUFA)
  >10 carbons
  Absorbed into mucosal cells by diffusion (requires re-esterification, formation into chylomicron, and transport to lymphatic system by lipoproteins)
  Believed to be important in brain and retinal development
Short and medium-chain triglycerides (MCT) easier to absorb (by passive diffusion)
  Easily hydrolyzed by pancreatic lipase to free fatty acids, which can be easily transported across the mucosal cell (i.e., easier to absorb than LCPUFA)

don't require bile salts
  MCTs are increased in breast milk for preterm infants, but there is still only a small fraction of fatty acids in breast milk
  Disadvantages to MCT as major source of fatty acids:
    Not as important for tissue building
    Increased MCT will decrease availability of long-chain fatty acids

Fat stores
  Body fat stores are formed by lipogenesis from glucose

Digestion begins in stomach
  Digestion of fatty acids by lipases and bile acid emulsification is often underdeveloped in newborns; therefore, neonates rely on intragastric lipases
  Improved digestion of fatty acids with decreased chain length and unsaturated form (presence of carbon to carbon double bonds)

Triene-to-tetraene ratio
  Increased ratio (> 0.4) suggests fatty acid deficiency
  In the presence of reduced linoleic acid and therefore, arachidonic acid (C20:4), the preferred biochemical reaction is to convert oleic acid to eicosatrienoic acid (C20:3)
  As a result, the concentration of trienes increases and the concentration of tetraenes decreases

Brain accounts for 75%
of fetal glucose consumption

VII. Carbohydrates 2nd major energy source

Lactose is the predominant carbohydrate in breast milk and many standard formulas Lactose in hindmilk
is ↑than colostrum

Lactose Reaches mature levels b/t 36-40wks
Other CHO digesting enzymes (disaccharides) are active 27-28 wks

* giving D10 alone → muscle catabolism for energy
glucose is stored as glycogen in the liver (in 3rd T)

[handwritten at top: glucose can be made f/ other CHO, PRO, Fats]
[handwritten: hyperglycemia may ↑ IVH]

Benefits of lactose
  Enhances absorption of calcium and magnesium
  Promotes intestinal growth of lactobacilli

Similar to fatty acids, short-chain glucose polymers are absorbed more easily than long-chain glucose polymers

Premature formulas often replace some of the lactose content with corn syrup and short-chain glucose polymers

VIII. Vitamins

[handwritten: Water — active transport]
[handwritten: Fat — Facilitated transport]

A. WATER-SOLUBLE VS FAT-SOLUBLE VITAMINS

Water-soluble vitamins	Fat-soluble vitamins
Vitamin B complex and vitamin C	Vitamins A, D, E, and K
Not formed by precursors (except niacin from tryptophan)	Synthesized from precursors
Daily intake required to prevent deficiencies	Daily intake not typically required except in specific circumstances (e.g., cystic fibrosis)
Does not accumulate in the body (except vitamin B12)	Not easily excreted, so can accumulate in the body and has the potential for toxicity
Most cross placenta by active transport	Placental transfer by simple or facilitated diffusion

Premature infants at risk for vitamin deficiency because:
  Likely to have low vitamin stores
  Increased requirement because of rapid growth
  Immaturity leading to ineffective metabolism

Premature infants also at increased risk of vitamin toxicity secondary to altered urinary excretion

B. VITAMIN B12 (COBALAMIN) AND FOLIC ACID (FOLATE) DEFICIENCY

Function   *[handwritten: DNA synthesis]*
  Vitamin B12 is endogenously synthesized by gastrointestinal (GI) microorganisms and required for folate metabolism
  Vitamin B12 is also important for CHO and fat metabolism
  Folate is a coenzyme for amino acids and nucleic acid metabolism

Risks
  Risk of B12 deficiency in breast-fed infants of vegetarian mothers who do not ingest eggs or dairy products *[handwritten: (should take supplement)]*
  Risk of folic acid deficiency in infants fed only evaporated milk or goat's milk

Clinical
  Vitamin B12 deficiency with anemia and associated with *[handwritten: (B12 deficiency)]* methylmalonic acidemia and homocystinuria
  Folate deficiency with poor weight gain, anemia; often coexists with iron deficiency

Laboratory values
  Vitamin B12 and folic acid deficiency evident by megaloblastic anemia with hypersegmented neutrophils

C. VITAMIN E (ALPHA-TOCOPHEROL) DEFICIENCY

Function
  Has antioxidant properties
  Vitamin E often recommended concurrently with iron administration to protect from iron-induced hemolysis (caused by
    the oxidant effect of iron)

Clinical
Increased sensitivity of red blood cells to H_2O_2 and hemolysis
Anemia and reticulocytosis
Thrombocytosis, acanthocytosis
Neurologic deficits

D. VITAMIN K DEFICIENCY   *may result in hemorrhagic disease of newborn*
Fat soluble

Function
Vitamin K required for carboxylation of prothrombin into active form
Vitamin K important for coagulation   *factor VII*

Risks
Newborns are predisposed to vitamin K deficiency because:
   Initial lack of GI microorganisms that synthesize vitamin K
   Immature newborn liver
Maternal medications can decrease neonatal vitamin K levels (e.g., anticonvulsants, warfarin, and antituberculosis medications)
Breast-fed infants have lower vitamin K levels compared with infants receiving cow's milk

Deficiency
Deficiency associated with hemorrhagic disease of newborns (see Hematology and Oncology & Bilirubin chapter)

E. OTHER VITAMIN DEFICIENCIES AND ASSOCIATED FEATURES

Vitamin	Associated features of vitamin deficiency
Vitamin A (retinol)	Important for pulmonary epithelial growth and cellular differentiation; deficiency may play a role in the development of chronic lung disease Photophobia, conjuctivitis Abnormal epiphyseal bone formation and tooth enamel Generalized scaling Failure to thrive
Vitamin B1 (thiamine)	Beriberi (symptoms include fatigue, irritability, constipation, cardiac failure) Associated with pyruvate dehydrogenase complex deficiency and maple syrup urine disease
Vitamin B2 (riboflavin)	Failure to thrive, photophobia, blurred vision, dermatitis, mucositis Associated with glutaric aciduria type I
Vitamin B6 (pyridoxine)	Dermatitis, mucositis Hypochromic anemia, possible seizures Associated with homocystinuria
Biotin	Alopecia, dermatitis, scaling, seborrhea Associated with biotinidase deficiency, β-methylcrotonyl glycinuria, propionic acidemia, and pyruvate dehydrogenase complex deficiency
Vitamin C (ascorbic acid)	Poor wound healing and bleeding gums Associated with transient tyrosinemia
Vitamin D	Rickets Failure to thrive Possible tetany

IX. Trace Elements

Trace element	Function	Clinical effects of deficiency
Chromium	Regulates glucose levels because of its role in insulin metabolism	In animals: diabetes In humans: unknown

(continued on following page)

Trace element	Function	Clinical effects of deficiency
Copper	Critical for production of red blood cells as well as hemoglobin formation Important for absorption of iron Associated with multiple enzyme activities	Anemia Osteoporosis Depigmentation of hair and skin Neutropenia Poor weight gain Hypotonia, ataxia later in life
Iron	Component of hemoglobin and myoglobin required for transport of oxygen and carbon dioxide	Anemia (microcytic, hypochromic) Failure to thrive
Manganese	Role in enzyme activation (e.g., superoxide dismutase) Important for normal bone stucture Role in CHO metabolism	Unknown
Selenium	Cofactor for glutamine peroxidase	In animals: muscle disease In humans: cardiomyopathy

Zinc	Important component of several enzymes (e.g., carbonic anhydrase and carboxypeptidase)
	Important for growth
		Acrodermatitis enteropathica
		    Autosomal recessive disorder in which there is an abnormality of zinc absorption or transport
		    Failure to thrive, alopecia, diarrhea, dermatitis (commonly perianal), ocular changes, rash (crusted, erythematous, involving face, extremities and anogenital areas), nail hypoplasia or dysplasia
		Acquired zinc deficiency
		    Premature infants receiving inadequate amounts of zinc
		    Maternal zinc deficiency can lead to fetal growth restriction, congenital anomalies
		    Infants with malabsorption, poor weight gain, poor wound healing, anemia (iron deficiency)

Modified from Behrman RE, Kliegman RM, and Arvin AM (eds): Nelson Textbook of Pediatrics (15th edition). Philadelphia, WB Saunders Co, 1996, p. 146-147.

X. Human Milk

Flouride – 6mo
Fe @ 4mo

A. PHYSIOLOGY

Prolactin secreted by maternal anterior pituitary gland throughout pregnancy

Prolactin important in establishing and maintaining lactation (including mammary gland production)

High levels of estrogen and progesterone throughout pregnancy inhibit milk production

At delivery, the decrease in estrogen and progesterone leads to increased milk production and milk delivery

Breast stimulation further increases production of prolactin and oxytocin

Milk ejection
   Mediated by oxytocin released from posterior pituitary gland
   Oxytocin leads to contraction of myoepithelium surrounding milk ducts

B. COMPOSITION OF BREAST MILK

↓ renal solute load ; improved gut motility
↑ absorption of Zinc : Fe, fat, AA : CHO

Immunologic and antibacterial factors
   Breast milk contains secretory IgA:
      With highest concentration in early breast milk
      Binds to viruses and bacteria
      Prevents invasion of mucosa
   Breast milk provides protective and bactericidal enzymes
   Lactobacilli growth increased by breast milk
   Colostrum has increased amounts of lymphocytes, macrophages, and immunoglobulins

Hormones
Cortisol and epidermal growth factor in breast milk

Enzymes
Breast milk contains bile salt–dependent lipase

Electrolytes
Breast milk has decreased sodium, calcium, potassium, choride, magnesium, and phosphorus compared with cow's milk

Protein
As breast milk matures, its protein levels decrease
Whey-to-casein ratio in colostrum is 80:20; changes to 55:45 in mature milk
Protein supplies ~75% of nitrogen in breast milk; remaining nitrogen is supplied by nonproteins
Most amino acids are lower in breast milk compared with cow's milk

Carbohydrates
Predominant carbohydrate is lactose

Fats
Fats provides 50% of calories of breast milk
Greater amount long-chain unsaturated fatty acids in breast milk compared with cow's milk
Breast milk provides other lipases to help fat digestion (thus, less fat in stool of breast-fed infants)
Breast milk fats are in globules, which contain cholesterol, phospholipids, and tryglycerides (85%)
With time, decreasing concentrations of cholesterol and phospholipids are present in breast milk
Tryglycerides are the most variable component of breast milk (varies by gestational age, time, and maternal diet)
There is an increased amount of easily digested palmitic acid in breast milk compared with type of palmitic acid contained in formulas
Increased amount arachnidonic acid in breast milk (most common LPUFA: long-chain polyunsaturated fatty acids) with greater amounts in milk for premature infants
Increased amounts of docohexanoic acid (DHA)
Colostrum has limited amount of cholesterol and phospholipids yet increased tryglycerides

Cholesterol
Cholesterol is necessary for tissue growth and is a precursor of bile salts and steroid hormones
Greater amount in breast milk compared with extremely minimal amount of cholesterol in formula
Amount of cholesterol in BM is independent of maternal diet

Carnitine
Decreased in premature infants (because of their decreased ability to synthesize it)
Increased amounts in breast milk
Supplemented in formulas

Inositol
Involved in membrane synthesis and activities; reduces retinal injury (unknown mechanism); and may enhance surfactant production
Greater amount in breast milk compared with formula

Choline
Important for development of central nervous system

Important component of acetylcholine and phosphatidylcholine
Unclear if required by infants exogenously
Low amounts in breast milk, formula, and cow's milk

Premature milk
Increased protein
Increased electrolytes
Inadequate protein, calcium, phosphorus, and vitamin D
To provide adequate growth and nutrition, need to supplement with human milk fortifier

C. BENEFITS OF BREAST FEEDING

Multiple, considered ideal form of nutrition for infants

Some examples of *possible* benefits include:
Decreased type I insulin-dependent diabetes, lymphoma, inflammatory bowel disease, obesity
Decreased infections
Improved neurodevelopment

D. CONTRAINDICATIONS TO BREAST FEEDING

Contraindications (in US)
Infection (maternal HIV, mother with herpes simplex virus lesions on breast, symptomatic mother with positive PPD and CXR [i.e., presumed active tuberculosis], active breast abscess)
Galactosemia (caused by lactose being the predominant carbohydrate in breast milk)
Drugs (cocaine, cyclosporine, lithium, methotrexate, phencyclidine, radioactive agents)

E. COMPARISON TABLE

Component	Human colostrum	Mature breast milk	Cow's milk
Protein (g/L)	22.9	10.6	32.5
Whey:casein	80:20	55:45	20:80
Lactalbumin (g/L)	–	3.6	2.4
Na (mg/dL)	48.0	15.0	58.0
K (mg/dL)	74.0	55.0	138.0
Cl (mg/dL)	85.0	43.0	103.0
Ca (mg/dL)	39.0	35.0	130.0
Fe (µg/dL)	70.0	100.0	70.0

Modified from Behrman RE, Kliegman RM, and Arvin AM (eds): Nelson Textbook of Pediatrics (15th edition). Philadelphia, WB Saunders Co, 1996, p. 158 and Lawrence RA and Lawrence RM. Breastfeeding: a guide for the medical profession (5th edition). St. Louis, Mosby, 1999, p. 128–129.

XI. Formulas

A. CLASSIFICATION BY CARBOHYDRATE SOURCE

Type of carbohydrate	Formula name
Lactose	Enfamil (standard, AR, Lipil, Enfacare, and Premature)
	Neosure (also contains glucose polymers)
	Similac (standard, 60/40, and Special Care)
Sucrose and glucose polymers	Alimentum
	Isomil
	Portagen
	(continued on following page)

Type of carbohydrate	Formula name
Glucose polymers	Enfamil Lactofree
	Neocate
	Neosure (also contains lactose)
	Nutramigen
	Pregestimil
	ProSobee
	Similac Lactose Free

Modified from Gunn VL, Nechyba C (ed): The Harriet Lane Handbook (16th Edition). Philadelphia, Mosby, 2002, p. 467.

B. CLASSFICATION BY PROTEIN SOURCE

Type of protein	Formula name
Cow's milk protein	Enfamil (standard, AR, Enfacare, Lipil, Premature)
	Portagen
	Similac (standard, Lactose Free, 60/40, Neosure, and Special Care)
Soy protein	Isomil
	ProSobee
Hydrolysate	Alimentum
	Nutramigen
	Pregestimil
Free amino acids	Neocate

Modified from Gunn VL, Nechyba C (ed): The Harriet Lane Handbook (16th edition). Philadelphia, Mosby, 2002, p. 470–47.

C. CLASSIFICATION BY FAT SOURCE

Type of fat	Formula name
Long-chain triglycerides	Enfamil (standard, AR, Lipil, Lactofree)
	Isomil
	Neocate
	Nutramigen
	ProSobee
	Similac (standard, 60/40 and Lactose Free)
Medium- and long-chain triglycerides	Enfamil (Enfacare and Premature)
	Neosure
	Portagen
	Pregestimil
	Similac (Special Care)

Modified from Gunn VL and Nechyba C (ed): The Harriet Lane Handbook (16th edition). Philadelphia, Mosby, 2002, p. 472.

XII. Parenteral Nutrition (PN)

Recommended 80 to 90 kcal/kg/day (fewer calories than enteral because of near-complete absorption of PN contents)

Most of the calories provided by lipids and glucose

A. COMPOSITION

complications → hyperosmolarity, hyperglycemia or glucosuria
↓
dehydration

1. Carbohydrates
Source mostly glucose (readily available to the brain)
1 g CHO provides 3.4 kcal

With increasing glucose concentration, increasing osmolarity

For positive nitrogen balance, 6 g of glucose should be provided for each g of protein

Carbohydrates should provide ~ 35% to 65% of total killocalories

Preterm CHO requirement: glucose utilization rate = 5 to 8 mg/kg/min

   Higher than full-term infants because of the increased brain-to-body weight ratio, decreased fat stores, increased total energy requirements

Full-term CHO requirement: glucose utilization rate = 3 to 5 mg/k/min

2. Fats   *0.5–1g/kg/d will prevent EFA defic.*

Common commercially available preparation is Intralipid solution

Components: neutral triglycerides (soybean oil), fatty acids (50% linoleic acid), egg yolk phospholipids (for emulsification), and glycerin (to regulate tonicity)

EFA compete c bili for plasma binding sites?

Intralipid does not provide omega oils or C20:4 arachidonic acid

20% versus 10% solutions: 10% solution has lower triglyceride content, lower calories per milliliter, and a higher phospholipid-to-triglyceride ratio (this increased ratio has been shown to impair lipid lipase activity in preterm infants, so 10% lipid preparation is not recommended)   *↳↑Tg level*

1 g fat provides 9 kcal (for 20% Intralipid solution: 1 mL = 2 kcals)

Fats should provide 30% to 50% of total daily calories (should not exceed 60% of total calories)

Limit to 3 g/kg/day

During intravenous fat administration, monitor serum triglyceride levels (recommended that value should be < 150 mg/dL)

Inadequate fat intake → thrombocytopenia, poor growth, dry skin

3. Proteins

Goal of protein administration is to prevent negative energy balance, negative nitrogen balance, and catabolism

Amino acid supplementation is required *early* in life to achieve above goals

Amino acid solutions have decreased tyrosine and cysteine levels because both have decreased solubility

1 g of protein provides 4 kcal

Protein should provide 7% to 15% of total kilocalories (to avoid negative nitrogen balance); 1 g protein = 1 g amino acid = 0.16 g nitrogen

Preterm protein requirement: 2.5 to 3.5 g/kg/day

Full-term protein requirement: 2 to 2.5 g/kg/day

4. Vitamins

Infants may receive a lower concentration of vitamins than intended because fat-soluble vitamins can be absorbed into the storage bag (~80% of vitamin A is lost); in addition, amounts can vary with light (vitamin A is light sensitive), O_2, and heat

5. Calcium (Ca) and phosphorus (P)

PN amounts are often lower than recommended levels

Difficult to administer both at high concentrations because of the increased risk of precipitation (increased risk of precipitation with increased temperature and lipid infusion)

Ca:P ratio should be in the 1.3:1 to 1.7:1 range; ratios < 1:1 are not recommended

Because of insufficient amounts, there is a risk of decreased bone mineralization with prolonged parenteral nutrition

6. Trace elements

Often present: zinc, copper, manganese, chromium, selenium

B. COMPLICATIONS

1. Cholestasis   *direct bili >2*

Pathogenesis:

   Both intracellular and intracannicular hepatic involvement, which leads to portal inflammation and bile duct proliferation

If prolonged, risk of partial fibrosis and later cirrhosis

Risks: GI surgery, hepatitis, visual Infections

Risk of cholestasis early in life is highest for lower birth weight infants [however, for prolonged PN (> 90 days), high risk of cholestasis independent of weight]

Clinical:

Jaundice

Laboratory values:

Direct hyperbilirubinemia, increased serum bile acids

Increased gamma-glutamyl transpeptidase (early and sensitive but nonspecific)

Increased liver function tests (late finding)

Management and prognosis:

Usually resolves with discontinuation of parenteral nutrition and initiation of enteral feedings

Limit amino acid load to 2 g/kg/day (may reduce hepatic toxicity from amino acids)

Phenobarbital and ursodeoxycholic acid have been shown to be effective for cholestasis in older children and adults; the benefits of these drugs for preterm infants with PN-associated cholestasis is unknown

2. Metabolic acidosis

Pathogenesis:

Metabolic acidosis caused by

Increased nonprotein metabolizable acids resulting in organic acidosis

Decreased nonmetabolizable base

Management:

Bicarbonate as needed

Consider administration of salts in acetate form

3. Hyperglycemia → dehydration

4. Metabolic bone disease: caused by imbalance in minerals, trace elements, and vitamin D

5. Nosocomial infections

Most common:

Staphylococcus epidermidis, Staphylococcus aureus, Candida albicans, Malassezia furfur

6. Complications of parenteral fat

Theoretical concern of pulmonary impairment because of potential risk of increased pulmonary artery pressure, decreased PaO_2, and accumulation of small lipid droplets within pulmonary capillaries (this has not been shown in newborns with graduated increases in fat delivery, an infusion rate of < 0.125 g/kg/h, and a maximum intake of 3 g/kg/d)

Possible impairment of host defense: lipid accumulation in macrophages of reticuloendothelial system

Competes with bilirubin for albumin-binding sites and theoretically may increase bilirubin levels (intakes of ≤ 3 g/kg/d do not appear to displace bilirubin)

May lead to hyperlipidemia, primarily from increased triglyceride administration or secondary to lowered lipoprotein lipase activity caused by trauma and infection

References

Committee on Nutrition. Pediatric Nutrition Handbook (4th edition). Elk Grove, IL, American Academy of Pediatrics, 1996.

Behrman RE, Kliegman RM, and Arvin AM (eds): Nelson Textbook of Pediatrics (15th edition). Philadelphia, WB Saunders Co, 1996.

Carb requir ↓ c̄ chronic lung disease
* more Lipids

Fanaroff, AA, Martin RJ (ed): Neonatal and Perinatal Medicine: Diseases of the Fetus and Newborn (7th edition). St. Louis, Mosby, 2001.

Gunn VL and Nechyba C (ed): The Harriet Lane Handbook (16th edition). Philadelphia, Mosby, 2002

Lawrence RA and Lawrence RM. Breastfeeding: a guide for the medical profession (5th edition). St. Louis, Mosby, 1999.

Polin RA and Fox WW. Fetal and Neonatal Physiology (2nd edition). Philadelphia, W.B. Saunders, 1998.

Porterfield SP. Endocrine Physiology (2nd edition). St Louis, Mosby, 2001.

Factors that ↑ fluid req → photo tx, radiant warmers, third spacing, temp (fever or cold stress), diarrhea, ostomy

↓ Fluid req → HIE, PDA, BPD, postop, CHF, meningitis, Renal failure

Ca, Phos : Mg
   — Nec for tissue structure: fxn, esp. bone mineralization
   — Ca, Phos retention: absorption are inter dependant

Fe
   — Impt for synthesis of Hgb, myoglobin
   — Difficult to achieve fetal accretion rate d/t poor enteral absorption
   — Physiologic anemia doesn't benefit f/supplementation
   — Supplement preterm @ 2mo to ↓ Fe defic. anemia

Transpyloric (tube below pyloric sphincter)
   — Fdg passes stomach → may result in fat malabsorption
   — Recommend if you have aspiration
   — Only continuous → duodenum & jejunum
Disadv. → ↑ risk of perf : fat malabsorption (stomach enzymes unable to aid digestn process)

Gastrostomy
   — cong anom
   — Inability to suck, swallow, breath
   — Adm. by gravity or pump (can be cont.)

CHAPTER 9

Gastroenterology

TOPICS COVERED IN THIS CHAPTER

Maternal polyhydramnios, vomiting, distention, failure to pass stool = suspect GI dysfunction

I. Embryology of the Gastrointestinal Tract

A. DEVELOPMENT OF THE GASTROINTESTINAL TRACT

GA (weeks)	Mouth, esophagus, and stomach (weeks)	Intestine (weeks)	Pancreas and liver (weeks)
3.5	Foregut and hindgut present		Liver bud
4	Derived from foregut	Single tube	Hepatobiliary system derived from foregut
	Esophagus and stomach separate		Pancreas derived from primitive midgut
5–9	In normal position (7)	Intestinal tube elongates and herniates into umbilical cord	
		Tube then undergoes a series of rotations	
		Formation of villi in jejunum (9)	
10		Tube re-enters abdominal cavity after rotating 270°	
		Formation of microvilli	
		Crypts of Lieberkühn appear	
12	Parietal cells in stomach	Muscularis and muscle layers well developed (13)	Formation of islet cells
	Mature taste buds		Bile secretion begins
		Disaccharidases	
16	Swallowing and sucking ability (not coordinated)	Villi present throughout intestine (14)	Lipase and trypsin activity
18		Meconium present	
		Ganglion cells	
		Crypts well developed (19)	
20–24	Mouth—amylase	Maltase, sucrase active	Pancreatic amylase (22)
	Ciliated columnar cells		
28		Disaccharidases reach adult levels (30)	
		Lactase increasing	
32	Normal gastric emptying		
	HCl detected in stomach		
34–36	Coordinated suck and swallow	Lactase at adult levels (36)	
	Rapid peristalsis		

GA = gestational age; Modified from: Fanaroff AA and Martin RJ (eds): Neonatal-Perinatal Medicine (6th edition). St Louis, Mosby, 1997, p. 1289–1290.

II. Digestion and Absorption

A. DIGESTION AND ABSORPTION BY NUTRIENT COMPONENT

Carbohydrate (CHO)	Overall, neonates have adequate CHO absorption because of (1) colonic salvage pathway; (2) normal glucosidases/disaccharidases (except for lactase); and (3) normal glucoamylase	
	Pancreatic amylase	Present at 22 weeks gestation
		Adequate amounts produced
		Decreased secretion at birth
	Glucoamylase	Normal action at birth
		Located in the intestinal brush border
		Removes glucose from the end of starch
	Intestinal disaccharidase	All except lactase reach adult levels at 28 weeks gestation
		Glucosidases = sucrase, maltase, isomaltase
	Colonic bacteria	Help ferment malabsorbed CHO to acids, which are absorbed in colon (system called colonic savage pathway)
	Glucose transport	Transport across intestine
		Less efficient in newborns, especially premature infants
	Lactase	Adult levels at 36 weeks gestation
		Colonic salvage pathway helps limit CHO malabsorption
Protein	Overall, adequate neonatal protein digestion secondary to (1) normal absorption of nitrogen and (2) increased intestinal uptake of intact protein (compared with adults) because neonates have increased secretory IgA levels and increased mucosal permeability	
	Gastric pH	Increased gastric pH in neonates (compared with adults) because of decreased HCl secretion
		Neonates also with increased buffering ability of stomach contents (thus, pH probes may underestimate gastrointestinal reflux because fluid is not very acidic)
	Pepsin	Pepsin is deactivated because of increased gastric pH
		No intragastric protein digestion first 5 to 8 days of life

(continued on following page)

	Chymotrypsin and trypsin	Present in duodenal fluid
		Decreased in both preterm and full-term infants
	Dipeptidase	In mucosa, well developed early in life
	Amino acid transport capacity	Well developed early in life
Fat	Fat digestion requires:	
	(1) bile acid emulsification of fat globules	
	(2) triglyceride hydrolysis by lipase	
	(3) solubilization of lipolytic products	
	(4) fatty acid transfer across intestinal mucosa	
	(5) triglyceride resynthesis from fatty acids in enterocytes	
	(6) chylomicron formation in enterocytes	
	(7) secretion of chylomicrons into portal blood or lymphatics	
	Despite reduced bile acid secretion and pancreatic lipase activity, fat malabsorption is minimized because of (1) lingual lipase, gastric lipase, and lipases in breast milk, which allows for triglyceride breakdown; (2) chylomicron formation; and (3) increased amounts of more easily digested medium chain fatty acids in breast milk	
	Bile acids	Made by liver from cholesterol
		Needed for fat digestion and absorption
		Form micelles of phospholipids, cholesterol, and bile acids, which help lipid absorption from intestines
		Decreased bile acid secretion in infants; adult values reached at age 2 months
	Pancreatic lipase	Reduced activity
		Adult values at age 4 to 5 months

B. DIGESTION AND ABSORPTION BY ANATOMICAL LOCATION

Location	Enzyme or hormone	Function	In Neonates
Mouth	**Salivary amylase**	Digests starch	
		Controlled by parasympathetics, taste, smell, and tactile stimulation	
	Lingual lipase		Well developed
Stomach	**Pepsinogen → pepsin** (regulated by acid)	Produced by chief cells	Pepsin downregulated secondary to increased pH
		Important for protein digestion	No intragastric digestion of protein for the first 5 to 8 days of life
		Stimulated by vagus nerve, histamine, gastrin	
	Acid	Produced by parietal cells	Increased gastric pH in neonates secondary to decreased HCl secretion (preterm infants >> term infants >adults)
		Stimulated by vagus nerve, histamine, gastrin	
	Chyme	= pepsin, H_2O, and acid	
	Intrinsic factor	Responsible for vitamin B12 absorption in distal ileum	
		Stimulated by vagus nerve, histamine, gastrin	
	Gastrin	Stimulated by the presence of food; stimulates enzyme pepsin and gastric acid secretion	Decreased
	Gastric lipase		Well developed
Pancreas	**Pancreatic amylase**	Carbohydrate digestion	Adequate production yet decreased secretion at birth
	Chymotrypsinogen → chymotrypsin	Reaction mediated by enterokinase (in the intestinal mucosa)	Decreased
		Protein digestion	
	Trypsinogen → trypsin	Reaction mediated by enterokinase (in the intestinal mucosa)	Decreased
		Protein digestion	
	Pancreatic lipase	Fat digestion	Decreased (age 4 to 5 months = adult values)
		Triglyceride → 3 fatty acids + 1 glycerol	
Liver	**Bile**	Synthesized from cholesterol	Decreased bile acids (age 2 months = adult values)
		Stored in the gallbladder	
		Released into the small intestine via bile duct	
		Fat digestion	
Small intestine	**Enterokinase**	In intestinal mucosa	
		Activates chymotrypsinogen and trypsinogen	
	Glucoamylase	Carbohydrate digestion located in intestinal brush border	
		Removes glucose from end of starch	

(continued on following page)

Location	Enzyme or hormone	Function	In Neonates
	Disaccharidases	In the brush border	
	Maltase	Maltose $\longrightarrow$ glucose + glucose	Adult levels at 28 weeks GA
	Sucrase	Sucrose $\longrightarrow$ glucose + fructose	Adult levels at 28 weeks GA
	Lactase	Lactose $\longrightarrow$ glucose + galactose	Decreased, adult levels at 36 weeks GA
	Aminopeptidases	Protein digestion	
	Dipeptidase	Protein digestion	Well developed
	Intestinal lipase		
	Cholecystokinin (CCK)	Hormone that triggers release of pancreatic juice and bile	
		Decreases gastrin secretion	
	Secretin	Hormone that stimulates pancrease to release bicarbonate, which slows gastric emptying	
	Gastrin inhibitory peptide (GIP)	Hormone that is stimulated by protein and fat	
		Slows gastric emptying	
		Decreases gastrin	
	Motilin	Hormone that increases gastric emptying (erythromycin is a motilin agonist)	
Large intestine	**Salvage pathway**	Important for carbohydrate digestion	
		Colonic bacteria helps ferment malabsorbed carbohydrates	

GA = gestational age.

III. Mouth and Pharynx

Sucking can be present at 16 weeks gestation

Coordination of suck, swallowing, and breathing at $\geq$ 34 weeks gestation; large variation with signs of dyscoordination or immaturity lasting until age 6 months

Conditions that lead to *absent or weakened suck* include maternal anesthesia, hypoxia, prematurity, congenital syndromes, neuromuscular disorders, sepsis, and hypothyroidism

Factors that mechanically *interfere with sucking* include macroglossia, cleft lip, cysts or tumors of mouth or gums, micrognathia

Conditions that lead to *disordered swallowing* include choanal atresia, cleft palate, micrognathia, postintubation irritation, dysautonomia

IV. Esophagus

A. ESOPHAGEAL DUPLICATION

Posterior mediastinal mass
If compresses trachea, respiratory difficulties and cyanosis
If compresses esophagus, feeding intolerance and emesis
Recurrent aspiration and pneumonias
Diagnose by ultrasound

B. ESOPHAGEAL CYSTS

Located within muscular wall
Lined by one or more cell types, including:
  Ciliated epithelium
  Squamous epithelium
  Gastric epithelium associated with acid secretion, leading to upper gastrointestinal hemorrhage, ulceration, and erosion
    into the neighboring bronchus or lung
Associated abnormalities:
  Abnormal cervical or thoracic vertebrae
  Pulmonary agenesis
  Tracheoesophageal fistula
  Intrabdominal cyst
Diagnose by barium swallow or computed tomography (CT) scan

C. TRACHEOESOPHAGEAL FISTULAE (TEF) AND ESOPHAGEAL ATRESIA (EA)

Incidence
  1/4500 births
  Most often isolated
  Rarely familial
  Possibly associated with a common teratogen
  30% to 40% of patients with additional anomalies
  Can be associated with VACTERL (vertebral, anal, cardiac, tracheo-esophageal, radial, renal, and limb abnormalities)

Etiology
  Abnormal formation during fourth week of gestation

Types

Esophageal atresia (upper pouch) with distal TEF just above carina	85% Distended abdomen Hypersalivation Potential to reflux gastric secretions into lung	*EA (upper pouch) distal TEF*
Isolated esophageal atresia with no tracheal communication	8% Scaphoid abdomen Hypersalivation	*EA isolated*

(continued on following page)

Isolated TEF (H type)	4% Abdomen not scaphoid Often asymptomatic; may present with coughing during feedings or aspiration pneumonias	
Double TEF, separate attachments with upper and lower esophagus	1% Distended abdomen Increased salivation into lungs Potential to reflux gastric secretions into lungs	
Upper pouch fistula	1% Scaphoid abdomen Hypersalivation Saliva may go into lungs	

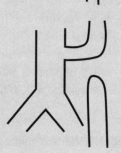

H-TEF

Double TEF

Clinical
  Prenatal:
    Fluid-filled stomach not visualized by fetal ultrasound
    Polyhydramnios (40%)
  Postnatal:
    Can present with excess salivation, nonbilious vomiting, feeding intolerance, respiratory distress with feedings, abdominal distention if fistula present, increased abdominal distention if ventilated (can try to block fistula with endotracheal tube), or intermittent periods of cyanosis

Diagnosis
  Place nasogastric tube and obtain chest and abdominal radiographs
  Will need other radiographic studies to rule out associated anomalies

Treatment
  Medical: upright positioning; catheter placed in upper pouch for frequent suctioning
  Surgical: three types of repair
    Primary: immediate end-to-end repair
    Delayed: correction of underlying complications before end-to-end repair
    Staged: gastrostomy to ventilate stomach; ligation of fistula; serial esophageal dilatations to reduce any gap between the upper and lower esophageal segments; end-to-end repair at age 2 to 3 months; if need to lengthen, esophagus, stomach, small intestines, or colon may be used

Prognosis
  Without associated anomalies, survival approaches 100%
  With anomalies, survival may approach only 50%

D. GASTROESOPHAGEAL REFLUX

Factors that place preterm and full-term newborns at risk
  Short lower esophageal sphincter (LES)
  Low LES pressure
  Prolonged LES relaxation
  Poor esophageal coordination of motility

Management options (some controversial)
  Upright positioning
  Thickened feedings
  Antireflux medications
  Surgical management considered if persistent symptoms and secondary complications (failure to thrive, recurrent
      pneumonias, esophageal bleeding, persistent vomiting, large hiatal hernia, esophageal stricture or ulceration)
    Nissen plication:
      Esophagogastric junction placed within abdomen and fundus wrapped around the esophagus
      85% successful
      Complications: small bowel obstruction (5% to 8%) displacement into chest (2% to 8%); wrap disruption (3% to 10%)

V. Stomach

A. SPONTANEOUS GASTRIC PERFORATION

Risks
  Increased with perinatal stress, prematurity, and postnatal steroid exposure
  20% without predisposing factor

Etiology
  Majority related to mechanical overdistention versus ischemia

Clinical
  Typically large and proximal
  Usually occurs at 2 to 7 days of life
  Presents with abrupt abdominal distension, marked respiratory distress, shock, or sepsis

Diagnosis
  Evident by plain abdominal radiograph

Management
  Paracentesis; surgical intervention

B. PYLORIC STENOSIS

Incidence
  3/1000 births
  Males greater than females (5:1); greater in first-born males
  Associated with blood groups O and B and maternal stress in last trimester

Risks
  If mother has pyloric stenosis, 19% risk of affected son; 7% risk of affected daughter
  If father has pyloric stenosis, 5.5% risk of affected son; 2.4% risk of affected daughter
  If one child has pyloric stenosis, 3% risk to next child (4% if male, 2.4% if female)

Etiology   "olive mass"
  Postnatal hypertrophy
  Congenital delay of pyloric sphincter development
  Unclear etiology

Clinical
  Presents during first week to age 5 months (average age 3 to 6 weeks)
  Nonbilious vomiting, dehydration
  Hypochloremic, hypokalemic metabolic alkalosis   ↓Cl ↓K M.alkalosis

Diagnosis
  Ultrasound preferred imaging choice
  "String sign" on barium enema

Management
  Correction of electrolyte abnormalities
  Pyloromyotomy

VI. Small Intestine

A. DUODENAL ATRESIA

Incidence
  1/10,000 births
  High rate of associated disorders:
     Trisomy 21 (31%), malrotation (20%), congenital heart disease (30%), esophageal atresia (10%), genitourinary
        anomalies (11%), annular pancreas (20%)

Etiology
  Failure of recannulization in the second month of gestation
  Usually occurs in the second part of the duodenum

Clinical
  In utero: polyhydramnios and fetal ultrasound may show a distended duodenum
  Postnatal: bilious vomiting in the first 24 hours of life
     Abdominal distention in the upper abdomen
     Can have meconium passage

Diagnosis
  Plain abdominal radiograph: double bubble, air–fluid level, no distal intestinal air

Management
  Abdominal decompression
  Surgery

B. JEJUNAL-ILEAL ATRESIA

Incidence
  Overall incidence greater than duodenal or colonic atresias
  Male = female
  Usually single atresia (multiple atresias occur in 6% to 20%)
    Distal ileum: 36%
    Proximal jejunum: 31%
    Distal jejunum: 20%
    Proximal ileum: 13%

Etiology
  In utero mesenteric vascular occlusion

Clinical
  Polyhydramnios in 1/3 of patients with jejunal atresia; more rare for those with ileal atresia
  Infants with jejunal atresia are often small for gestational age
  Bilious vomiting
  Abdominal distention: greater with more distal atresias
  Can fail to pass meconium

Diagnosis
  Plain abdominal supine and lateral radiographs: dilated loops with air-fluid levels
  The greater amount of air, the lower the obstruction
  If peritoneal calcifications are observed, suggests *in utero* perforation and meconium peritonitis

Management
  Surgery

C. MALROTATION   Ladd's Bands

Incidence
  Can be isolated or associated with other malformations, including congenital diaphragmatic hernia, abdominal wall
    defects, intestinal atresias, and Beckwith-Wiedemann syndrome

Etiology
  Failure of normal rotation with abnormal fixation
  Presence of *Ladd's bands:* fibrous bands form between the cecum and right posterior retroduodenal peritoneum

Clinical
  80% with symptoms in the first month of life
  Bilious vomiting
  If concurrent volvulus, may have acute ischemia with acute episode of rectal bleeding and shock

Diagnosis
  Plain abdominal radiograph: decreased air because lesion is proximal
  Barium enema: cecum seen in the right *upper* quadrant rather than the usual location of the right *lower* quadrant;
    corkscrew appearance of the proximal jejunem

Management
  Surgery: Ladd's procedure

D. MECONIUM ILEUS

Incidence

10% to 15% of patients with cystic fibrosis (CF) also have meconium ileus

90% of patients with meconium ileus have CF

Etiologies

Obstruction caused by hyperviscous secretions from the mucous glands of the small intestine

Meconium with decreased water and adheres to intestinal lining

Clinical

Symptoms within 24 to 48 hours

No passage of meconium

Increased abdominal distention at birth (in contrast to jejunal atresia, which usually presents 12 to 24 hours later)

Bilious vomiting

Palpable bowel loops

Associated findings: volvulus, intestinal necrosis, perforation, meconium peritonitis

Diagnosis

Plain abdominal radiograph—distended intestinal loops without air-fluid levels (similar to ileal atresia)

Can appear granular or "bubbly" (because of meconium)

Management

If uncomplicated, treat with enema (hypertonic barium enema, gastrografin, or Hypaque); this is effective because hyperosmolality draws fluid into the intestines and allows for disimpaction; successful in 60% of cases

E. MECONIUM PERITONITIS

Etiology

In utero intestinal perforation with meconium spillage into the peritoneal cavity

Usually a secondary complication of meconium ileus; can also be a result of intestinal atresia, volvulus, or gastroschisis

Most often associated with intestinal obstruction or mesenteric vascular occlusion

Types

Meconium pseudocysts: wall of fibrous tissue surrounds meconium; may occur if meconium accumulates over a long period

Adhesive meconium peritonitis: widespread contamination of peritoneal cavity days to weeks before birth; scattered calcifications seen on abdominal radiograph; vascular adhesions observed with exploratory laparotomy; often associated with intestinal obstruction

Meconium ascites: perforation only a few days before birth; large amount meconium-stained ascitic fluid; no calcifications

Infected meconium peritonitis: intestinal perforation that does not seal, allowing for seeding of microorganisms into peritoneal cavity

Management

If perforation has sealed and there is no intestinal obstruction, specific treatment may not be necessary

However, a majority of patients require surgical intervention for the following associated complications:

Intestinal obstruction

Persistent peritonitis and sepsis

Abdominal mass

Abdominal wall cellulitis
Test for cystic fibrosis

VII. Large Intestine

A. SMALL LEFT COLON SYNDROME OR MICROCOLON

Incidence
Associated with:
Maternal diabetes (most common)
Maternal hypothyroidism
Maternal toxemia (maternal magnesium exposure)
Prematurity
Rare complication of cecal perforation

Etiology
Functional immaturity of the ganglion cells
Primarily affects the descending and rectosigmoid colon
Transient functional obstruction

Clinical
Abdominal distention
Failure to pass meconium

Diagnosis
Plain abdominal radiograph: multiple dilated loops of bowel
Barium enema: small colon segment with dilated bowel proximal to the involved segment
Rectum is normal (unlike Hirschsprung disease)

B. COLONIC ATRESIA

Incidence
1/1500 to 1/20,000 births
Often associated with skeletal anomalies (polydactyly, absent radii, club foot), ocular abnormalities, or congenital heart disease

Etiology
Secondary to vascular compromise

Clinical
Bilious vomiting; absent stools

Diagnosis
Plain abdominal radiograph: multiple, large distended loops
Barium enema: distended proximal bowel, collapsed rectum (no air)

Management
Surgery

C. HIRSCHSPRUNG DISEASE

Incidence
1/5000 births
If one child has Hirschsprung disease, there is a 3% to 5% risk to next child
1/3 have a relative with Hirschsprung disease
80% are male   *↗ difference in coloration*
Associations: trisomy 21, heterochromia, Waardenburg syndrome, congenital deafness, 13q deletion,
pheochromocytoma, neurofibromatosis, neuroblastoma
          ↖ neuroendocrine tumor of adrenal gland

Etiology
Failure of complete cranial to caudal migration of neural crest cells at 8 to 10 weeks gestation
Aganglionic, so there is no parasympathetic innervation to distal colon
Abnormal peristalsis leading to functional constipation

Pathology
75% to 80%: only rectosigmoid involved
5% to 10%: complete colon involved
Normal proximal intestine becomes thickened because of excess stimulation attempting to overcome distal functional
obstruction
Transition zone: area between the end of the normal proximal zone and beginning of the abnormal distal zone

Clinical
No meconium in first 24 hours
Abdominal distention
Constipation or foul-smelling liquid stool seepage
Bloody diarrhea
Failure to thrive
Urinary obstruction because of mechanical obstruction by large colon
Complication:
Acute bacterial enterocolitis
Rapidly progressive with abdominal distention, vomiting, foul-smelling bloody stools, ulceration of intestinal
mucosa, necrosis of bowel wall, sepsis
25% to 30% mortality rate
Differential diagnosis: distal ileal atresia, colonic atresia, meconium ileus (barium enema [BE] shows small or
microcolon in all of the above, but those with Hirschsprung disease have a normal or dilated colon)

Diagnosis
50% diagnosed by age 1 month
Plain abdominal radiograph: large colon with absence of air in rectum
BE: to assess for transition zone (also, retention of barium 24 hours after study suggests disease in full-term infants); a
negative BE result does not rule out disease
Biopsy to detect the absence or presence of ganglionic cells by pattern of acetylcholinesterase staining

Management
Diverting colostomy proximal to transition zone with definitive treatment at age 1.0 to 1.5 years or weight > 10 kg
Daily anal dilations followed by laparoscopy-soave pullthrough of colon through anus
Monitor for signs of enterocolitis
Hearing screen

VIII. Rectum and Anus

A. IMPERFORATE ANUS

Incidence

1/5000 births

Includes wide spectrum of anorectal abnormalities (anal stenosis, genitourinary abnormalities)

Associated with other anomalies:

Genitourinary (28% to 50% if high imperforate anus), gastrointestinal (13%), cardiac (7%), skeletal or central nervous system (6%), VACTERL

Usually no familial pattern, but there have been reports of autosomal recessive or dominant inheritance

Etiology

Anorectum derives from cloaca

Failure of the normal separation and division of the cloaca into the anterior urogenital sinus and the posterior intestinal canal; this results in a constellation of findings, including imperforate anus

Types

Types	General Features	Male Features	Female Features
High	Blind end of rectum ends above levator muscle More common in boys Most complex	Anorectal agenesis with or without rectoprostatic-urethral fistula Rectal atresia	Anorectal agenesis with or without rectovaginal fistula
Intermediate	Manage similar to high type	Rectobulbar urethral fistula Agenesis without fistula	Rectovaginal fistula Rectovestibular fistula Agenesis without fistula
Low	Male = female	Anocutaneous fistula Anal stenosis (uncommon)	Anovestibular fistula Anal stenosis Anocutaneous fistula

Modified from Fanaroff, AA and Martin RJ (eds): Neonatal-Perinatal Medicine (6th edition). St. Louis, Mosby-Year Book, 1997, p. 1325.

Clinical

High lesions and intermediate lesions often without anal opening

If rectal atresia: anal opening appears normal

Rocker bottom perineum suggests sacral agenesis and has a poor prognosis for fecal continence

Sacral deformities are predictive of higher incidence of incontinence

Urinary reflux if rectourinary fistula

In high lesions: 10% tethered cord

Diagnosis

Physical examination

Prone lateral plain abdominal radiograph

In the past, a Wangensteen-Rice invertogram was used to delineate level

Management

Anal dilation surgery

IX. Pancreas

A. PANCREATIC INSUFFICIENCY

Inability to break down fats, leading to watery diarrhea, steatorrhea

Diagnosis
  Assess daily fecal fat loss, test stool for trypsin, and assess for cystic fibrosis

Etiology
 Schwachmann-Diamond syndrome
   Pancreatic insufficiency, bone marrow dysfunction (neutropenia), short stature, diarrhea, normal bicarbonate
    secretion
   Normal sweat test result
   Management: oral pancreatic enzymes; increased calories; increased protein; vitamin A, D, E, and K supplements;
    growth colony stimulating factor
 Cystic fibosis
   Incidence: 1/2500, more common in white populations
   Pathophysiology: majority with mutation in 508 position, chromosome 7
    Protein abnormality necessary for chloride transport = cystic fibrosis transmembrane regulator (CFTR); leads to
     thick mucus in lumens of pancreas, lungs, intestines, biliary tract, and appendix
   Clinical:
    Meconium ileus
    Diarrhea, edema, failure to thrive, vitamin K malabsorption (bleeding), hypocalcemia, cholestasis, rectal prolapse,
     pulmonary complications, nasal polyps, peptic ulcer, pancreatitis
   Studies:
    Increased chloride in sweat (> 50 mEq/L); sweat test not reliable until infant > 2 kg
    Hyponatremic, hypochloremic metabolic alkalosis
    Newborn screening: tests for increased immunoreactive trypsinogen (not specific), need to confirm with
     mutational analysis
   Management:
    Supportive, pulmonary toilet, supplementation of fat-soluble vitamins and pancreatic enzymes

X. Abdominal Wall Defects

Abnormal Fusion of Abdominal Folds	Disorder
Lateral cephalic folds	Pentalogy of Cantrell (cleft sternum, anterior midline diaphragmatic abnormality, pericardial defect, ectopic cordis, upper abdominal omphalocele)
Lateral abdominal folds	Omphalocele
Caudal and lateral folds	Cloacal or bladder exstrophy
	Hypogastric omphalocele

A. GASTROSCHISIS

Incidence
  1/4000 to 1/20,000 births

Etiology
  Controversial; several mechanisms have been proposed:
   Involution of right umbilical vein creates a potential weak spot at the junction of the right aspect of the umbilical ring
    and the abdominal wall; this may allow for rupture and bowel herniation

Teratogenic exposures such as solvents, colorants, aspirin, ibuprofen, pseudoephedrine, and cocaine have been associated with an increased risk of gastroschisis; many of these substances are vasoconstrictive agents, supporting a vascular contribution to the pathogenesis of gastroschisis

Genetic influences have been implicated, with several reports of familial occurrences, including multiple affected siblings and vertical transmission from mother to son

Clinical
  Prenatal:
    Elevated α-fetoprotein levels are associated with abdominal wall defects
    Antenatal ultrasound can accurately diagnose gastroschisis in the second trimester; the finding of dilated loops of bowel on antenatal ultrasound has been found to correlate with presence of bowel edema, longer repair time, and higher rate of postoperative complications
    An amniocentesis is not necessary because of the very low incidence of associated chromosomal abnormalities in infants with gastroschisis
    High incidence of oligohydramnios, fetal growth restriction, and meconium-stained amniotic fluid; if intestinal atresia is present, the patient may develop polyhydramnios
    Preferred route for delivery remains controversial; elective cesarean section has been advocated to reduce additional bowel injury that may occur during passage through the birth canal; however, delivery by elective cesarean section has not been shown to be advantageous in multiple recent studies; currently, cesarean section is recommended for rare, large lesions with the liver exposed (to avoid bleeding and damage to the liver)
  Postnatal:
    Eviscerated intestinal loops without a covering sac through an abdominal wall defect located to the right of umbilical cord
    Intact umbilical cord
    Intestinal loops may be thickened, foreshortened, or covered with a fibrous peel
    Associated defects:
      All infants with gastroschisis have abnormal rotation and fixation of the intestines (malrotation)
      16% of these infants have other gastrointestinal anomalies, including midgut volvulus, intestinal atresia, intestinal stenosis, or intestinal perforation
      Chromosomal or nongastrointestinal structural anomalies are rare (in contrast to an omphalocele)

Management
  Surgical correction

Prognosis
  Survival rate is > 90%; most patients experience good long-term health and growth
  Prematurity, low birth weight, staged silo repair, and the presence of intestinal atresia are all associated with longer time to full enteral feedings and prolonged hospital stays
  Minority of patients have cholestasis
  Reported long-term complications include nonspecific abdominal pain and need for additional abdominal surgery to repair strictures and revise scars

B. OMPHALOCELE

Incidence
  1/3000 to 1/10,000 births
  Higher incidence of prematurity and fetal growth restriction
  3:1 male to female predominance
  Associated defects are present in as many as 80%

Chromosomal (50%)—trisomy 13, 18, 21

Cardiac (28%)—septal defects, patent ductus arteriosus, dextrocardia, tetralogy of Fallot, bicuspid aortic valve

Genitourinary (20%), craniofacial (20%), diaphragmatic hernia (12%), musculoskeletal (vertebral and limb deformities), pulmonary hypoplasia secondary to thoracic maldevelopment

Associated syndromes:

Pentalogy of Cantrell

Beckwith-Wiedemann syndrome

OEIS complex (*o*mphalocele, *e*xstrophy of the bladder, *i*mperforate anus, *s*pinal deformity)

Etiology

Occurs if the intestinal loops fail to return to the abdominal cavity at 11 weeks gestation or the somatic folds fail to complete formation of the abdominal wall by 18 weeks gestation

Because of abnormal embryologic development, there is a high rate of associated defects and chromosomal anomalies

Clinical

Prenatal:

Elevated α-fetoprotein levels

Accurately diagnosed by antenatal ultrasound in the second trimester

Careful examination of other organ systems (including a fetal echocardiogram) because of the high rates of additional anomalies

Amniocentesis is recommended to rule out chromosomal abnormalities

Infants with small lesions may be delivered vaginally; cesarean sections are recommended in those with large lesions that contain liver

Postnatal:

Amniotic sac and peritoneum protect the intestinal loops; covering sac may be ruptured

Umbilical cord inserts onto the amniotic sac

Abdominal wall musculature is normal

Defect can vary in size; larger lesions (giant omphalocele, $>$ 5 cm) may contain liver as well as intestinal loops, but smaller lesions contain only bowel

All infants with omphalocele have malrotation of the intestines; in contrast to gastroschisis, it is rare to have other intestinal anomalies with omphalocele

Management

Surgical correction

Prognosis

Mortality can be as high as 30% to 40% in the presence of multiple underlying complications; factors that affect survival include large defect, ruptured sac, low birth weight, presence of additional congenital anomalies, and early respiratory failure

Survival rate is 90% in patients with isolated omphalocele

Potential complications include:

Decreased gastrointestinal motility (although to a lesser extent than with gastroschisis)

Bowel obstruction

Perforated viscus

Gastroesophageal reflux

Sepsis

TABLE 1. Clinical distinction between gastroschisis and omphalocele

Characteristic	Gastroschisis	Omphalocele
Incidence	1/4000 to 20,000	1/3000 to 10,000
Maternal age	Younger	Older
Male: female ratio	1:1	3:1
Location of defect	Right of the umbilical cord	Within umbilical ring
Umbilical cord	Intact, normal insertion	Insertion onto covering sac
Size of defect	Usually < 4 cm	Usually > 4 cm
Organs extruded in addition to bowel	Stomach	Liver, spleen, bladder, uterus, ovaries
Covering sac	Absent	Present; may be ruptured
Appearance of bowel	Matted, foreshortened, edematous	Usually normal
Additional anomalies	10% to 20%	45% to 80%
Gastrointestinal, other than malrotation	16%, intestinal atresia, midgut volvulus, intestinal stenosis	Rare
Nongastrointestinal	Rare	Common
		Cardiac (28%), genitourinary (20%), craniofacial (20%), diaphragmatic hernia (12%), musculoskeletal
Chromosomal	Rare	50%, trisomies common
Syndromes	None	Pentalogy of Cantrell
		Beckwith-Wiedemann syndrome
		OEIS complex
Surgery	Primary closure in 80%	Often primary closure for lesions < 5 cm; multistaged for larger lesions
Bowel function after surgery	Usually slow	Normal to slow
Survival	> 90%	90% in absence of associated anomalies, 60% to 70% in presence of multiple associated anomalies

OEIS = omphalocele, exstrophy of the bladder, imperforate anus, spinal deformity.

Printed with permission from Hansen A and Puder M (eds): Manual of Surgical Neonatal Intensive Care. Hamilton, Ontario, BC Decker, 2003.

XI. Necrotizing Enterocolitis (NEC)

Incidence

1 to 3/1000

1% to 5% of all infants admitted to the neonatal intensive care unit

10% of infants < 1,500 g

Premature infants tend to get NEC later compared with full-term infants:

Age	Age of Onset (Days)
26 weeks GA	23
> 31 weeks GA	11
Full-term infant	3

Increased risk after gastroschisis

Pathophysiology

Precise pathogenesis remains unknown

Multifactorial:

  Prematurity: immature host defense, immature regulation of circulation, abnormal bacterial colonization

  Formula: 90% to 95% affected neonates had been fed formula; decreased risk with breast milk

  Intestinal ischemia

  Abnormal bacterial colonization: reduced number of bacterial species after antibiotic therapy; reduced anaerobic species

Final pathway to injury (despite inciting event) appears to be activation of the inflammatory cascade

Most commonly located in the terminal ileum and proximal colon

Clinical — Bright Red bloody stools

Abdominal distention, feeding intolerance, emesis, hematochezia, loose stools, abdominal wall erythema, systemic instability

Laboratory values

Leukopenia (more common than leukocytosis), thrombocytopenia, hyponatremia, hypokalemia, metabolic acidosis, disseminated intravascular coagulopthay (DIC), glucose instability

Diagnosis

Plain abdominal radiographs (preferably two views, prone with lateral or decubitus): pneumotosis intestinalis, dilated loops, thickened bowel wall, ileus, pneumoperitoneum

Modified Bell staging criteria for NEC

	Signs		
Stage	**Systemic**	**Intestinal**	**Radiographic**
I Suspected	Temperature instability, apnea, bradycardia	Elevated gastric residuals, mild abdominal distention, occult blood in stool	Normal or mild ileus
IIA Mild	Similar to stage I	Prominent abdominal distention +/− tenderness, absent bowel sounds, grossly bloody stools	Ileus, dilated bowel loops with focal pneumotosis
IIB Moderate	Mild acidosis and thrombocytopenia	Abdominal wall edema and tenderness, +/− palpable mass	Extensive pneumotosis, early ascites, +/− portal venous gas,
IIIA Advanced	Respiratory and metabolic acidosis, mechanical ventilation, hypotension, oliguria, DIC	Worsening wall edema and eryhthema with induration	Prominent ascites, persistent bowel loop, no free air
IIIB Advanced	Vital signs and laboratory evidence of deterioration, shock	Evidence of perforation	Pneumoperitoneum

DIC = disseminated intraracular coagulopathy;
Printed with permission from Kleigman RM, Walsh MC: "Neonatal necrotizing enterocolitis: pathogenesis, classification, and spectrum of disease." *Curr Prob Pediatr.* 1987; 17:213.

Management

Medical: supportive based on clinical presentation

Abdominal decompression, bowel rest, broad-spectrum antibiotics, hyperalimentation

Surgical: 34% to 50% of patients require surgical intervention

Penrose drain placement, exploratory laparotomy with resection of diseased bowel, enterostomy, and stoma formation

Complications and prognosis

Intestinal strictures, short bowel syndrome (25% postoperatively), parenteral nutrition-induced cholestasis, neurodevelopmental delay (50%)

Mortality 30% to 40%

XII. Allergic Gastroenteropathy

A. COW'S MILK PROTEIN INTOLERANCE

Clinical: symptoms within first 6 months of life; usually in infants fed cow's milk or cows milk–based formulas (although can also be observed in breast-fed infants if mother consumes cow's milk)

Diarrhea, anemia, hematochezia, edema, eczema, vomiting, increased white blood cells, decreased platelets

Pathology: jejunal biopsy shows inflammation, eosinophils, lacteal dilation

Management: delay introduction of cow's milk until after age 6 months; symptoms may decrease after changing to a non-cow's milk formula or formula with hydrolyzed protein (soy protein can also be sensitizing)

Prognosis: can usually tolerate cow's milk after age 9 to 12 months

Alimentum
Nutramigen
Pregestimil

B. ALLERGIC COLITIS

Closely related to above, but less severe symptoms
Blood and mucus in stool
Manage by removing offending formula

XIII. Short Bowel Syndrome

Pathophysiology
  Malabsorption secondary to bowel resection (caused by small intestinal atresias, NEC, volvulus, gastroschisis, Hirschsprung disease)
  A small section of intestines removed may lead to severe chronic diarrhea and failure to thrive

Complications
  Intestinal hyperplasia when exposed to enteral nutrition (ileum > jejunal)
  Gastric hypersecretion
  Bacterial overgrowth (leads to vitamin B12 deficiency and lactic acidosis)
  Colitis or ileitis
  Watery diarrhea
  Cholestasis
  Failure to thrive

Management
  Hyperalimentation
  Enteral formula to mimic normal physiology
  Antibiotics for bacterial overgrowth
  Monitor for dumping and electrolyte or fluid loss

Prognosis
  Better if intact ileum because of its role in bile acid absorption
  Intact ileocecal valve important because it delays transit time, so there is more time for digestion and absorption; the value also acts as a barrier to prevent overgrowth of colonic bacteria in small intestine
  Worse prognosis if colon resected, no ileocecal valve, > 25 cm bowel resected with ileocecal valve, or > 40 cm without ileocecal valve
  Infants with as little as 15 cm and intact ileocecal valve have survived
  If no ileocecal valve, require ~30 to 45 cm of intestinal length

XIV. Liver

A. CONJUGATED HYPERBILIRUBINEMIA

Etiology
  Increased direct fraction of serum bilirubin levels caused by abnormal bilirubin excretion
  Differential diagnosis

Hepatocellular:
  Neonatal idiopathic hepatitis*
  Infectious hepatitis
  Hyperalimentation
  Intestinal obstruction
  Hematologic disorders
  Metabolic disorders
Ductal disorders:
  Biliary atresia*
  Non-syndromic paucity of bile ducts
  Alagille syndrome (paucity of intrahepatic bile ducts with extrahepatic ducts, unusual facies, vertebral anomalies)
  Choledochal cyst
  Bile plug syndrome
  *Biliary atresia and idiopathic neonatal hepatitis together account for 60% to 70% of cases

Pathology
  Biliary atresia: bile duct proliferation
  Idiopathic neonatal hepatitis: multinucleated giant cells, increased α-fetoprotein

Clinical
  Conjugated hyperbilirubinemia, jaundice, hepatomegaly, acholic stools, colorless meconium at age 2 weeks

Diagnosis
  Ultrasound to assess for choledochal cyst
  HIDA or isotope scan (normal if isotope excreted in bile and in intestine)
  Consider liver biopsy

Management
  Treat underlying disorder
  Ursodeoxycholic acid, phenobarbital

XV. Congenital Diaphragmatic Hernia (CDH)

Incidence
  1/4000 births
  Left defect (85%) > right; bilateral (1%)

Pathology
  Herniation of intestines through diaphragm secondary to failure of closure of pleuroperitoneal canal at 8 weeks gestation
  Most often occurs at left posterior lateral region = foramen of Bochdalek

Clinical
  Polyhydramnios, scaphoid abdomen, mediastinal displacement, 5% present later with intestinal obstruction
  Right-sided CDH sometimes associated with group B *Streptococcus pneumoniae* infection
  Hernia sac (21% to 47%) most often contains intestine and spleen; more severe if contains liver and stomach
  Pulmonary hypoplasia (worse if large and early defect) because of decreased concentration of pulmonary arteries/cm^2 and arteriolar muscle hyperplasia

Diagnosis
Abdominal contents in thoracic cavity, evident on plain radiographs

Management
Respiratory support and possible extracorporeal membrane oxygenation
Surgical correction

Prognosis
Poor; 20% to 30% survival rate

XVI. Radiology

A. ESTABLISHMENT OF AIR PATTERN ON PLAIN RADIOGRAPH

Hours	Air Pattern
3	To small intestine
6–8	Through large intestine
24	In rectum

B. RADIOGRAPHIC FINDINGS OF SPECIFIC GASTROINTESTINAL DISORDERS

Disorder	Radiologic features
Diaphragmatic hernia	Plain radiograph: bowel loops in thoracic cavity
Duodenal atresia	Plain radiograph: double-bubble
Hirschsprung disease	Plain radiograph: distended bowel loops, absence of rectal gas Barium enema: lack of transition zone
Ileal atresia	Plain radiograph; triple-bubble or multiple dilated loops with air-fluid levels
Malrotation	Barium swallow: corkscrew appearance
Meconium ileus	Plain radiograph: varying distended small bowel loops; bubbly appearance of contents (meconium mixed with air); may have air-fluid levels
Meconium peritonitis	Plain radiograph: peritoneal calcifications
Microcolon	Barium enema; small left colon with dilated bowel proximal to involved segment
Necrotizing enterocolitis	Plain radiograph; pneumotosis intestinalis
Pyloric stenosis	Barium enema: "string sign"

C. FETAL ULTRASOUND

Stomach visible at 13 to 15 weeks gestation

Small intestine not clearly visualized except in the center of abdomen during the third trimester

Large intestine visible at 22 weeks gestation

Echogenic bowel majority are normal but can be associated with:
Chromosomal abnormalities (e.g., trisomy 21)
Congenital infection (e.g., cytomegalovirus)
Meconium ileus

Meconium peritonitis
Atresia or volvulus
Swallowed maternal blood
Proximal bowel obstruction associated with polyhydramnios

D. CONTRAST STUDIES

Barium	Good for opacifying stomach and intestines
	Good for diagnosis of malrotation or Hirschsprung disease
	Inert
	Inexpensive
Gastrografin	Good for meconium plug because the increased osmolality draws water into the lumen and helps release the plug
	Water-soluble
	Need to monitor fluid and electrolytes
Iodide-containing contrast	e.g., iohexol, iopamidol
	Low osmolality
	Water-soluble
	Good if suspect perforation because readily absorbed from peritoneal surface and can visualize intestines for longer periods of time

References

Bianchi DW, Crombleholme TM, D'Alton ME: Fetology. New York, McGraw-Hill, 2000.

Caplan MS, Jilling T: The pathophysiology of necrotizing enterocolitis. *NeoReviews.* 2001; 2(5): c103–c108.

Dimmitt RA, Moss RL: Clinical management of necrotizing enterocolitis. *NeoReviews.* 2001; 2(5): c110–c116.

Fanaroff AA, Martin RJ (eds): Neonatal-Perinatal Medicine (6th edition). St Louis, Mosby, 1997.

Hansen A, Puder M (eds): Manual of Surgical Neonatal Intensive Care. Hamilton, Ontario, BC Decker, 2003.

Kirpalani H, Mernagh J, Gil Gerald (eds): Imaging of the Newborn Baby. Edinburgh, Churchill Livingstone, 1999.

Kleigman RM, Walsh MC: Neonatal necrotizing enterocolitis: Pathogenesis, classification, and spectrum of disease. *Curr Prob Pediatr.* 1987;17:213.

Jaundice
1. Biliary atresia — conjugated bilirubin unable to pass to duodenum for excretion in stool.

2. Intestinal atresia
3. Meconium Ileus   } enterohepatic circulation exaggerated as
4. Hirschbrungs   stasis of luminal contents promotes intest.
                           Reabsorption

CHAPTER 10

Hematology/Oncology and Bilirubin

TOPICS COVERED IN THIS CHAPTER

I. Hematopoiesis

Hematopoiesis = production of circulating blood cells

Stem cells originate from mesoderm

The *secondary yolk sac* is the early active site of hematopoiesis
  Blood cells appear as early as 16 to 19 days gestation
  Hematopoiesis declines after 8 weeks gestation
  Secondary yolk sac begins to regress by week 10

Fetal *liver* hematopoiesis begins at 5 to 6 weeks gestation
  Becomes primary site between 6 to 22 weeks gestation

The *bone marrow* in developing long bones start hematopoiesis between 8 to 19 weeks gestation
  Becomes primary site after 22 weeks gestation

Erythropoiesis exceeds granulopoiesis at 10 to 11 weeks gestation; however, granulopoiesis exceeds erythropoiesis by week 12

Hematopoiesis by fetal location		
Location	GA (weeks)	Cell types (% of total cells)
Yolk sac	2.5–10	Primitive erythrocytes
		Mature macrophages
Fetal liver	4–5	Primitive erythrocytes
	5–6	Mature macrophage is the predominant cell
	6–10	Mature or definitive erythroblast; megakaryocytes detected at 8 weeks
	5–22	Megakaryocytes; granulocytes; lymphocytes (low amounts)
Bone marrow	8–9	Primitive erythrocytes; granulocytes
	10–13	Neutrophils (30–40); lymphocytes (12); eosinophils (1); basophils (0.3)
	10–16	Peak numbers of macrophages; peak monocytes
	11–14	Increasing definitive erythroblasts
	14+	All definitive erythroblasts (20–30)
	21	Neutrophils (60); lymphocytes (20–30); eosinophils (5); basophils (few)

GA = gestational age.

Change in red blood cell (RBC) indices over gestational age	
RBC indices	Change with increasing gestational age
RBC number ($\times 10^6$)	Increases
Hematocrit (%)	Increases
Mean corpuscular volume (MCV) (μm^3)	Decreases
Reticulocytes (%)	Peaks at 26 to 27 weeks gestation and then declines
Nucleated RBC	Decreases

II. Hemoglobin

Alpha globin genes on chromosome 16

Beta globin genes on chromosome 11

Globin chain expression is not fixed throughout human maturation

Hb F favors transfer of oxygen from maternal to fetal blood; in term newborns, composition 80% Hb fetal; at 6 months, ~ 5%

Hemoglobin production throughout fetal life and early infancy

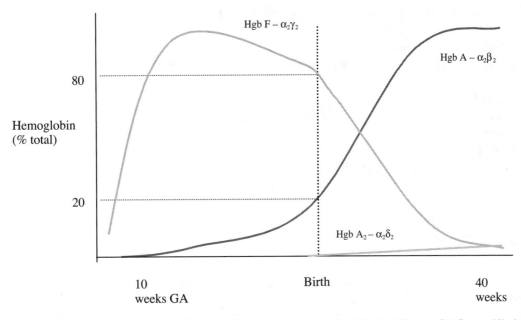

Hgb=hemoglobin (denoted as Hb in text). Modified from Fanaroff AA, Martin RJ (eds): Neonatal and Perinatal Medicine: Diseases of the Fetus and Newborn (6th edition). St. Louis, Mosby, 1997, p. 1205.

Globin chain production throughout fetal life and early infancy

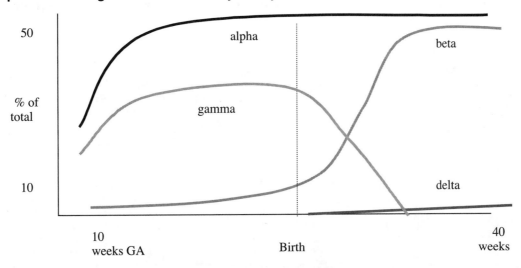

Modified from Fanaroff AA, Martin RJ (eds): Neonatal and Perinatal Medicine: Diseases of the Fetus and Newborn (6th edition). St. Louis, Mosby, 1997, p. 1205.

Human hemoglobins expressed during development			
Hemoglobin	Globin chain composition	Expression	Production
Hb Gower 1	$zeta_2$-$epsilon_2$	Embryonic	Yolk sac
Hb Gower 2	$alpha_2$-$epsilon_2$	Embryonic	Yolk sac
Hb Portland	$zeta_2$-$gamma_2$	Embryonic	Yolk sac
Hb F	$alpha_2$-$gamma_2$	Fetal	Liver
Hb A_2	$alpha_2$-$delta_2$	Adult	Bone marrow
Hb A	$alpha_2$-$beta_2$	Adult	Bone marrow

Printed with permission from Fanaroff AA, Martin RJ (eds): Neonatal and Perinatal Medicine: Diseases of the Fetus and Newborn (6th edition). St. Louis, Mosby, 1997, p. 1204.

III. Hemoglobinopathies

A. THALASSEMIA

Hereditary anemias from quantitative defect of globin chain synthesis
Four genes for alpha-globin production
Two genes for beta-globin production
Clinical syndrome depends on the number of defective genes and the degree of deficient or absent alpha or beta globin chains

Alpha-thalassemia
  Prevalent in Chinese subcontinent, Malaysia, Indochina, Africa
  May be detected at birth

Beta-thalessemia
  Prevalent in Mediterranean region, Africa, China, Pakistan, India, Middle East
  Usually not diagnosed until after age 6 months, when anemia persists beyond what is expected for the physiologic nadir
  Microcytic
  Historically, severe beta-thalassemia was called Cooley anemia
  (see chart for further details)

Alpha-thalassemia and beta-thalassemia characteristics		
Type	Hemoglobin (Hb)	Clinical
Alpha (α)-Thalassemia: severity based on the number of genes expressed		
Absence of one gene = silent carrier $-\alpha/\alpha\alpha$	Normal	Normal
Absence of two genes = alpha-thalassemia trait $-\alpha/-\alpha$, or $--/\alpha\alpha$	Normal to increased Hb Barts (4% to 6%)	Mild microcytosis; hypochromia; erythrocytosis May be asymptomatic
Absence of three genes = Hb H (four β chains) disease $-\alpha/--$	Infant 20% to 30% Barts Child 4% to 20% Hb H	Moderately severe hemolytic anemia Heinz bodies May require splenectomy
Absence of four genes = Barts Hb (four γ chains) or homozygous alpha-thalassemia $--/--$	80% to 90% Hb Barts (gamma$_4$) No Hb A No Hb F	Rare Very severe Hydrops fetalis $P_{50} << P_{50}$ adult
Beta (β)-Thalassemia – not usually detected in first month because β not necessary for fetal Hb		Blood smear—mild microcytic, hypochromic anemia; target cells
β-thalassemia trait		
$\beta/\beta°$	Mild increased A$_2$ ($\alpha_2\delta_2$), F	
$\beta/\beta+$	Mild increased A$_2$, F	
β-thalassemia disease		
β zero	Increased Hb F (>90%) Increased Hb A$_2$ No or decreased Hb A	Severe anemia in first year of life; splenomegaly; poor growth; thalassemia bony changes; chronic transfusions
β plus	20% to 40% A 60% to 80% F	Moderate anemia; may not require transfusions

Modified from Behrman RE, Kliegman RM, Arvin AM (eds): Nelson Textbook of Pediatrics (15th edition). Philadelphia, WB Saunders, 1996, p. 1399, 1403.

B. SICKLE CELL DISEASE

Incidence: 1/600
  Autosomal recessive
  8% of African-Americans
  2% of Mediterranean region

Etiology:
Inherited qualitative abnormality of the beta-globin chain gene
Valine for glutamic acid at position 6

Clinical:
Diagnosis may be suggested by newborn screening with hemoglobin electrophoresis results of Hb S and Hb F, but no Hb A (needs confirmation testing)
Hemolytic anemia with reticulocytosis
Usually present after age 6 months (as fetal hemoglobin reduces and abnormal beta-globin chains are produced):
    In neonates: fever, splenomegaly, hyperbilirubinemia
    Other: dactylitis, pain crisis, infection, acute chest syndrome, stroke
Variant of HbSS with HPFH (hereditary persistence of fetal hemoglobin): asymptomatic with normal blood counts
Blood smear with sickle-shaped red blood cells

Management:
Supportive
Prophylactic antibiotics with penicillin secondary to splenic dysfunction
Folate

C. HEMOGLOBIN E

Most common hemoglobinopathy in the world

Abnormal transcription message in the beta-globin gene results in decreased production of beta chains, resulting in chronic, mild, microcytic anemia

High incidence in Southeast Asia (Laos, Cambodia, Thailand)

Nucleotide substitution of the beta-globin gene (^{26}GLU $\longrightarrow$ LYS)

Can still form tetramer with α_2 with potentially normal function

If one inherits Hb E allele with a beta-thalassemia allele, will have more severe anemia

IV. Red Blood Cell (RBC) Disorders

A. ANEMIA

Definition: 2 standard deviations below the mean for age

Differential diagnosis:
1. *Blood loss:* sequestered blood: subdural hematoma (see Neurology chapter), cephalohematoma (see Neurology chapter), ecchymosis, hemangiomas; coagulation defect; maternal–fetal: placental, delayed umbilical cord clamping, twin-to-twin transfusion (see Maternal-Fetal Medicine chapter), fetal–maternal hemorrhage
   Fetal-maternal hemorrhage
      Detectable to some degree in 50% to 75% of pregnancies
      Degree of transfer
         Most very small amount of 0.01 to 0.10 cc
         1/400 of pregnancies transfer > 30 cc
         1/2000 of pregnancies transfer > 100 cc

Clinical: decreased fetal movement, sinusoidal fetal heart rate pattern, physical examination results negative for hepatosplenomegaly, pallor, tachypnea

Diagnostic tests:

Kleihauer-Betke

Test done on maternal blood, detects fetal blood

Blood is treated with citric acid–phosphate buffer (pH 3.3)

At this pH, adult Hb is soluble and is dissolved out of the RBC

Hb F remains precipitated and is stained with eosin on a slide; Hb A or mother's blood appears as "ghosts" and Hb F (baby's) stain red

%Hb F = # fetal cells / # maternal cells $\times$ 100

1% Hb F $\sim$ 50cc of fetal blood

Vials of Rhogam = mL of fetal blood / 1.5

1 vial = 300 mcg

False (+) results = anything that increases maternal Hb F (thalassemia minor, sickle cell, HPFH)

False (−) results = blood group incompatibility that leads to accelerated clearance of fetal cells from maternal circulation

Apt Test

Test done on fetal sample (bloody aspirate, stool), detects maternal blood

Treat blood with NaOH

Fetal Hb is resistant to alkali denaturation, unlike adult Hb

On slide, fetal Hb pink, adult Hb yellow-brown

2. *Congenital erythrocyte underproduction:* hypothyroidism, adrenal insufficiency, hypopituitarism, osteopetrosis, congenital hypoplastic anemia (see below), congenital aplastic anemia (see below)

Congenital hypoplastic anemia (Diamond-Blackfan)

Also referred to as "congenital erythroid aplasia"

Incidence:

Rare

Genetic disorder: can be either autosomal dominant or recessive

Etiology: pure red cell aplasia, fetal Hgb present, I antigen present

Clinical:

Symptoms present in first few months of life; most by 4 months

Median age of diagnosis: 2 months

Macrocytic anemia with reticulocytopenia in the first year of life; leukocyte and platelet counts normal to slightly elevated; bone marrow examination with absent erythroid precursors; increased serum erythropoietin; increased RBC adenosine deaminase levels; increased RBC Hb F and I antigen

Associated features: low birth weight, short stature, abnormal facies, abnormal musculoskeletal (abnormal, triphalangeal thumbs), cardiac, and renal systems

Management: chronic transfusion therapy, steroids, bone marrow transplant

Prognosis: increased risk for aplastic anemia, myelodysplastic syndrome, acute leukemia

Constitutional aplastic anemia (Fanconi's anemia) *chromosomal breaks*

Incidence:

Autosomal recessive

Etiology: chromosomal instability with breaks common; test chromosomes with mitomycin C $\longrightarrow$ increased chromosomal breaks

Clinical and associated features:

Musculoskeletal abnormalities (abnormal thumbs, radial hypoplasia, short stature, small cranium)

Hyperpigmentation, microcephaly, and mental deficiency, strabismus, abnormal ears, renal anomalies

Marrow hypoplasia (eventual pancytopenia) progressive after age 5 years (median age, 7 years)

Macrocytosis, increased Hb F and I antigen

Diagnosis: chromosomal breaks

Management: bone marrow transplant

Prognosis: predisposition to leukemia, lymphoma

3. *Acquired erythrocyte underproduction:* erthyroid aplasia (parvovirus B19); aplastic anemia (maternal drug ingestion: azathioprine), chloramphenicol; infectious (hepatitis, HIV, syphilis); treatment with growth factors; bone marrow transplant; iron, folic acid, and vitamin B12 deficiency; lead toxicity

Transient erythroblastopenia of childhood (TEC)

Incidence: common

Etiology: no known etiology

Clinical: usually second year of life (range 0.5 to 4 years); normocytic anemia; absent fetal hemoglobin and I antigen; no associated anomalies

Management: no specific treatment; transient disorder

Prognosis: resolves within several months

4. *Increased destruction:*

Isoimmunization: rhesus (Rh) incompatability, ABO incompatibility

Minor blood group incompatibilities

Structural abnormalities of erythrocytes: hereditary spherocytosis, hereditary elliptocytosis, infantile pyknocytosis

Erythrocyte biochemical defects: G6PD deficiency, pyruvate kinase deficiency, hexokinase deficiency, congenital erythropoietic porphyria

Infection: bacterial, viral, protozoal

Differential diagnosis of anemia and associated laboratory findings

Type of anemia	Cell morphology	Reticulocytes	MCV
Vitamin B12 and folate deficiency	Hypersegmented neutrophils; macrocytes	↓	↑
Iron deficiency	Microcytes; hypochromasia	↓	↓
Blood loss	Normal or polychromasia	Normal or ↑	Normal
Hemolysis	Polychromasia; microspherocytes	↑	Normal
Anemia of Prematurity	Normal	↓	Normal

MCV = mean corpuscular volume.

Differential diagnosis by size of RBC (MCV)

Size of red blood cell	Differential diagnosis
Normocytic	*Low reticulocyte count*
	Parvovirus B19
	Transient erythroblastopenia of childhood
	Chronic disease
	Immune hemolytic anemia
	Drugs
	Leukemia
	Hemoglobinopathy
	Normal or high reticulocyte count
	Red cell enzyme defects
	Blood loss
	Sequestration
Microcytic*	Thalassemia
	Iron deficiency
	Lead poisoning
	Infection
Macrocytic	Methylmalonic aciduria
	Folate or vitamin B12 deficiency
	Acquired aplastic anemia
	Diamond-Blackfan anemia

(continued on following page)

Fanconi anemia
Drugs
Hypothyroid

*Mentzer index = MCV/#RBC, > 13.5 = iron deficiency, < 11.5 = thalassemia major.
Printed with permission from Fanaroff AA, Martin RJ (eds): Neonatal and Perinatal Medicine: Diseases of the Fetus and Newborn (6th edition). St. Louis, Mosby, 1997, p. 1209.

Differential diagnosis by RBC morphology

Red blood cell morphology	Differential diagnosis
Hypochromia	Iron deficiency
	Thalassemia
	Lead poisoning
Target cells	Hemoglobin C, S, E
	Thalassemia
	Liver disease
	Abetalipoproteinemia
Basophilic stippling	Iron deficiency
	Lead poisoning
	Hemolytic anemia
	Thalassemia
Heinz bodies	Hemolytic anemias
Precipitated denatured Hb in RBC; usually occurs when Hb is unstable; can be normal in newborns	Enzymatic defects
Howell-Jolly bodies	Presence represents spleen dysfunction or absence of spleen
Nuclear RBC remnants usually destroyed by the spleen	
Spherocytes	Hemolysis
	G6PD deficiency
	RBC membrane defects
Elliptocytes	RBC membrane defects
Schistocytes	Microangiopathic hemolytic anemia
Polychromasia	Can be normal in newborns, proliferative response to anemia

Hb = hemoglobin.
Printed with permission from Fanaroff AA, Martin RJ (eds): Neonatal and Perinatal Medicine: Diseases of the Fetus and Newborn (6th edition). St. Louis, Mosby, 1997, p 1209.

B. ANEMIA OF PREMATURITY

Pathophysiology:
  Factors predisposing preterm infants:
    Preterm infants deprived of third trimester hematopoiesis and Fe transport
    Transition to adult hemoglobin
    Shorter life span of red blood cells
    Hemodilution caused by rapidly increasing body mass
    Phlebotomy
  Physiologic drop caused by *low erythropoietin (EPO) output* in response to anemia (of note, progenitor cells are quite responsive to EPO *in vitro*)
  Normocytic, normochromic anemia
  Considered "nutritionally insensitive": does not respond to exogenous administration of iron, vitamin E, or folate

Physiologic hemoglobin nadir: preterm versus term newborns

	Hemoglobin level (mg/dL)	Age
Term	9	10–12 weeks
Preterm	7 (< 1.0 kg)	Earlier at age 8 weeks
	8 (1.0–1.5 kg)	

Erythropoietin (EPO)

Predominant source of EPO in fetus is liver; switch to kidneys about third trimester; however, hepatic source still $>$ renal source at birth

Human EPO mRNA detected at 17 weeks gestation

Hepatic EPO allows the liver to be insensitive to tissue hypoxia (low output), avoiding marked erythrocytosis

Hepatic and renal EPO have identical biochemistry

Pharmacokinetics of EPO in neonates vs adults; in neonates,

Plasma EPO levels drop rapidly post exogenous administration

Increased volume of distribution

Increased metabolism or clearance

EPO increased by iron supplementation

 Clinical:

Tachycardia, increased apnea and bradycardia, increased oxygen requirement, poor weight gain

Management: limit phlebotomy, give blood transfusion, routine practice of EPO administration remains controversial

Prognosis: resolves over 3 to 6 months

C. HEMOLYTIC DISEASE

1. Blood type incompatibilities and isoimmunization

Direct versus indirect Coombs

Direct

Antibodies directly on RBC

Patient's RBCs are mixed with anti-human globulin antibody (Ab) (raised in rabbits)

Indirect

Detects antibodies in sera

Sera suspected of containing Ab is reacted with indicator RBCs having a known antigen on their surface

ABO incompatibility

Incidence: ~ 3%

May occur in first pregnancy; subsequent pregnancies are *not* more severely affected

Etiology: maternal production and placental transfer of blood group antibodies against different fetal blood type, resulting in hemolysis of fetal blood cells

Clinical:

Mothers with A or B blood types tend to produce antibodies mostly of the IgM class; in contrast, mothers with the O blood type produce antibodies mostly of the IgG class (only IgG crosses the placenta and plays a causative role in isoimmune hemolytic anemia; therefore, infants born to mothers of type A or B tend to have a milder hemolysis)

Hemolysis tends to be milder than Rh incompatibility because A and B antigens are expressed in all tissues in the body, including placenta, therefore diluting and neutralizing the maternal antibody

Direct Coombs usually weakly positive or negative; indirect Coombs generally positive

Microspherocytes, polychromasia, spherocytes, reticulocytosis, and increased nucleated red blood cells on blood smear

If severe, may have anemia in the first 24 hours of life with hyperbilirubinemia; can also have late anemia after the first month

B/O incompatibility can also have thrombocytopenia because B antigen is also expressed on platelets

Management: phototherapy, exchange transfusion

Rh incompatibility

Incidence: before RhoGAM, 1% of pregnancies developed alloimmunization; currently incidence is approximately 11/10,000 total births (9% need fetal therapy)

Etiology: Rh negative = homozygous absence of D antigen; if mother is negative and fetus is positive, and transplacental hemorrhage occurs, mother will produce and placentally transfer anti-D antibodies into the fetal circulation, resulting in hemolysis

The maternal primary immune response is the production of IgM antibodies

This is followed by production of IgG antibodies

With a repeat exposure, IgG antibodies are made more swiftly

ABO incompatibility may be protective against a primary Rh sensitization, because of the rapid clearance of the fetal red blood cells by the maternal circulation, limiting the potential of a Rh response by the mother

Clinical: direct and indirect Coombs' positive; elevated nucleated RBCs; spectrum of hyperbilirubinemia in an otherwise healthy infant to severe hydrops fetalis

Management:

Maternal–fetal: prophylactic RhoGAM (Rh immunoglobulin) at 28 weeks gestation and delivery, after any invasive procedures, and within 72 hours of delivery of Rh-positive infant; after mothers' serum antibody titers, fetal monitoring by plotting amniotic fluid samples against a Liley curve; intrauterine transfusions

Neonate: monitor serum bilirubin; phototherapy; exchange transfusion

Minor blood group incompatibilities

Alloimmunization can occur with other fetal RBC antigens:

Other Rh antigens (c, E): next most common after D

Kell (K and k): infrequent

Duffy (Fya)

Kidd (Jk^a and Jk^b)

Lewis: antigen not on RBC surface, but do get positive Coombs' result; hemolytic disease of the newborn is not an issue

2. RBC membrane defects or structural abnormalities (e.g., hereditary elliptocytosis; pyropoikilocytosis; hereditary spherocytosis)

Hereditary spherocytosis

Incidence: 1/5000

Majority autosomal dominant; may have spontaneous mutations; rarely autosomal recessive

Etiology: defect in membrane proteins (spectrin, ankyrin, band 3, protein 4.2) leading to membrane instability and membrane loss; splenic sequestration of abnormal RBCs

Clinical: spherocytes not always present; anemia; neonatal jaundice; splenomegaly; can lead to aplastic crisis

Jaundice may be more pronounced in infants positive for the *UDPGT1* gene polymorphism

Diagnosis: osmotic fragility test: exposure of RBCs to hypo-osmolar solutions; spherocytes lyse with high saline solutions because the membrane defect prevents normal compensatory swelling

Management: if severe, splenectomy; vaccination against encapsulated organisms; penicillin prophylaxis

3. RBC biochemical defects

Glucose-6-phosphate dehydrogenase (G6PD) deficiency

Incidence:

Most frequently inherited enzyme defect

Prevalence maintained by selection of heterozygotes that are protected against infection with *Plasmodium falciparum* (malaria species)

X-linked recessive; male > female in severity because female expression modified by Lyon hypothesis

Mediterranean, Greek, African-American (especially A negative), and Asian populations

Etiology:

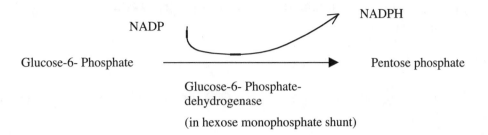

NADP   NADPH

Glucose-6- Phosphate   Pentose phosphate

Glucose-6- Phosphate-
dehydrogenase

(in hexose monophosphate shunt)

RBCs must make glucose via the Embder-Meyerhoff pathway and the hexose monophosphate shunt

NADPH is needed to maintain the antioxidants catalase and glutathione within the RBC

Laboratory values:

Normal shape of RBC

Normal osmotic fragility test

Shorter RBC life span

Heinz bodies

Anemia, reticulocytosis, hyperbilirubinemia

Diagnose by testing for enzymatic activity: young, newly formed red blood cells have normal levels of enzymatic
    activity, so if the test is done at a time of crisis with reticulocytosis, you may get a false-negative result

Clinical:

Heterogeneous

Decreased NADPH levels

Exacerbation with exposure to oxidant stress: acidosis, hypoglycemia, drugs, sulfa, moth balls

Increased risk of methemoglobinemia, anemia, hyperbilirubinemia (similar to hereditary spherocytosis, positive
    UDPGT1 polymorphism is an additive risk for the development of jaundice)

Management: avoid substances that may promote oxidant stress; monitor newborns carefully for development of
    anemia and hyperbilirubinemia

Pyruvate kinase deficiency

Incidence:

Second most common inherited RBC enzyme defect (after G6PD)

Autosomal recessive

Northern European ancestry

Pathophysiology: Embden-Myerhof pathway and pentose phosphate shunt

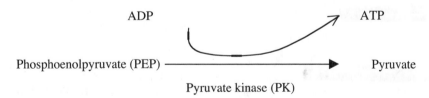

ADP   ATP

Phosphoenolpyruvate (PEP)   Pyruvate

Pyruvate kinase (PK)

Pyruvate kinase converts PEP to pyruvate, generating ATP in the process; with PK deficiency, lack of ATP leads to
    chronic anemia, increased 2,3-DPG

Diagnosis: enzyme assay

Clinical: variable; anemia, hyperbilirubinemia

Blood smear: normocytic, normochromic, abnormal RBC shapes, reticulocytosis

Management: monitor for anemia, hyperbilirubinemia, potential role for splenectomy

D. POLYCYTHEMIA

Definition: hemoglobin > 20 gm/dL or hematocrit $> 65\%$ based on a peripheral venous sample; due to increased RBC mass or decreased plasma volume

Newborn hematocrit concentrations peak at 2 hours of life, then steadily decline over the next 6 to 24 hours of life

Capillary measurements usually yield higher values than venous or arterial measurements; venous and arterial values correlate well with each other

Incidence: 1% to 5%; however, newborns less frequently show clinical symptoms

Pathophysiology: primary—caused by increased fetal production of erythropoietin; secondary—caused by transfer of RBC mass to fetus

At high hematocrits levels, plasma viscosity is increased, posing a potential risk to the newborn of secondary symptoms (usually when the level is greater than 70%)

Clinical:
Newborn risks:
Primary: fetal growth restriction, maternal insulin-dependent diabetes, neonatal thyrotoxicosis, trisomy 21, Beckwith-Wiedemann syndrome
Secondary: twin-to-twin transfusion, maternal–fetal transfusions, delayed cord clamping, perinatal asphyxia
Symptoms potentially secondary to polycythemia and hyperviscosity: plethora, lethargy, tachypnea, hepatomegaly, hypoglycemia, hypocalcemia, thrombocytopenia

Management: partial volume exchange transfusion
Blood volume exchanged $=$

$$\text{Blood volume} \times \frac{(\text{observed hematocrit} - \text{desired hematocrit})}{\text{Observed hematocrit}}$$

Blood volume $=$ weight $\times$ 80 to 100 cc/kg
Desired hematocrit $=$ 55% to 60%

Prognosis: remains controversial as to what extent short and long-term outcomes are adversely affected by polycythemia

E. METHEMOGLOBINEMIA (MET)

Pathophysiology:
Iron in hemoglobin is normally in reduced or ferrous state (Fe^{++})
With MET, Hb is in oxidized or ferric state (Fe^{+++})
MET Hb does not complex with oxygen, resulting in decreased blood oxygen capacity and transport
Normally, MET Hb is 3% of total hemoglobin
Increased formation of MET Hb with exposure to:
Nitrates, nitrites, very high doses of inhaled nitric oxide, aniline dyes, local anesthetics such as prilocaine
Congenital causes include:
NADH-MET Hb reductase deficiency: autosomal recessive, Navajo Indians
Abnormal hemoglobins that stablize heme iron in the ferric state (hemoglobin M disorders): autosomal dominant disorders, amino acid substitutions; can be resistant to methylene blue treatment

Clinical:
Cyanosis without evidence of cardiac or respiratory disease
Blood can be brownish in appearance

Management:
Methylene blue increases activity of NADPH-MET Hb reductase; after treatment, urine becomes blue-green

V. Platelets

Derived from megakaryocytes; only comprise 0.03% to 0.1% of the total cells in the bone marrow

Detected in liver and circulatory system at 8 weeks gestation

Fetal megakaryocytes are smaller than adult megakaryocytes; however, there are a larger number circulating in fetuses compared with the adults

Counts $> 150 \times 10^9$ /L, achieved after 17 weeks gestation

A. THROMBOCYTOPENIA

Definition: platelet count less than 150 K/μL; severe if less than 50 K/μL

Incidence:
Congenital thrombocytopenia rare, $< 1\%$
Thrombocytopenia in a sick infant is a much more common event; incidence: $\sim 35\%$

Differential diagnosis:
1. Increased platelet destruction (or consumption): predominant etiology
   Shortened platelet survival; increased mean platelet volume, normal number of megakarocytes; inadequate response to platelet transfusion
   Etiologies: drug-induced, maternal idiopathic thrombocytopenia purpura (ITP), disseminated intravascular coagulation (DIC), thrombosis, necrotizing enterocolitis (NEC), maternal pregnancy-induced hypertension (PIH) and HELLP syndrome, Kasabach-Merritt, systemic infections, sequestration (hypersplenism), neonatal alloimmune thrombocytopenia (see below), neonatal autoimmune thrombocytopenia (see below)
   Neonatal alloimmune thrombocytopenia (NAIT) *(Normal maternal plt. count)*
      Incidence: 1/1800
      Pathophysiology: production and placental transfer of maternal alloantibodies against paternally inherited antigens on fetal platelets (similar to Rh disease)
         Human platelet antigen (HPA)-1a is the most common implicated antigen (80% to 90% of cases)
         98% whites have HPA-1a antigen expressed, other ethnicities have HPA-2a
      Clinical: can have severe thrombocytopenia
         Platelets are low at birth, decline over the first several days, then start to increase over the next 4 weeks
         Maternal history of human platelet antigen (HPA)-1a negative
         Mother has normal platelet count
         May have history of thrombocytopenic infant; increased incidence with second or subsequent children
         May have intrauterine intracranial bleeding and death
         Infant may present with bleeding diathesis and petechiae
         Overall 20% mortality
      Management: administer platelets from the mother or HPA-1a negative platelets; may need to give random donor if neither is available
         Head ultrasound if platelet count < 50 K/μL
         Consider intravenous gamma-globulin, corticosteroids
   Neonatal autoimmune thrombocytopenia *(maternal low plt count)*
      Maternal antiplatelet antibodies caused by idiopathic thrombocytopenia purpura, lupus, other autoimmune diseases

In contrast to NAIT, mother's platelet count is also low (unless the primary condition has been successfully treated)

Generally, infants have milder thrombocytopenia compared with infants with NAIT

Even if mother's ITP is well-controlled or after splenectomy, infant may still have thrombocytopenia because of persistent platelet antibodies passing across the placenta; therefore, maternal platelet count is not a good indicator of neonatal platelet count and severity

Management may include platelet transfusion, intravenous gamma-globulin, and corticosteroids

2. *Diminished platelet production*

Decreased number of clonogenic megakaryocyte progenitors; low levels of thrombopoietin

Etiologies:

Congenital viral syndromes

Marrow infiltrative disease: congenital leukemia, congenital neuroblastoma, Letterer-Siwe disease

Mixed: congenital infections (TORCH), acquired infections (bacterial sepsis), erythroblastosis fetalis

Miscellaneous: exchange transfusion, ECMO, polycythemia, chromosomal abnormalities (trisomy 21), neonatal cold injury, mechanical ventilation, pulmonary hypertension, phototherapy

Underlying congenital syndrome: thrombocytopenia with absent radii (TAR) syndrome (see below), Fanconi's anemia, amegakaryocyte thrombocytopenia (see below), Wiskott-Aldrich syndrome, Chediak-Higashi syndrome

Thrombocytopenia with absent radii (TAR) syndrome

Genetics: autosomal recessive; male: female = 1:2

Clinical:

Severe thrombocytopenia with absent or reduced megakaryocytes: most by age 4 months; other hematologic findings include leukemoid reactions and eosinophilia

Bilateral absent radii and ulnar abnormalities (usually thumbs and digits are developed normally, in contrast to Fanconi's anemia)

30% to 35% with associated cardiac disease: tetrology of Fallot, atrial septal defect

25% mortality, most within the first 4 months of life; leading cause of death is intracranial hemorrhage

If survive first 4 months, gradual increase in platelet count with normalization by school age

Management: platelet transfusions until spontaneous resolution

Amegakaryocyte thrombocytopenia

Genetics: rare; male:female = 2:3; suspected X-linked transmission

Clinical: severe, isolated thrombocytopenia; no other abnormalities; bone marrow demonstrates absent or scarce megakaryocytes; 50% develop aplastic anemia; risk of developing leukemia; high mortality (hemorrhage, opportunistic infection)

Management: some success with bone marrow transplant

Differential diagnosis of neonatal thrombocytopenia		
Infant	**PT/PTT**	**Differential Diagnosis**
Sick	Normal	Infection without DIC
		Hypersplenism
		Marrow infiltration
		Necrotizing entercolitis
	Increased	DIC
		Sepsis
		Hypoxia
		Acidosis
		Cold stress
		Severe liver disease
		(continued on following page)

Infant	Maternal platelet count	Differential Diagnosis
Well	Normal	Neonatal alloimmune Neonatal drugs Hemangioma Congenital thrombocytopenia Maternal ITP in remission
	Decreased	Maternal ITP: autoimmune, increased platelet associated IgG levels Maternal drugs Pregnancy-induced hypertension Familial

Modified from Cloherty JP, Stark AR (ed): Manual of Neonatal Care (4th edition). Philadelphia, Lippincott-Raven, 1998, p. 471.

B. THROMBOCYTOSIS

Definition: counts > 450 to 600 K/μL

Differential diagnosis: normal physiologic response seen in preterm infants at 4 to 6 weeks of life, reactive process seen with infections or inflammation, iron deficiency, drugs, trisomy 21, and vitamin E deficiency

VI. Hemostasis and Clotting Disorders

A. HEMOSTASIS

Maternal clotting factors do not cross the placenta; therefore, fetal levels depend on endogenous production

Clotting proteins are synthesized by the fetus beginning in the first trimester (measurable at 5 to 10 weeks gestation), with concentrations gradually increasing throughout gestation

Most levels become comparable to adult levels at age ~ 6 months

Neonatal factor levels compared to the adult	
Factors	**% Adult**
Contact (factor XI, XII, prekallikrein, and high-molecular-weight kininogen)	< 70
Vitamin K–dependent (II, VII, IX, X)	<70
V, VIII, XIII, von Willebrand, fibrinogen	> 70
ATIII, protein C, protein S	30
Thrombomodulin	3× greater

Coagulation cascade

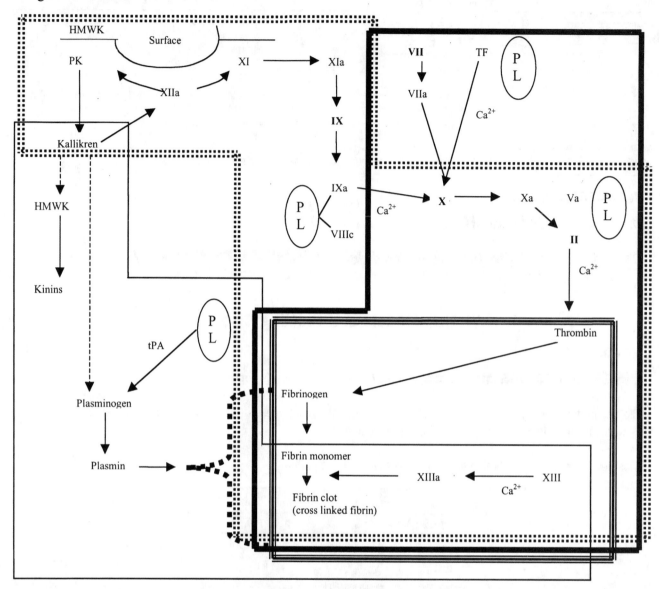

Single thick line—coagulation pathway measured by Prothrombin Time (PT); Double dotted line—coagulation pathway measured by Partial Thromboplastin Time (PTT); Triple line—coagulation pathway measured by Thrombin Time (TT); Single thin line—part of the coagulation system that is not assessed by a coagulation or bleeding screen (defects of increased fibrinolysis and deficiency/abnormality of factor XIII).

Factors in bold—Vitamin K dependent: II, VI, IX, X.

PL = platelet; HMWK = high-molecular-weight kininogen; PK = prekallekrein; TF = tissue factors; tPA = tissue plasminogen activator

Modified from lecture notes: DiMichele D. An approach to the clinical and laboratory diagnosis of the bleeding child. Resident Core Lecture Series. Children's Memorial Hospital, Chicago, IL, 1992.

Differential diagnosis for abnormal coagulation test results	
Test (normal values*)	Differential diagnosis
Bleeding time	Platelet count < 100 K
	Platelet function
	Von Willebrand's disease
	Other platelet/vessel interaction factors
Platelet count	Increased MPV found in ITP
(≥ 150 K/μL)	DIC
	Inherited platelet defects of adhesion or aggregation

(continued on following page)

Test (normal values*)	Differential diagnosis
Prothrombin time (PT) (10–16 sec) = Extrinsic pathway	Inherited factor VII deficiency Liver disease DIC Vitamin K deficiency (Vitamin K-dependent factors: II, VII, IX, X) Inherited/acquired factor V, X, II defect if also with prolonged PTT (e.g., Coumadin or Warfarin)
Partial thromboplastin time (PTT) = Intrinsic pathway (Term: 25-60 sec; preterm: 26-80 sec)	Contact factor deficiency (XI, XII, PK, HMWK) hemophilia A (VIII), or B (IX) Von Willebrand if along with prolonged bleeding time Inherited or acquired factor V, X, II defect Vitamin K deficiency Liver disease if along with prolonged PT DIC if also with thrombocytopenia, increased fibrin split products or D-dimers Heparin Lupus anticoagulant
Thrombin time	Heparin contamination of sample Decreased fibrinogen (< 100 mg%) Abnormal fibrinogen Increased fibrin split products (FSPs)
Fibrinogen activity level	Inherited fibrinogen deficiency Type I: actual deficiency Type II: dysfibrinogenemia Acquired fibrinogen deficicency DIC if also with prolonged PTT, increased FSPs, decreased platelets Fibrinolysis caused by liver disease or thrombolytic therapy if along with increased FSPs and decreased plasminogen

*Normal ranges vary among laboratories; general estimates from Christensen RD (ed): Hematologic Problemes in the Neonate. Philadelphia, W.B. Saunders, 2000, p. 244–245. Modified from lecture notes: DiMichele D. "An approach to the clinical and laboratory diagnosis of the bleeding child". Resident Core Lecture Series. Children's Memorial Hospital, Chicago, IL, 1992.

Differential diagnosis of bleeding in neonates

Clinical	Platelets	PT	PTT	DDx
Sick	Decreased	Increased	Increased	DIC
Sick	Decreased	Normal	Normal	Platelet consumption: infection, NEC, renal vein thrombosis
Sick	Normal	Increased	Increased	Liver disease
Sick	Normal	Normal	Normal	Compromised vascular integrity: hypoxia, acidosis
Healthy	Decreased	Normal	Normal	ITP, occult infection, thrombosis, bone marrow hypoplasia or infiltration
Healthy	Normal	Increased	Increased	Vitamin K deficiency
Healthy	Normal	Normal	Increased	Hereditary clotting factor deficiencies
Healthy	Normal	Normal	Normal	Local bleeding (trauma), platelet abnormalities, factor XIII deficiency

Printed with permission from Cloherty JP, Stark AR (ed): Manual of Neonatal Care (4th edition). Philadelphia, Lippincott-Raven, 1998, p. 462.

B. HEMOPHILIA A (FACTOR VIII DEFICIENCY) 8 defic.

Genetics: X-linked recessive; ~ 70% of hemophilia

Clinical: can present in the neonatal period (10%); may see increased bleeding after blood draws, circumcision, hemarthrosis (rarely), intracranial hemorrhage
Most develop symptoms by age 18 months
Prolonged PTT
Grading by plasma Factor VIII levels:

Severe	< 1%
Moderate	1% to 5%
Mild	> 5%

Management: factor VIII replacement

C. HEMOPHILIA B (FACTOR IX DEFICIENCY OR CHRISTMAS DISEASE) 9 def / Chnstmas

Genetics: X-linked recessive; ~ 30% of hemophilia

Clinical: similar to hemophilia A

Management: factor IX replacement

D. HEMOPHILIA C (FACTOR XI DEFICIENCY)

Genetics: autosomal recessive; greater incidence among Ashkenazi Jews

Clinical: associated with Noonan syndrome; increased risk of genitourinary bleeding; no degree of correlation between level of deficiency and symptoms (unlike hemophilia A or B)

Management: fresh frozen plasma

E. FACTOR XIII (FIBRIN STABILIZING FACTOR) DEFICIENCY

Genetics: autosomal recessive

Clinical: normal routine clotting studies; prolonged bleeding from umbilical stump or several days after circumcision; intracranial hemorrhage; wound dehiscence

Management: cryoprecipitate or factor XIII concentrate

F. VON WILLEBRAND (vWF) DISEASE

Genetics: autosomal dominant or recessive

Clinical: vWF is a component of factor VIII functioning as a ligand between platelet and vessel; rarely presents in newborn period; mucus membrane bleeding; abnormal bleeding time; +/− prolonged PTT; usually normal PT and platelets; diagnose by checking ristocetin factor

Management: cryoprecipitate; factor VIII with vWF, DDAVP (= desmopressin acetate)

G. HEMORRHAGIC DISEASE OF THE NEWBORN

Pathophysiology: vitamin K is an essential cofactor for factors II, VII, IX, and X and for protein C and S; deficiency of vitamin K leads to a bleeding diathesis

Neonatal risks for vitamin K deficiency: maternal anticonvulsant therapy; liver disease; malabsorption; antibiotics; coumadin; breast-fed infants

Clinical:

Prolonged PT; normal platelet count	
Type	**Features**
Early	Onset within first 24 hours of life Secondary to placentally transferred maternal drugs affecting vitamin K production (e.g., carbamazepine, phenytoin, barbiturates, cephalosporins, rifampin, isoniazid, and warfarin)

(continued on following page)

Type	Features
Classic	Onset between 2 and 7 days of life Inadequate vitamin K (increased risk in breast-fed infants taking inadequate amounts) Gastrointestinal bleeding, umbilical cord bleeding, intracranial hemorrhage, prolonged bleeding after phlebotomy and circumcisions
Late	Onset between 2 weeks and 6 months of life Caused by inadequate intake or hepatobiliary disease High risk for intracranial hemorrhages and death More common in boys; more common in the summer

Laboratory findings: prolonged PT, normal platelet count

Management: vitamin K; symptoms typically resolve $\sim$ 4 hours after administration of vitamin K

VII. Thrombosis

Newborn infants are at greater risk of thrombosis compared with older children; fibrinolysis diminished because of moderately low plasminogen levels

Newborn factors that increase the risk for thrombosis: umbilical vessel catheterization; asphyxia; sepsis; polycythemia or hyperviscosity (dehydration, infant of a diabetic mother, growth restriction, congenital heart disease); shock; deficiencies in protein C, S, ATIII, factor V Leiden

Clinical syndromes: renal vein thrombosis (flank mass, hematuria, hypertension, thrombocytopenia), renal artery thrombosis, sagittal sinus thrombosis, stroke (newborn seizures)

Management: antithrombolytic therapy usually reserved for massive or life-threating thromboses
  Options include tissue active plasminogen activator or heparin (intravenous or subcutaneous low-molecular-weight form)

VIII. Oncology

A. CONGENITAL LEUKEMIA

Incidence:
  Rare, $< 5/1,000,000$
  Increased risk if infant has Fanconi's anemia, Diamond-Blackfan syndrome, trisomy 21

Clinical: can present in newborn period; often with decreased platelets and anemia caused by bone marrow invasion; increased WBC > 100 K ; infiltration of non-bone marrow organs by blasts; palpable cutaneous nodules

Management: chemotherapy

B. HISTIOCYTOSIS

Pathophysiology: tissue infiltration by monocytes or macrophage cell line

Letterer-Siwe disease or Langerhan cell histiocytosis: present in infants younger than age 2 years, fever, pancytopenia, multiorgan infiltration

Malignant familial histiocytosis: autosomal recessive, fever, pancytopenia, hepatosplenomaegaly, adenopathy, fatal

Virus-associated hemophagocytic syndrome: fever, pancytopenia, hepatosplenomegaly, implicated viruses: cytomegalovirus, Epstein-Barr virus, herpes simplex virus, adenovirus

C. SOLID TUMORS

Teratoma	Most common solid tumor in the neonatal period 50% sacrococcygeal; next major site is the head and neck Malignant potential < 10% in neonates (compared with 50% to 60% in older children)
Neuroblastoma	>50% of all tumors in neonates Adrenal primary site (70%): neural crest origin; sites anywhere along sympathetic chain Better prognosis if presents in infantile period (< age 12 months) Symptoms: Horner's syndrome, heterochromia iridis, hypertension, flushing, diarrhea, abdominal mass, opsomyoclonus, subcutaneous nodules ("blueberry muffin spots"), orbital ecchymoses ("raccoon eyes") Prognosis dependent on stage, age, N - myc amplification Stage IV-S = primary abdominal with metastases except to bone (favorable prognosis)
Pheochromocytoma	Increased catecholamine secretion (also with neurogenic tumors) Location: adrenal, periadrenal; may also arise form the walls of the ureter or bladder Associated with neurofibromatosis, von Hippel-Lindau disease, islet cell adenomas, medullary cancers of the thyroid
Wilms	Associated with congenital anomalies: GU, nonfamilial aniridia, hemihypertrophy Bilateral (5%) Metastasis to lung, liver, bones, opposite kidney Good prognosis
Hepatoblastoma	Associated with hemihypertrophy, renal abnormalities Abdominal mass with thrombocytosis Increased alpha-fetoprotein
Retinoblastoma	Most frequent eye tumor 1/20,000 to 30,000 births Autosomal dominant (40%); sporadic (60%): an inherited or bilateral retinoblastoma survivor has a 45% chance of having an affected child; a unilateral retinoblastoma survivor has a 6% chance of having an affected child; parents of a bilaterally affected child have a 3% chance of having another affected child; parents of a unilaterally affected child have a 0.4% chance of having another affected child Unilateral (70%) and bilateral (30%) Symptoms: leukokoria, strabismus, decreased vision, secondary glaucoma Secondary malignancies: osteosarcoma, pinealoblastoma (in inherited form)
Rhabdomyosarcoma	Sriated muscle cell origin Rare in neonates Abdominal and pelvic tumors Botryoid sarcoma variant protrudes from the bladder or vagina

GU = genitourinary.

IX. Transfusions and Component Therapy

Blood component therapy		
Product	**Indications**	**Components**
PRBC (packed RBCs)	Hypovolemia Severe anemia	Red blood cells Some white cells No immunoglobulins or clotting factors
FFP (fresh frozen plasma)	Bleeding DIC Vitamin K deficiency Factor IX deficiency	All clotting factors Fibronectin Gamma-globulins Albumin Plasma proteins
Cryoprecipitate	VIII deficiency von Willebrand	VIII vWF Fibrinogen XIII Fibronectin
Platelets	Thrombocytopenia Bleeding	Platelets Some white cells

X. Bilirubin

Fetal and neonatal bilirubin metabolism
Bilirubin (IXα) derived from heme
75% from catabolism of circulating RBCs
25% from ineffective erythropoiesis (red cell catabolism in bone marrow) and turnover of heme protein and free heme
No known physiologic function, possible antioxidant function
Placenta can remove indirect bilirubin but not biliverdin, so fetal advantage to make bilirubin

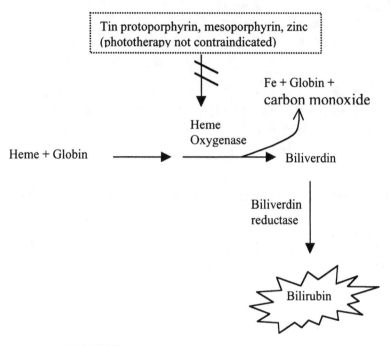

Heme oxygenase converts heme to biliverdin

Biliverdin reductase converts biliverdin to bilirubin

Bilirubin forms:
Free unconjugated bilirubin: the form that most readily crosses the blood–brain barrier (BBB)
Unconjugated bilirubin: bound to albumin; disruption of this bond by certain drugs, hypothermia, hypoxia, acidosis
Conjugated bilirubin: water-soluble
Conjugated bilirubin bound covalently to albumin: remains water-soluble

Bilirubin is unconjugated and nonpolar

In plasma: bilirubin rapidly and tightly binds to albumin
Bilirubin bound to albumin does not cross the BBB
Some drugs can displace bilirubin from albumin such as rapid infusion of ampicillin, sulfa drugs, ceftriaxone, free fatty
acids
Benzyl alcohol can alter BBB

Liver: bilirubin binds to ligandin and other binding-proteins, enters hepatocyte, and is transported to the smooth
endoplasmic reticulum (SER)
Glucuronosyl transferase conjugates bilirubin to a polar, water-soluble substance, bilirubin glucuronide
This is excreted in bile and then into the small intestines

Then one of two pathways:

1. Reduced by bacteria to urobilinogen and excerted in the stool (minimal in newborns, because of decreased bacteria and because other pathways are favored)
2. Deconjugated by beta glucuronidase and then reabsorbed into the blood (increased *enterohepatic circulation*)

Physiologic jaundice

Newborn risks: increased RBC volume, increased RBC turnover, increased enterohepatic circulation (delayed establishment of feedings), decreased glucuronyl transferase activity

Clinical jaundice develops in 25% to 50% of all newborns

Only 3% develop serum bilirubin levels > 15 mg/dL

Peak at age 3 to 5 days (6 to 8 mg/dL) with clearance over the next 5 to 10 days for term infants

Premature infants have higher levels with later peak (10 to 12 mg/dL; peak at 5 days)

Exaggerated physiologic jaundice

Factors that may enhance or worsen normal physiologic course but are not themselves pathologic processes:
Prematurity, sequestered blood, delayed establishment of feedings, maternal drugs (e.g., oxytocin, diazepam, promethazine), delayed cord clamping

Breastfeeding jaundice

Higher levels for a longer period of time; can reach 20 to 30 mg/dL by age 2 weeks and then begin to fall and normalize over age 4 to 12 weeks

Levels fall rapidly over 48 hours with cessation of breastfeeding (BF)

When BF is resumed, levels increase 2 to 4 mg/dL but do not reach previously high levels

Kernicterus has been reported

Incidence: 1/200

Nonphysiologic or pathologic jaundice

Characteristics:

Onset before age 24 hours

Rate of increase > 0.5 mg/dL/h

Evidence of underlying illness (gastrointestinal (GI), hematologic, infectious)

Jaundice that persists greater than 8 days in term infants and 14 days in preterm infants

Broad diagnostic categories:

Increased "load" of bilirubin:

Hemolytic disease: ABO incompatibility, Rh incompatibility, minor group incompatibility, non-immune

Enzyme deficiencies: G6PD, PK

Membrane defects: spherocytosis, elliptocytosis, pyknocytosis

Decreased hepatic ligandin

Decreased activity of glucuronyl transferase:

Gilbert's, Crigler-Najjar

Increased enterohepatic circulation:

GI obstruction: intestinal atresia, meconium ileus, Hirschsprung's disease

Multifactorial:

Congenital hypothyroidism, inborn errors, liver failure, sepsis (increased hemolysis, decreased uptake, decreased excretion)

Bilirubin toxicity

Kernicterus: acute bilirubin encephalopathy, yellow staining of the brain generally involving basal ganglia, cranial nerve nuclei, hippocampus

Staining correlates microscopically with necrosis, neuronal loss, and gliosis

Three phases:

Jaundice, hypotonia, lethargy, poor feeding, poor suck

After few days, hypertonia, opisthotonus, high-pitched cry, fever, seizures

After about 1 week, hypertonia replaced by hypotonia, long-term neuronal injury

Surviving children develop extrapyramidal disturbances (choreoathetosis), hearing loss, gaze palsies, dental dysplasia, mild intellectual deficits

Greatest risk with rapid rate of increase (hemolytic processes)

Diagnosis:

History

Family history of jaundice, anemia, splenectomy, gallbladder, or liver disease

Ethnicity (East Asians, Greeks, and American Indians have higher levels of physiologic jaundice)

Maternal illness or drugs (infection, diabetes, sulfas, nitrofurantoin, antimalarials, G6PD)

Labor and delivery (trauma, asphyxia, delayed cord clamping)

Stooling pattern (enterohepatic circulation)

Physical examination

Jaundice visible when bilirubin > 7 mg/dL (in adults > 2 mg/dL); visual inspection does not demonstrate good predictive ability

Cephalocaudal progression

Evaluate for prematurity, SGA (polycythemia, congenital infection), extravascular blood (cephalohematoma or other bruising), pallor (hemolysis, extravascular blood), petechiae (congenital infection, sepsis, erythroblastosis), HSM (hemolytic disease with CHF, congenital infection, liver disease), evidence of sepsis, evidence of hypothyroidism

Studies

Bilirubin level (total and direct)

Infant's blood type and direct Coombs test

Mother's blood type and antibody screening

Peripheral smear for RBC morphology

Hematocrit level (polycythemia, anemia)

Reticulocyte count

Others depending on course: G6PD, PK enzyme levels, osmotic fragility, liver function tests, sepsis evaluation, metabolic tests, thyroid function tests

Management:

Phototherapy

Converts to products less lipophilic that can be excreted without further metabolism

Configurational isomerization (isomer changes from 4Z, 15Z to 4Z, 15E, which is less toxic)

Structural isomerization (Lumirubin): the formation and excretion of lumirubin is the major reason for decline in serum bilirubin levels

Wavelength of 425 to 475 nanometers most effective

Possible side effects: increased insensible water loss, dehydration, watery stools, hypocalcemia, retinal damage (animal), increased skin perfusion (rash), mutation DNA strand breaks (cover gonads), alteration in amino acids (protect peripheral nutrition)

Contraindications: high direct bilirubin level ("bronze baby" syndrome)

Exchange transfusion

Double volume

Fresh irradiated whole blood or reconstituted PRBC with fresh frozen plasma, hematocrit of replacement blood should equal 40% to 50%

5 to 20 cc aliquots

Replaces 87% of blood volume

Removes bilirubin and any free antibody

Decrease in serum bilirubin level by 45% (although may get a rebound to 60% of original level)

Collect infant's blood before transfusion for potential diagnostic studies

Monitor heart rate, blood pressure, pH, K^+, glucose, Ca^{++}, Mg^{++}

Side effects: hypocalcemia, thrombocytopenia, necrotizing enterocolitis

Experimental pharmacotherapy

Phenobarbital: increases concentration of ligandin, increasing uptake, induces enzymes, increases bile flow

Agar: decreases enterohepatic circulation

Metalloporphyrins (tin): inhibit heme oxygenase

IVIG: in severe Rh hemolytic disease

References:

Behrman RE, Kliegman RM, Arvin AM (eds): Nelson Textbook of Pediatrics (15th edition). Philadelphia, WB Saunders, 1996.

Christensen RD (ed): Hematologic Problemes in the Neonate. Philadelphia, WB Saunders, 2000.

Cloherty JP, Stark AR (eds): Manual of Neonatal Care (4th edition). Philadelphia, Lippincott-Raven, 1998.

DiMichele D. An approach to the clinical and laboratory diagnosis of the bleeding child. Resident Core Lecture Series. Children's Memorial Hospital, Chicago, IL, 1992.

Fanaroff AA, Martin RJ (eds): Neonatal and Perinatal Medicine: Diseases of the Fetus and Newborn (7th edition). St. Louis, Mosby, 2001.

Manco-Johnson M, Nuss R. Neonatal Thrombotic Disorders. *NeoReviews*. 2000; 1(10): e201–e205.

Spitzer AR (ed): Intensive Care of the Fetus and Neonate. St. Louis, Mosby, 1995.

Walker WA, Durie PR, Hamilton JR, Walker-Smith JA, Watkins JB (eds): Pediatric Gastrointestinal Disease (2nd edition). St. Louis, Mosby, 1996.

CHAPTER 11

Endocrinology

TOPICS COVERED IN THIS CHAPTER

I. Thyroid Gland

A. EMBRYOLOGY

Anatomic development of thyroid gland begins at 3 weeks gestation

Thyroid gland develops from a median *endodermal* thickening in the primitive pharyngeal floor

Thyroid follicles form and begin thyroglobulin production at ~8 weeks gestation

Fetal thyroid can accumulate iodide at ~10 weeks gestation

Thyroid-stimulating hormone production from pituitary gland begins ~12 weeks gestation

B. THYROID HORMONE LEVELS IN FETUS AND NEONATE

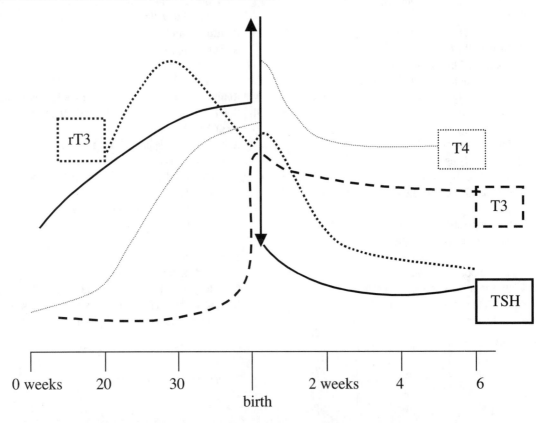

Modified from Sperling MA. Pediatric Endocrinology (2nd edition). Philadelphia, WB Saunders, 2002, p 163.

T4 (thyroxine)
  Low amounts until about 18–20 weeks gestation and then increases proportionally with gestational age
  Increases dramatically at birth (~2–6 x); peak ~24–36 hours of age

T3 (triiodothyronine)
  Low until about 30 weeks gestation when fetus is able to convert T4 to active T3
  Increases dramatically at birth (~2–6 x); peak ~24–36 hours of age
  T3 levels increase postnatally due to neonate's increased ability to convert T4 to T3

rT3 (reverse T3)
  Fetus metabolizes T4 $\rightarrow$ reverse T3

TSH (thyroid-stimulating hormone or thyrotropin)
  Large increase at birth (peak ~30 minutes of age) due to extrauterine cold exposure, which leads to an increase in T4
    and some increase in T3
  Remains elevated for 3–5 days after birth

Premature infants ($<$ 30 weeks gestation): lower T3, T4, and TSH levels compared with full-term infants; these levels are
    indirectly proportional to birth weight and gestational age

C. PLACENTAL ROLE IN THYROID HORMONES

Placenta produces estrogens that increase maternal thyroxine-binding globulin (TBG), T4, and T3; in addition, placenta
    produces human chorionic gonadotropin (hCG) that induces maternal T4 and T3 production since hCG is structurally
    similar to TSH; despite these changes, a euthyroid state is maintained during pregnancy

T4 and T3 are partially permeable across placenta:
  Although there is a limited amount of thyroid hormone transferred to fetus, maternal thyroid hormones are critical for
    fetal development during the 1st trimester when the hypothalamic-pituitary axis is not yet developed
  Transfer of maternal thyroid hormones later in gestation may be neuroprotective for a fetus with hypothyroidism

Placenta degrades maternal T4 to reverse T3 and maternal T3 to T2; T3 and diiodothyronine (T2) then cross to fetal side

Thyroid-releasing hormone (TRH) crosses placenta to fetus (yet only small amount to fetus due to low TRH in maternal
    serum); iodide also crosses placenta to fetus

Maternal thyroid-stimulating immunoglobulins (TSI) and TSH-binding inhibitory immunoglobulins (TBII) also cross the
    placenta

TSH does *not* cross placenta

D. THYROID HORMONE PRODUCTION

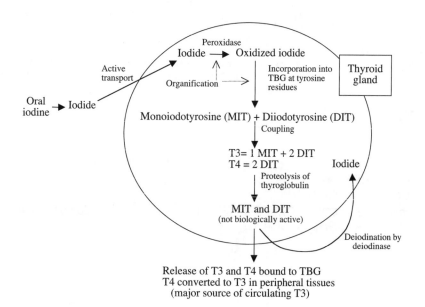

TRH (majority produced in the hypothalamus) acts on the anterior pituitary gland to induce TSH synthesis and secretion

TSH (produced by anterior pituitary gland) increases all steps in TH production and is regulated by peripheral TH levels (mostly T4)

E. T3 VS T4

Characteristic	Comparison between T3 and T4		
Secretion from thyroid gland	9% is T3 and 1% is rT3		90% of T4
Potency	T3	>	T4
Concentration in blood	T3	<	T4 (50-100x)
Protein-binding affinity	T3	<	T4
Percentage in free form	0.4% T3		0.04% T4
Plasma half-life	T3	<	T4
Localization	T3 mostly intracellular		T4 mostly extracellular

F. THYROID HORMONE FUNCTION

Maintains basal metabolic rate and stimulates both anabolic and catabolic pathways
Stimulates normal growth
Important in bone mineralization and skeletal muscle activity
Increases heart rate, contractility, and cardiac output
Role in central nervous system maturation both prenatally and postnatally

G. TESTS OF THYROID FUNCTION

Total T4	= bound + free T4 Bound T4 binds to TBG (70-75%), transthyretin (15%), and albumin (10%)
Total T3	= bound + free T3 Bound T3 binds to TBG and albumin
Free T4	Good measure of thyroid function since only free form can enter cells
Reverse T3	Inactive metabolite of T4
TBG	Prematurity, glucocorticoids, and malnutrition will decrease TBG levels Phenytoin decreases TBG binding affinity
TSH	Most sensitive and specific test of hypothyroidism if determined after TSH surge
T3 resin uptake	Used to assess if low total T4 level is due to low levels of TBG or free T4 Radioactive T3 is added to serum and can bind to TBG present in the serum; resin is then added to bind to labeled T3 that is not bound to TBG; following, unbound, radioactive T3 is measured If low radioactive T3, suggests many empty TBG binding sites; if this is associated with low total T4 → hypothyroidism If high radioactive T3, suggests few empty TBG binding sites; if this is associated with low total T4 → free T4 is normal and TBG is low

H. CONGENITAL HYPOTHYROIDISM

Types
  Thyroid dysgenesis: ~75%, 1:4000
    Due to thyroid aplasia, hypoplasia, or ectopy
  Thyroid dyshormonogenesis: ~10%, 1:40,000
    Defect in synthesis of thyroid hormone (TH) due to TSH unresponsiveness, iodide transport defect, organification defect, thyroglobulin abnormality, or deiodinase deficiency

Hypothalamic-pituitary defect: 5%, 1:100,000

Panhypopituitarism, hypothalamus or pituitary abnormality, isolated TSH deficiency, or TH resistance

Transient hypothyroidism: ~10%, 1:40,000

May be due to maternal anti-thyroid medications (e.g., propylthiouracil crosses placenta) or maternal antibodies (e.g., TSH receptor-blocking antibodies); can also be due to neonatal iodine exposure (since excess iodine inhibits the iodination of TBG)

Usually spontaneously resolves quickly (by age 2 weeks); may take longer (up to age 12 weeks) if associated with maternal blocking antibodies

Transient hypothyroxinemia of prematurity

Occurs in 30% to 80% of premature and low birth weight infants

Etiology is unknown and may be due to infant's immature hypothalamic-pituitary axis or variant of sick euthyroid

Closely monitor infant's thyroid function

Sick euthyroid

Acute or chronic illness leading to abnormal thyroid tests yet normal thyroid function

Clinical

Can be subtle or severe

Prolonged physiologic jaundice (> 7 days), large posterior fontanel (> 1cm diameter), umbilical hernia, macroglossia, hoarse cry, distended abdomen, hypotonia, difficulty feeding, lethargy, mottled skin, hypothermia, goiter (especially if iodide transport defects, organification defects, thyroglobulin abnormalities, or deiodase deficiency)

Possible long-term effects include delayed bone and body growth, mental deficiency (due to delayed myelination and abnormal neuronal cell membrane synthesis), and delayed puberty

May have Pendred syndrome (autosomal recessive organification defect with congenital eighth nerve abnormality leading to deafness, goiter during childhood)

Diagnosis

Newborn screen (majority initially measure T4; if low T4, then TSH levels are determined)

Ideal to sample at 3–5 days of age to avoid high TSH from appropriate physiologic TSH surge (earlier screening will increase false-positive rate)

Newborn screen results	Possible etiologies
Low T4 and high TSH	Thyroid dysgenesis Dyshormonogenesis Transient hypothyroidism
Low T4 and normal TSH	Transient hypothyroxinemia of prematurity Sick euthyroid syndrome TBG deficiency TSH deficiency
Normal T4 and high TSH	Transient hypothyroidism Thyroid dysgenesis

If abnormal screen, repeat T4 and TSH to confirm and measure free T4, T3 and TBG

Consider testing antithyroid antibodies, TRH level, and urinary iodine excretion

Ultrasound to assess for presence or absence of thyroid gland

Bone age may be helpful to assess degree of severity of hypothyroidism

Radionuclide scanning with iodine[123] to assess degree of radioactive iodine uptake (RAIU) if thyroid dysgenesis is suspected

Disease	T4	TSH	Other
Thyroid dysgenesis	Low or normal	High	RAIU can detect ectopic thyroid tissue
			If absence of RAIU, suggests agenesis of thyroid gland
Organification, thyroglobulin defects, and deiodase deficiency	Low	High	Thyroglobulin defects usually with low thyroglobulin and/or limited thyroglobulin response to TSH
			Often with history of familial congenital thyroid disease
			Increased RAIU
Thyroid hormone resistance	High	Normal or high	Autosomal dominant or sporadic
TSH deficiency	Low	Normal or low	Abnormal response to TRH
			If due to panhypopituitarism, also with low cortisol and growth hormone levels
TRH deficiency	Low	Low	Low TRH, normal response to TSH (with increase in T4)
Transient hypothyroidism	Low or normal	Variably high	May have history of autoimmmune thyroid disease in family
			If due to maternal antibodies, can measure neonatal TSH receptor antibodies
TBG deficiency	Low	Normal	Low TBG levels
Transient hypothyroxinemia of prematurity	Low	Normal or low	Low free T4
			Normal response to TRH and TSH
Sick euthyroid	Low or normal	Normal	Low T3
			Normal or high free T4

Management

Treat with levothyroxine sodium as early as possible once diagnosis is confirmed to minimize neurological effects of hypothyroidism

TSH levels may remain elevated for some time despite corrected T4 levels

If transient hypothyroidism, treat if persists > 2 weeks (to suppress TSH production)

If transient hypothyroidism of prematurity → controversial if need to treat (if TSH levels increase, consult endocrinologist since treatment may be warranted for 1st 3 years of life)

I. CONGENITAL HYPERTHYROIDISM DUE TO MATERNAL GRAVES DISEASE

Incidence

Uncommon since low incidence of thyrotoxicosis in pregnancy (1–2/1000) and neonatal disease in 1–5% of thyrotoxic pregnancies

Etiology

Mother with Graves disease leading to transplacental passage of TSH receptor-*stimulating* antibodies and TSH receptor-*blocking* antibodies

If fetus or neonate has greater amount of stimulating antibodies compared to blocking antibodies, will have increased TSH leading to increased thyroid hormone and *transient* hyperthyroidism

However, if fetus or neonate has greater amount of blocking antibodies, transient hypothyroidism may develop due to inhibition of TSH

Fetal effects can be present even if mother with inactive Graves disease (due to removal or destruction of thyroid gland) since fetus is still exposed to maternal antibodies

[Note: *permanent* hyperthyroidism due to pituitary resistance to thyroid hormone or TSH receptor mutations (sporadic or autosomal dominant) will lead to constitutive receptor activation and permanent hyperthyroidism]

Clinical

Can present in utero and up to 6 weeks of life

In utero: fetal tachycardia, growth restriction, goiter, advanced bone maturation or craniosynostosis, increased risk of premature birth

Postnatally: symptoms can last 3–12 weeks (due to thyroid receptor-stimulating antibodies with half-life ~4 weeks) and can include goiter, exophthalmos, tachycardia, bounding pulses, congestive heart failure, hypertension, arrhythmia, irritability, poor weight gain despite hyperphagia and hepatosplenomegaly

Labs may demonstrate thrombocytopenia or hyperbilirubinemia

Diagnosis

Cord blood with extremely low TSH levels and normal or elevated T4 and T3

Postnatally, high T4, free T4 and T3 levels, and low TSH

Neonate will have abnormal TSH-receptor antibodies

Management

Closely monitor for fetal tachycardia in utero

If evidence of fetal hyperthyroidism, treat mother with propylthiouracil and monitor for fetal goiter and growth restriction (Small studies suggest methimazole may be associated with aplasia cutis but this has not been proven in larger studies)

If elevated maternal or neonatal TSH-receptor antibodies, monitor neonate's thyroid function tests every 1–2 weeks for 4–6 weeks of life

If asymptomatic neonate: check newborn screen; consider checking cord TSH and T4 levels; consider repeating thyroid function tests by 2 weeks of age; monitor clinically for 4–6 weeks

Postnatal management should include consideration of:

Consultation with pediatric endocrinologist; supportive care

Iodide (Lugol's solution) to rapidly inhibit thyroid hormone release and decrease vascularity of thyroid gland

PTU (propylthiouracil) to inhibit organification and block conversion of T4 to T3

β-blockade (propranolol) to control tachycardia

Can administer *glucocorticoids* if severe hyperthyroidism to decrease TH secretion and inhibit conversion of T4 to T3

[Note: if hyperthyroidism due to mutation of TSH receptor, may require near-total thyroidectomy with radioiodine ablation of remaining thyroid tissue]

Prognosis

Majority with improvement in 3–12 weeks as maternal antibody levels decrease

Long-term effects include decreased growth, craniosynostosis, and intellectual/developmental impairment

~15% mortality

II. Adrenal Gland

A. EMBRYOLOGY AND ANATOMY

Adrenal cortex is derived from mesoderm and adrenal medulla is derived from neuroectodermal cells of the neural crest

~5-6 weeks gestation, development of gonadal ridge that gives rise to steroidogenic gonadal cells and adrenal cortex cells; following, gonadal cells migrate caudally and adrenal cells migrate retroperitoneally

At 7–8 weeks gestation, sympathetic neural cells invade adrenal cells and form adrenal medulla

By 8 weeks gestation, adrenal gland becomes encapsulated

The fetal adrenal gland is dramatically larger than adult adrenal gland and contains a large inner fetal zone that involutes during the first few months of life

The fetal adrenal gland plays an important role in fetal adrenal steroidogenesis and leads to the production of dehydroepiandrosterone (DHEA) sulfate; DHEA sulfate is then converted to DHEA in the placenta and serves as a precursor for placental estrogen production

While the adrenal medulla produces catecholamines (epinephrine, norepinephrine and dopamine), the adrenal cortex produces mineralocorticoids, glucocorticoids, and sex hormones

B. PATHWAYS OF ADRENAL CORTEX

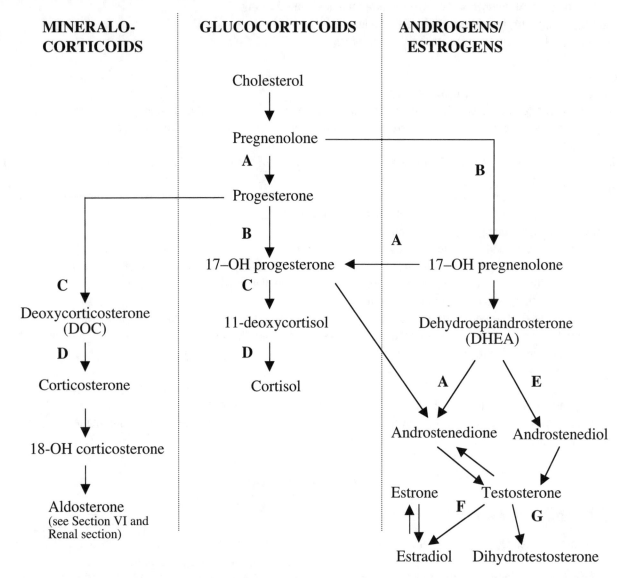

MINERALO-
CORTICOIDS

GLUCOCORTICOIDS

ANDROGENS/
ESTROGENS

Cholesterol

Pregnenolone

Progesterone

17–OH progesterone

11-deoxycortisol

Cortisol

Deoxycorticosterone
(DOC)

Corticosterone

18-OH corticosterone

Aldosterone
(see Section VI and
Renal section)

17–OH pregnenolone

Dehydroepiandrosterone
(DHEA)

Androstenedione   Androstenediol

Estrone   Testosterone

Estradiol   Dihydrotestosterone

A   3β-hydroxysteroid dehydrogenase
B   17α-hydroxylase
C   21-hydroxylase
D   11β-hydroxylase
E   17β-hydroxysteroid dehydrogenase
F   aromatase
G   5α-reductase

C. 21-HYDROXYLASE DEFICIENCY

Incidence
 #1 cause of congenital adrenal hyperplasia, 1:14,000
 Linkage with human major histocompatibility complex (HLA)

Pathophysiology
  Aldosterone deficiency since cannot convert progesterone to DOC *deoxy corticosterone*
  Cortisol deficiency since cannot convert 17-OH progesterone to 11-deoxycortisol
  Increased testosterone production due to increased precursors of 17-OH progesterone

Clinical
  Broad spectrum of clinical manifestations including:
    Salt-wasting that typically presents in the 2nd week of life with vomiting, diarrhea, dehydration, hyperkalemia, and hyponatremia; may progress to hypotension and shock
    Males have normal external genitalia and if no salt-wasting, may present later in life with precocious puberty and advanced bone age
    Females may have ambiguous external genitalia (ranging from mild cliteromegaly to complete labioscrotal fusion) and normal ovaries, fallopian tubes, and uterus; in milder cases, females present later in life with hirsutism, menstrual irregularities, and decreased fertility
  Classic form with salt-wasting, female pseudohermaphroditism, and virilization
  Nonclassic form is milder with premature adrenarche, menstrual irregularities, hirsutism, and decreased fertility

Diagnosis
  Prenatal
    Elevated 17-OH progesterone in amniotic fluid if severe salt-losing form
    If parents are heterozygous and fetus at risk, can diagnose by HLA typing of fetal amniocytes yet prior linkage analysis of family is required
  Postnatal
    Abnormal newborn screen with elevated 17-OH progesterone; ideal to measure after 24 hours of age; often falsely elevated in premature infants
    Confirm with elevated 17-OH progesterone following intravenous adrenocorticotropic hormone (ACTH) administration
    Cortisol response to ACTH can be absent or low; ACTH levels may be high or normal
    Increased serum androgens

Management
  Prenatal: experimental and controversial therapy with maternal glucocorticoid administration (to suppress fetal ACTH and thus suppress adrenal steroidogenesis); this may prevent masculinization of female fetus if administered prior to 6th week of gestation
  Postnatal: glucocortiocoid and mineralocorticoid replacement, salt supplementation, reconstructive surgery of abnormal female genitalia, monitor growth and bone age

D. 11-β HYDROXYLASE DEFICIENCY

Incidence
  Second most common cause of congenital adrenal hyperplasia (especially in Moslem and Middle Eastern Jewish population)

Pathophysiology
  Cortisol deficiency since cannot convert 11-deoxycortisol to cortisol
  Increased testosterone production due to increased precursors of 11-deoxycortisol
  Able to retain sodium despite aldosterone deficiency since DOC functions as a mineralocorticoid

Clinical
  No salt-wasting (note that may have some salt-wasting in neonatal period due to normal newborn resistance to mineralocorticoids)

Males have normal external genitalia and postnatal virilization

Females with ambiguous external genitalia

Diagnosis

Postnatal: high DOC and 11-deoxycortisol levels with increased response to ACTH; normal or decreased renin activity, increased serum androgens

Management

Glucocorticoid replacement

Reconstructive surgery of abnormal female genitalia

E. COMPARISON OF ENZYME DEFICIENCIES

Enzyme Deficiency	Effect on Males	Effect on Females	Effect on Blood Pressure (BP) and Salt Retention	Laboratory
21-hydroxylase deficiency	Normal external genitalia May have rapid growth or virilization	Ambiguous external genitalia Milder form may present later in life with hirsutism, menstrual irregularities and decreased fertility	Normal BP (some may have low BP) Salt-wasting	Elevated 17-OH progesterone Elevated 17-OH progesterone following ACTH administration
11β-hydroxylase deficiency	Normal external genitalia Postnatal virilization	Ambiguous external genitalia Postnatal virilization	High BP No salt-wasting (note: may have salt-wasting in neonatal period)	Increased DOC and deoxycortisol
17α-hydroxylase deficiency	Ambiguous male genitalia	Normal external genitalia but there is no development of secondary sexual traits	High BP No salt-wasting	Elevated DOC and corticosterone Low 17-OH progesterone and low 17-OH pregnenolone
3β-hydroxysteroid dehydrogenase deficiency (rare)	Incomplete male development with small phallus and severe hypospadias	Ambiguous external genitalia (clitoromegaly, mild virilization)	Normal BP Salt-wasting	Elevated 17-OH pregnenolone, pregnenolone, and DHEA

F. CORTISOL

Production

Produced in the zona fasciculata and reticularis of adrenal cortex

Hypothalamus secretes corticotropin-releasing hormone (CRH) that induces anterior pituitary gland to secrete ACTH, which leads to the production of cortisol by adrenal gland

Cortisol exerts negative regulation on CRH and ACTH secretion

Function

Induces gluconeogenesis and antagonizes insulin in muscle and fat tissue, both leading to increased serum glucose levels; cortisol also increases lipolysis

Increases calcium and phosphate release from bone

Critical for vascular responses to catecholamines

Decreases inflammation and suppresses immune system

Inhibits antidiuretic hormone, increases gastric acid secretion, increases production of red blood cells

Disorders

Cortisol deficiency—leads to hypoglycemia, hypotension, anemia and poor weight gain

Cortisol excess—leads to hyperglycemia, polycythemia, poor wound healing, decreased growth, hypertension, hypokalemia, and increased risk of infections

III. Sexual differentiation

A. NORMAL SEXUAL DIFFERENTIATION

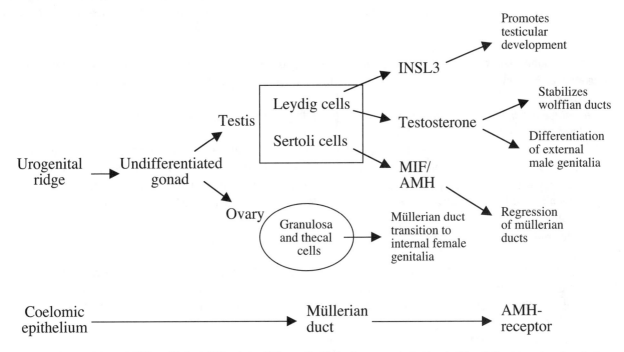

INSL3 = insulin–like growth factor-3; MIF = müllerian inhibiting factor; AMH = anti-müllerian hormone; note that female differentiation does not require estrogen production while male differentiation requires testosterone production; Modified from Sperling MA. Pediatric Endocrinology (2nd edition). Philadelphia, WB Saunders, 2002, p 112 and Fanaroff AA and Martin RJ (eds): Neonatal-Perinatal Medicine (6th edition). St Louis, Mosby–Year Book Inc, 1997, p 1505.

Male Development	Female Development
Wolffian duct (derived from excretory mesonephros duct) develops into epididymis, vas deferens, ejaculatory duct, and seminal vesicles	Müllerian duct (or paramesonephric duct, derived from coelomic epithelium) develops into fallopian tubes, uterus, cervix, and upper third of vagina
	Lower portion of vagina from canalization of vaginal plate
Urethral folds fuse → corpus spongiosum and penile urethra	Urethral folds do not fuse → labia minora
Genital tubercle → corpora cavernosa of penis/phallus	Genital tubercle → clitoris
Labioscrotal folds fuse → scrotum	Labioscrotal swellings do not fuse → labia majora

B. ABNORMAL SEXUAL DIFFERENTIATION

1. Gonadal disorders

True hermaphrodite: rare disorder in which one individual with both ovarian tissue (with follicles) and testicular tissue (with seminiferous tubules); typically sporadic and > 50% with genotype 46, XX; usually with ambiguous external genitalia; majority raised as males

Turner syndrome (see Genetics chapter): 45, X; female with gonadal dysgenesis (cortical); usually doesn't develop secondary sexual traits and majority are infertile; normal external female genitalia

Klinefelter syndrome (see Genetics chapter): 47, XXY; male with hypogonadism, hypogenitalia, infertility due to atrophy of seminiferous tubules, gynecomastia (~1/3, increased risk of breast cancer)

2. Female pseudohermaphrodite = 46, XX karyotype with ambiguous external genitalia due to excess androgens

Congenital adrenal hyperplasia (refer to II above, due to 21-hydroxylase, 11β-hydroxylase and 3β-hydroxysteroid dehydrogenase deficiency)

Maternal androgen and progesterone therapy

Exposure between 8–13 weeks gestation → fetus with posterior fusion of vagina, scrotalization of labia, and some fusion of urethral folds

Exposure after 13 weeks gestation → clitoromegaly

Aromatase deficiency: inability to convert testosterone to estradiol and androstenedione to estrone

Females with müllerian duct structures and absent wolffian duct structures; female exam significant for ambiguous genitalia or clitoromegaly; females may have multicystic ovaries, tall stature, virilization at puberty, delayed bone age

3. Male pseudohermaphrodite = 46, XY karyotype with ambiguous external genitalia due to undervirilization

Congenital adrenal hyperplasia (refer to II above, due to 17α-hydroxylase and 3β-hydroxysteroid dehydrogenase deficiency)

5α-reductase deficiency: autosomal recessive disorder leading to inability to convert testosterone to dihydrotestosterone

Males have ambiguous genitalia with appropriately differentiated wolffian structures, absence of müllerian-derived structures, *small phallus,* urogenital sinus with perineal *hypospadias* and *blind vaginal pouch;* later in life, males with progressive virilization yet may have decreased facial hair and smaller than normal prostate; infertile

Has been referred to as "testicles at twelve" due to virilization and descent of testes to labial location at time of puberty

Females with normal phenotype

Androgen resistance or insensitivity

Complete form (previously denoted as testicular feminization) due to impaired activation of the androgen receptor

Normal female phenotype at birth, may have unilateral or bilateral inguinal hernias or labial masses, cryptorchidism, blind vaginal pouch, hypoplastic labia majora, no uterus or oviducts, underdeveloped wolffian structures

Have elevated leutinizing hormone and normal follicle-stimulating hormone, increased testosterone

Increased risk of testes developing malignancy after puberty

Partial form (~10%)—similar laboratory findings as complete form; some virilization at time of puberty (unlike complete form)

4. Hypospadias   *urethral opening @ base or along shaft*

Occurs in ~1 in 500 births

Failure of urethral differentiation leading to meatus that is proximal to tip of glans penis; majority are glandular or coronal

Eiologies include idiopathic (most common, especially if mild and no other abnormalities), hermaphroditism, gonadal dysgenesis, male or female pseudohermaphroditism, and syndrome-associated (e.g., Smith-Lemli-Opitz)

If bilaterally undescended testes, need to rule out congenital adrenal hyperplasia

Delay circumcision since foreskin required for repair later in life

Controversial about ideal timing of repair (usually prior to 18 months of age)

5. Cryptorchidism

Failure of testicular descent (normally occurs in the 7th month of gestation)

Right testes more often undescended compared with left

Majority are inguinal and 1/4 are intra-abdominal

If unilateral cryptorchidism, the contralateral testes usually becomes hypertrophied

If both hypospadias and cryptorchidism, increased risk of congenital adrenal hyperplasia

May be an isolated finding

10-fold increased risk of developing carcinoma (probably due to damage of testes in elevated temperature of abdomen) and thus orchipexy recommended early in life

IV. Glucose Metabolism

A. FETAL CARBOHYDRATE PHYSIOLOGY

Fetal glucose is maintained entirely by placental transfer from mother; this transfer is mediated by facilitated diffusion using glucose transporters as carriers

Levels of fetal glucose concentration are dependent on maternal glucose concentration and maternal-fetal glucose gradient across placenta

Acute hypoglycemia or hyperglycemia in the fetus does not alter fetal insulin or glucagon levels; in contrast, fetus is able to respond to *chronic* states of abnormal glucose levels (i.e. during chronic hyperglycemia, fetus insulin levels will increase and glucagon levels will decrease; during chronic hypoglycemia, fetal insulin levels will decrease and glucagon levels will increase)

Fetus can respond to an increase in catecholamines with mobilization of fetal glucose and free fatty acids

B. NEONATAL CARBOHYDRATE PHYSIOLOGY

At birth, the maternal glucose supply is acutely interrupted and the neonate accommodates by increasing glucagon levels (3- to 5-fold) within minutes-hours after birth, decreasing insulin production, and rapidly increasing catecholamine secretion; all of these changes lead to an increase in glycogenolysis, gluconeogenesis, lipolysis, and ketogenesis

Glucose concentration is lowest 30–90 minutes after birth in full term-infant

Glucose production in full-term infant is ~4–6 mg/kg/min (this is greater than adult glucose production); premature infant often with higher glucose production

C. NEONATAL HYPOGLYCEMIA

Definition
  Decrease in glucose plasma level
  The precise limit in neonate is controversial with range between 40 and 60 mg/dL

Measurement of glucose levels
  Whole blood glucose levels are 10–15% lower than plasma glucose levels
  Blood samples that are not processed quickly will undergo glycolysis and lead to lower glucose levels (ideal if glycolytic inhibitors are present in collection tubes)
  Hospital glucose monitors are less precise than laboratory methods
  Falsely elevated glucose levels if sample drawn from indwelling lines without appropriate pre-flushing

Etiology
  Prematurity (due to inadequate glycogen stores and immature enzymes)
  Hyperinsulinism due to infant of a diabetic mother, small or large for gestational age infant, discordant twin, perinatal depression, Beckwith-Wiedemann syndrome, pancreatic islet adenoma, erythroblastosis fetalis
  Hormone abnormalities due to panhypopituitarism, growth hormone deficiency, cortisol deficiency (e.g., 21-hydroxylase deficiency, 11β-hydroxylase deficiency, adrenal hemorrhage)
  Hereditary abnormalities including galacatosemia, glycogen storage disease, hereditary fructose intolerance, maple syrup urine disease, propionic acidemia, methylmalonic acidemia, β-methylcrotonyl glycinuria, glutaric aciduria type I and type II, mevalonic aciduria, long chain 3-hydroxyacyl-CoA deficiency

Clinical

Numerous clinical manifestations and thus maintain high index of suspicion

Symptoms include irritability, hypothermia, cyanotic episode, apnea, myoclonic jerks, seizures, and lethargy

Diagnosis

Identify underlying etiology by obtaining history, identify timing of hypoglycemia (hyperinsulinism and glycogen storage disease usually demonstrate hypoglycemia within a few hours after eating while fatty acid oxidation disorder with hypoglycemia 10–12 hours after eating), and examining for anomalies

Laboratory studies can include insulin level, pH, and lactate level

Further evaluation may include free fatty acid and ketone levels, tests of pituitary, thyroid and adrenal function, and glucagon stimulation test

Management

Immediate treatment

If asymptomatic, consider treatment with oral glucose (especially if transient etiology)

If symptomatic, treat intravenously with bolus followed by infusion (or increase in maintenance infusion)

May require diazoxide if prolonged hypoglycemia due to hyperinsulinism

If possible, treat underlying etiology

D. MATERNAL DIABETES

Incidence

~2% of pregnant women develop gestational diabetes

1 in 1000 pregnant women with insulin-dependent diabetes

Screening

Typically screen all women at 24–28 weeks gestation

2 possible screening methods:

1. Measure plasma glucose 1 hour after 50 grams oral glucose and if abnormal, repeat and measure glucose 1, 2 and 3 hours after 100 grams

2. Measure plasma glucose 1 hour after 100 grams oral glucose

Classification of diabetes during pregnancy

	Class	Onset	Vascular disease	Management
LGA	A_1	Gestational	None	No insulin, diet-controlled
	A_2	Gestational	None	Small amount of insulin
	B	> 20 years old	None	Insulin-dependent
	C	10–19 years old	None	Insulin-dependent
SGA	D	< 10 years old	Mild retinopathy	Insulin-dependent
	F	Any age	Nephropathy	Insulin-dependent
	R	Any age	Proliferative retinopathy	Insulin-dependent
	H	Any	Heart disease	Insulin-dependent

LGA=large for gestational age infant; SGA=small for gestational age infant; Modified from Cunningham FG, Gant NF, Leveno KJ, Gilstrap LC, Hauth JC and Wenstrom KD (eds): Williams Obstetrics (21st edition). New York, McGraw-Hill, 2001, p 1361.

Possible fetal and neonatal effects (effects are due to fetal hyperinsulinemia in response to elevated fetal glucose; greater risk with uncontrolled, severe maternal diabetes; risk of congenital malformations correlates with degree of elevated glycosylated hemoglobin levels)

May have stillbirth, polyhydramnios, or premature birth

Large for gestational age (note: if mother with severe vascular effects of diabetes, can have small for gestational age infant due to uteroplacental insufficiency); macrosomic infants with greater risk of birth trauma

Transient hyperinsulinism and neonatal hypoglycemia that typically resolves in 1–2 days

Hyperplasia and hypertrophy of pancreatic islet cells

Organomegaly

Hyaline membrane disease

Congenital heart disease including hypertrophic cardiomyopathy, ventricular septal defect and transposition of great vessels

Polycythemia leading to hyperbilirubinemia

Early neonatal hypocalcemia (due to decreased placental Ca transfer, decreased PTH secretion, hypercalcitonemia, hypomagnesemia, and decreased Ca absorption)

Caudal regression, hydrocephalus, neural tube defects, anencephaly, anal atresia, situs inversus, small left colon, renal anomalies, and renal vein thrombosis

Management

Initially attempt maternal euglycemia by diet-control accompanied by exercise

If unable to manage maternal hyperglycemia by diet, treat with insulin

During labor, avoid maternal hyperglycemia to prevent fetal hyperglycemia and the associated greater risk of severe hypoglycemia from acute hyperinsulinemia

Monitor neonate for evidence of above effects, initiate early feeds, and treat hypoglycemia as noted above

Prognosis

> 1/2 of women with gestational diabetes will develop diabetes within 20 years

Women with gestational diabetes with greater risk of cardiovascular disease

Pregnancy does not alter long-term course of diabetes

V. Pituitary Gland

A. EMBRYOLOGY AND ANATOMY

Pituitary gland is derived from ectodermal tissue

The adenohypophysis (anterior lobe) of the pituitary gland originates from the primitive oropharynx called Rathke's pouch and the neurohypophysis (posterior lobe) is derived from the floor of the forebrain; this lobe synthesizes and secretes the majority of hormones including TSH, luteinizing hormone, follicle-stimulating hormone, prolactin, growth hormone (GH), ACTH, and pro-opiomelanocortin

The supraoptic and paraventricular nuclei of the hypothalamus produce vasopression and oxytocin and the posterior pituitary gland stores and secretes these hormones

The blood supply of the anterior pituitary communicates closely with the blood supply of hypothalamic neurons while the blood supply of the posterior lobe is separate from the hypothalamus since it is mediated by neural stimuli

By 12 weeks gestation, while all anterior pituitary gland and hypothalamic hormones are detectable, the hypothalamus/pituitary axis develops later (by ~18 weeks gestation)

Although fetal hormone production occurs in utero, the fetal pituitary is not required for the early development of endocrine organs

B. PANHYPOPITUITARISM

Clinical
   Males with microphallus
   Midline facial malformations including cleft lip/palate
   May have other midline malformations (e.g., septo-optic dysplasia)
   Increased risk of holoprosencephaly
   Often with liver dysfunction similar to cholestatic liver disease
   If significant growth hormone deficiency, may have severe short stature later in life

Labs
   Hypoglycemia (due to decreased growth hormone and cortisol)
   May have prolonged physiologic jaundice
   Varying low levels of hormones secreted by pituitary gland

Evaluation and management
   MRI if suspect diagnosis
   May require thyroid hormone, hydrocortisone, and/or testosterone supplementation
   If significant GH deficiency, treat with recombinant human GH as soon as possible after diagnosis is made

C. ANTI-DIURETIC HORMONE (ADH)

Production
   ADH or arginine vasopressin is produced in the paraventricular and supraoptic nuclei of the hypothalamus, transported
      via axons to the posterior pituitary gland where it is stored and released into the circulation
   When the osmolality of the extracellular fluid (ECF) is high, fluid moves out of osmoreceptor cells (precise location is not
      known) and the posterior pituitary gland increases ADH secretion; this leads to increased water reabsorption by the
      kidneys and a decrease in ECF osmolality (the opposite also occurs: when osmolality of ECF is low, ADH secretion is
      inhibited)
   Cardiovascular volume receptors can induce ADH secretion when blood volume is low

Function
   Controls water homeostasis by increasing the permeability of the distal nephron to H_2O, leading to increased H_2O
      absorption and increased urine osmolality
   Also acts as a vasoconstrictor and functions to stimulate renal mesangial cell contraction, decrease renin secretion, and
      increase ACTH secretion

Disorders of ADH
   1. Diabetes insipidus (DI)

Nephrogenic DI	Neurogenic DI (or Central DI)
Increased urine output due to failure of kidneys to respond to ADH	Increased urine output due to inadequate production of ADH
Increased plasma osmolality	Increased plasma osmolality
Decreased urine osmolality	Decreased urine osmolality
Normal to high ADH levels	Low ADH levels
No change in urine osmolality after fluid restriction	No change in urine osmolality after fluid restriction
Increase in ADH levels after fluid restriction	No change in ADH levels after fluid restriction
No change in urine osmolality after ADH administration	Increase in urine osmolality after ADH administration

Modified from Porterfield SP. Endocrine Physiology (2nd edition). St Louis, Mosby, 2001, p 55.

2. Syndrome of inappropriate ADH (SIADH)

Inappropriately high concentration of ADH relative to the plasma osmolality; this results in an increased blood volume, which induces atrial natriuretic peptide levels and leads to increased renal Na excretion

Can be associated with central nervous system abnormalities (e.g., subarachnoid hemorrhage, hydrocephalus, meningitis), pulmonary processes (e.g., pneumonia, pneumothorax), and induction by medications

Diagnosed by hyponatremia (note that Na is still excreted in urine despite hyponatremia), increased weight gain, higher than appropriate urine osmolality in setting of low plasma osmolality, often with hypouricemia

Treat by fluid restriction; sodium replacement is not effective for increasing serum sodium levels since it will continue to be rapidly excreted in urine; treat underlying disease

VI. Renin, Angiotensin, and Aldosterone Pathway (see Renal section as well)

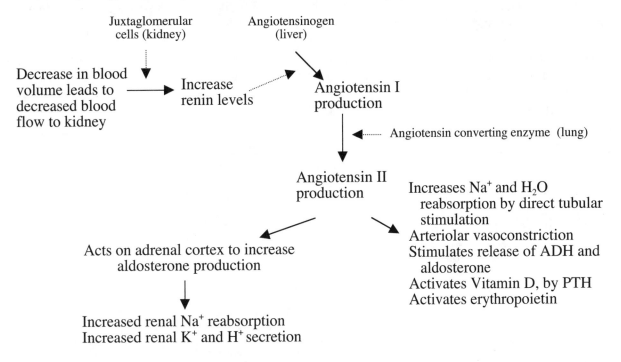

Juxtaglomerular cells (kidney)   Angiotensinogen (liver)

Decrease in blood volume leads to decreased blood flow to kidney → Increase renin levels ⋯→ Angiotensin I production

Angiotensin converting enzyme (lung) ⋯→

Angiotensin II production

Acts on adrenal cortex to increase aldosterone production

Increased renal Na⁺ reabsorption
Increased renal K⁺ and H⁺ secretion

Increases Na^+ and H_2O reabsorption by direct tubular stimulation
Arteriolar vasoconstriction
Stimulates release of ADH and aldosterone
Activates Vitamin D, by PTH
Activates erythropoietin

VII. Calcium (Ca), Phosphate (P), and Magnesium (Mg) Metabolism

A. CALCIUM, PHOSPHATE, AND MAGNESIUM HOMEOSTASIS IN UTERO

Maternal: significant increase in PTH-related hormone (PTHrP), which increases calcitriol [= 1,25(OH)₂ vitamin D] production; this increase in calcitriol increases maternal intestinal absorption of Ca; thus, maternal serum Ca levels can remain normal despite loss from placental transfer of Ca to fetus

Placental transfer: Ca, P and Mg cross placenta via active transport; calcidiol [= 25 (OH) vitamin D] crosses placenta

Fetus: fetal skeletal growth and cell/tissue growth depend upon maternal Ca and P supply; Ca increases throughout gestation with the greatest increase during 3rd trimester

The high fetal serum calcium level leads to increased calcitonin and suppressed fetal parathyroid function

Fetal kidney capable of converting calcidiol to calcitriol (active form)

Premature infants: increased risk of low mineral levels due to peak placental transfer occurring during late pregnancy

This deficiency continues postnatally due to low mineral intake, low Ca stores, increased Ca and P renal losses, abnormal Ca intestinal absorption, and *physiologic hypoparathyroidism*

Postnatally: Ca levels decrease rapidly in first 6 hours after delivery and are at lowest levels at ~24 hours of age
Following the initial decrease in Ca, PTH increases during the 1st day of life and peaks at ~48 hours of age; calcitriol levels similarly increase initially and then remain constant after ~24 hours of age
Phosphate is high in first few days of life and slowly declines with age
Calcitonin increases immediately after birth and then slowly decreases

B. POSTNATAL FUNCTIONS OF CALCIUM, PHOSPHATE AND MAGNESIUM

Ca function: role in bone mineralization and blood clotting; regulates cell membrane permeability, controls neuromuscular excitability, important in cellular signal transduction, muscular contraction, and cardiac rhythm; also functions as a 2nd messenger for many hormones

P function: important buffer and component of numerous compounds including adenosine triphosphate, deoxyribonucleic acid and ribonucleic acid

Mg function: cofactor for many intracellular enzymatic reactions, important role in Na/K pump, decreases excitability of muscle and nerve cells, antagonist of Ca entry in vascular system and thus modulates vascular tone

C. REGULATION OF CALCIUM AND PHOSPHATE METABOLISM

	Intestine	Kidney	Bone
Ca (tightly-regulated)	~20-60% absorption Majority occurs in proximal small intestine	Filters free Ca and ~98% reabsorbed (~60% in proximal tubule, ~25% in loop of Henle and fine regulation in distal nephron)	Enters bone when Ca levels are high and exits when Ca levels are low Cortisol and thyroid hormones increase release from bone
P (daily levels vary widely)	~70-90% absorption	Filters free P and ~90% reabsorbed (majority in proximal tubule)	Cortisol and thyroid hormones increase release from bone
PTH action	Increases renal production of active form of vitamin D (or calcitriol) and thus indirectly increases Ca and P intestinal absorption	Increases Ca reabsorption in thick ascending loop of Henle Decreases P reabsorption (this is PTH's greatest effect on P) Decreases renal HCO_3 reabsorption (and thus increases Cl reabsorption) Increases renal calcitriol production	Increases release of Ca and P from bone (i.e. increases bone resorption) Also increases bone remodeling Requires vitamin D for these actions
Vitamin D action	1, 25 $(OH)_2$ vitamin D increases absorption of Ca and slightly increases intestinal absorption of P	Conversion of inactive form to active form [25 (OH) vitamin D/calcidiol to 1,25 $(OH)_2$ vitamin D/calcitriol] PTH and low serum P levels increase calcitriol production	Calcitriol increases PTH effect on bone
Calcitonin action	No direct effect	Small increase in Ca and P renal excretion Site of inactivation of calcitonin	Calcitonin inhibits release of Ca and P from bone (i.e. decreases bone resorption) No effect on bone remodeling

D. HYPOCALCEMIA

Etiology
  Early neonatal hypocalcemia (birth–72 hours of age):
    Maternal illness (diabetes, preeclampsia, hyperparathyroidism)
    Prematurity, growth restriction, perinatal depression, infection, hypomagnesemia, transfusion of blood products (particularly exchange transfusion; due to compounds such as citrate that form complexes with Ca); reports of low Ca associated with phototherapy
  Late neonatal hypocalcemia (after 72 hours of age):
    Hypoparathyroidism (can be due to DiGeorge syndrome; familial with autosomal dominant, autosomal recessive, or X-linked recessive inheritance; transient neonatal pseudohypoparathyroidism due to blunted phosphaturic response to PTH)

Hypomagnesemia, vitamin D deficiency, renal insufficiency, high-phosphate milk diet, osteopenia of prematurity (typically occurs later at 2–4 months of age), malabsorption

Other: alkalosis (HCO_3 leads to increased Ca binding to albumin and thus *decreases* free ionized Ca), liver renal disease, drug-induced (e.g., diuretics, corticosteroids)

Clinical

May be asymptomatic (especially if early hypocalcemia); if symptomatic, may have seizures, jitteriness, laryngospasm, high-pitched cry, positive Chvostek and Trousseau sign, irritability, tetany

EKG with prolonged QT interval

Management

Evaluation to determine etiology including total serum Ca, ionized Ca (better indicator of physiologic functional ability of Ca), phosphate, creatinine, alkaline phosphatase, urine Ca excretion, calcitriol, CD4 count (low if decreased thymic function), skeletal radiographs, chest radiograph to assess for presence or absence of thymus

Administer Ca (intravenous if severe hypocalcemia or presence of seizures or tetany)

Supplement with vitamin D (in form of calcitriol) if hypoparathyroidism suspected; supplement with ergocalciferol if parathyroid function is normal

Feed with low-phosphate formula to maximize calcium absorption

During treatment, monitor for iatrogenic hypercalcemia, hypercalciuria, nephrocalcinosis, nephrolithiasis, and renal insufficiency

If possible, treat underlying cause

E. HYPERCALCEMIA

Etiology

Maternal illness (hypoparathryoidism, increased vitamin D intake)

Hyperparathyroidism, Williams syndrome, idiopathic, excessive vitamin D or Ca intake, hypophosphatemia, drug-induced (e.g., thiazide diuretics)

Subcutaneous fat necrosis (due to reabsorption of precipitated Ca and macrophage calcitriol synthesis with increased intestinal Ca absorption)

Infantile hypophosphatasia (due to decreased alkaline phosphatase activity)

Familial hypocalciuric hypercalcemia

Clinical

Symptoms are typically nonspecific and include poor feeding, emesis, lethargy, irritability, polyuria, constipation

Management

Evaluation to determine etiology including total serum Ca, ionized Ca, phosphate, alkaline phosphatase, urinalysis and urine Ca/P/creatinine; if prolonged, can measure PTH, calcidiol, and calcitriol

If severe, treat with intravenous normal saline (to treat dehydration) followed by furosemide (to increase Ca excretion) with monitoring of electrolytes; hydrocortisone (particularly if chronic hypercalcemia; decreases intestinal Ca absorption)

Feed with low-calcium formula

Avoid sunlight to limit vitamin D

If possible, treat underlying cause (e.g., if severe primary hyperparathyroidism, may require subtotal or total parathyroidectomy)

F. DISORDERS OF MAGNESIUM

Hypomagnesemia

Etiology: maternal illness (diabetes, preeclampsia), growth-restricted fetus, prematurity, malabsorption, chronic diarrhea, renal tubular disorders, drug-induced (e.g., amphotericin B); also can be associated with liver disease, hypoparathyroidism, hyperphosphatemia, perinatal depression

Clinical: may have irritability, tremors, seizures, hyperreflexia, muscle weakness (particularly respiratory muscle); may have prolonged QT interval

Management: depending on severity of hypomagnesemia—intravenous, intramuscular, or oral Mg supplementation; monitor for hypocalcemia

Hypermagnesemia

Etiology: excess maternal Mg supplementation (to manage premature labor, preeclampsia, or toxemia), prematurity, perinatal depression, renal failure

Clinical: majority of neonates without symptoms

　　May have hypotonia, flaccidity, decreased respiratory effort, hypotension, may develop rickets

　　Gentamicin therapy in presence of high magnesium levels increases risk of severe apnea

Management: hydrate to maximize urinary Mg excretion

　　Most infants will have spontaneous resolution in 24–48 hours if renal function is normal

　　May require Ca supplementation (to decrease neuromuscular action of Mg), consider loop diuretics (to increase Mg excretion)

　　If life-threatening hypermagnesemia, may require exchange transfusion

G. OSTEOPENIA, OR RICKETS OF PREMATURITY

Pathophysiology

　　Decreased bone mineralization primarily due to inadequate Ca and P; this leads to weak bones and increased risk of fractures

　　Increased risk with greater degree of prematurity and severity of illness

Etiology

　　Premature neonates develop rickets due to:

　　　　Low initial Ca levels (from insufficient placental transfer)

　　　　Decreased Ca and P intestinal absorption

　　　　Insufficient Ca and P in parenteral nutrition (partly due to incompatibility of Ca and P in high amounts)

　　　　Insufficient Ca and P intake relative to premature infant's requirements (e.g., if unsupplemented breast milk)

　　　　Increased risk of necrotizing enterocolitis and/or malabsorption

　　　　Increased risk of liver disease, renal disease, and other chronic illnesses

　　　　Greater risk of exposure to specific medications

Clinical

　　Majority present with fractures (peak time of presentation at ~2-4 months of age)

　　May have craniotabes, rachitic rosary (widened costochondral junctions of ribs), enlarged anterior fontanel

Labs (variable)

　　Alkaline phosphatase may be increased with low or low-normal P

　　Ca is typically normal (since PTH is functional) yet may also be decreased or even increased

　　Normal or elevated PTH, normal calcitonin

　　While 25 (OH) vitamin D may be low, normal or high, levels of 1,25 $(OH)_2$ vitamin D are typically increased

　　May have increased renal Ca excretion and increased tubular reabsorption of P

　　X-ray abnormalities include fractures, delayed ossification, demineralization of bones

Management

　　Attempt to prevent in premature infants by administering maximal daily requirements of Ca, P, and vitamin D, initiate oral feeds as soon as possible, and supplement breast milk

　　Treat with Ca and P supplementation to maximize bone deposition and avoid hypocalcemia to prevent bone resorption

Gentle with cares to prevent fractures

Monitor for fractures and immobilize as needed

H. LABORATORY RESULTS IN DISORDERS ASSOCIATED WITH ABNORMAL CA AND P METABOLISM

Disease	Serum Ca	Serum P	Other
Osteopenia of prematurity	Usually normal (but can be decreased or even increased)	Decreased or normal	Increased 1,25 $(OH)_2$ vitamin D Alkaline phosphatase may be increased
Primary hyperparathyroidism	Increased	Decreased	May have hyperchloremic acidosis due to renal effect of PTH
Primary hypoparathyroidism	Decreased	Increased	Low PTH levels Decreased calcitriol synthesis Alkalosis
Pseudohypoparathyroidism	Decreased	Increased	Due to tissue resistance to PTH Increased PTH levels Low calcitriol
Chronic renal failure	Decreased	Increased	Increased PTH levels to compensate for low serum Ca
Malabsorption	Decreased	Decreased	Multiple nutrient deficiency

REFERENCES

Buckingham B: The hyperthyroid fetus and infant. *Neo Reviews,* 2000; 1(6):e103–9.

Cloherty JC and Stark AR (eds): Manual of Neonatal Care (5th edition), Thyroid Section. Philadelphia, Lippincott–Raven Publishers, in press.

Cunningham FG, Gant NF, Leveno KJ, et al (eds): Williams Obstetrics (21st edition). New York, McGraw-Hill, 2001.

Fanaroff AA and Martin RJ (eds): Neonatal-Perinatal Medicine (6th edition). St Louis, Mosby–Year Book Inc, 1997.

Gordon C: Neonatal Core Conference: Neonatal Thyroid Development and Disease. Children's Hospital, Boston, April 1997.

Porterfield SP: Endocrine Physiology (2nd edition). St Louis, Mosby, 2001.

Sperling MA: Pediatric Endocrinology (2nd edition). Philadelphia, WB Saunders, 2002.

CHAPTER 12

Inborn Errors of Metabolism and Thermal Regulation

Urea Cycle
⊗ 1. Ornithine transcarb defic.
2. carbamyl
3. Transient hyperamm.
4. Arginosuccinate synthetase def.
5. Argininolyase defic.
6. N. Acctly glutam. synthetase

TOPICS COVERED IN THIS CHAPTER

I. **Clinical Presentation of Neonates with Inborn Errors of Metabolism**

II. **Carbohydrate Disorders**
   A. Galactosemia
   B. Galactokinase deficiency
   C. Glycogen storage disease
   D. Hereditary fructose intolerance

III. **Protein Abnormalities**
   A. Urea cycle defects
   B. Maple syrup urine disease
   C. Phenylketonuria
   D. Tyrosinemia
   E. Homocystinuria
   F. Non-ketotic hyperglycinemia
   G. Histidinemia
   H. Cystinuria
   I. Lysinuric protein intolerance
   J. Hartnup disease

IV. **Organic Acidemias**
   A. Isovaleric acidemia *sweaty feet*
   B. β-methylcrotonyl glycinuria
   C. Propionate pathway abnormalities
   D. Mevalonic aciduria
   E. Glutaric aciduria type I
   F. Hydroxymethyl glutaryl-CoA lyase deficiency

V. **Fatty Acid Abnormalities**
   A. Medium chain acyl-CoA dehydrogenase deficiency
   B. Long chain 3-hydroxyacyl-CoA dehydrogenase deficiency

↓ Hallmark ⊗
Non-Ketogenic.
hypoglycemia

   C. Carnitine deficiency
   D. Glutaric aciduria type II

VI. **Lysosomal Storage Diseases**
   A. Mucopolysaccharidosis
   B. Lipidoses
   C. Mucolipidoses

VII. **Mitochondrial Disorders**
   A. Pyruvate dehydrogenase complex deficiency
   B. Pyruvate carboxylase deficiency
   C. Respiratory chain disorders

VIII. **Cofactor Abnormalities**
   A. Biotinidase deficiency

IX. **Other Metabolic Diseases**
   A. Wilson disease
   B. Menkes disease
   C. Zellweger syndrome
   D. Defects of bile acid synthesis

X. **Differential Diagnosis of Hyperammonemia**

XI. **Clinical Traits Associated with Metabolic Diseases**

XII. **Laboratory Blood Tests Associated with Metabolic Diseases**

XIII. **Urine Tests Associated with Metabolic Diseases**

XIV. **Neonatal Temperature Regulation**
   A. Heat maintenance
   B. Heat loss: neonate vs adult
   C. Heat gain: neonate vs adult
   D. Neonatal hypothermia and hyperthermia
   E. Types of neonatal heat loss
   F. Incubators

Hyperammonemia
1. Urea Cycle
2. Organic acidemia
3. Fatty Acid Oxidation

I. Clinical Presentation of Neonates with Inborn Errors of Metabolism

Overall incidence is as high as 1:2000

Majority present after first 48 hours of age

Consider diagnosis of metabolic disease if:
  Family history: neonatal death of unclear etiology, history of child with neurological deterioration (note: majority of metabolic diseases are autosomal recessive and thus typically no family history)
  Clinical: infant with decreased oral intake, vomiting, lethargy, coma, seizures, changes in tone, hepatosplenomegaly, cardiomegaly, dysmorphic features, cataracts, developmental delay, or failure to thrive (FTT)
  Labs: infant with hypoglycemia of unexplained etiology, metabolic acidosis of unexplained etiology, respiratory alkalosis, abnormal liver function tests (LFTs), hyperbilirubinemia that is not consistent with physiologic jaundice or other causes, ketonuria, abnormal urine odor, hyperammonemia, urine reducing substances

II. Carbohydrate Disorders

A. GALACTOSEMIA

Pathway

$$\text{Lactose} \xrightarrow{\ \textbf{A}\ } \substack{\text{Galactose} \\ \text{+ glucose}} \xrightarrow{\ \textbf{B}\ } \substack{\text{Galactose 1-phosphate} \\ \text{+ UDP glucose}} \xrightarrow{\ \textbf{C}\ } \substack{\text{Uridine diphospho-} \\ \text{galactose +} \\ \text{glucose-1 phosphate}}$$

  A Lactase (intestinal)
  B Galactokinase; if absent → galactokinase deficiency
  C Galactose-1-phosphate-uridyltransferase

Clinical
  Autosomal recessive
  Typically presents soon after feeds are introduced
  Poor feeding, vomiting typically within first 2–3 days of life, lethargy, hepatomegaly, liver failure, renal tubular dysfunction (acidosis, glycosuria, amino aciduria)
  Cataracts at birth due to fetal exposure to galactose (formation due to excess galactitol in lens, regresses with good control of dietary lactose)
  Increased risk of neonatal infection (especially *E. coli sepsis*)
  If mild neonatal symptoms, can present later with failure to thrive (FTT)
  Older children with learning disabilities despite therapy

Labs
  Elevated LFTs, increased indirect bilirubin, later—elevated direct bilirubin, *low glucose,* decreased coagulation factors produced by liver, albuminuria
  Increased galactose in urine (represented *by reducing substances* and negative glucose oxidase or *negative Clinistix*)
    Hyperchloremic *metabolic acidosis* due to renal tubular dysfunction, normal lactate, and normal pyruvate

Diagnosis

Newborn screen: measures galactose in blood (limited screening tool if severe neonatal disease since infant may die prior to results), some measure galactose-1-phosphate uridyltransferase levels

Decreased erythrocyte galactose-1-phosphate uridyltransferase with elevated precursor (galactose-1-phosphate)

Management

Emergent treatment

Eliminate all galactose/lactose in diet (not needed in diet since humans can produce galactose endogenously)

Decreasing dietary galactose in pregnant female with previous child with galactosemia to try and prevent cataract development (note—fetus can synthesize galactose-1-phosphate and thus may not be beneficial)

B. GALACTOKINASE DEFICIENCY

Pathway (see galactosemia section)

Due to deficiency of galactokinase leading to excess galactose

Clinical

Autosomal recessive

Cataracts (due to excess galactitol in lens)

Increased intracranial pressure

Labs

Elevated blood glucose, increased urine reducing substances

Low galactokinase activity in blood, liver, or fibroblasts

Management

Eliminate galactose intake for entire life

C. GLYCOGEN STORAGE DISEASE

Glycogen metabolism

Glycogen is the stored form of glucose, found mostly in the liver

Also found in muscle (anaerobic work)

Insulin increases glycogen storage

Glycogenolysis stimulated by epinephrine and/or glucagon

Pathway

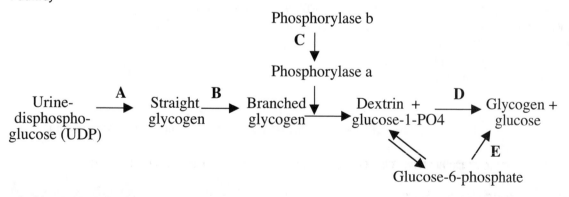

A Glycogen synthetase

B Branching enzyme; deficiency $\longrightarrow$ type IV (Andersen)

C Phsophorylase b kinase; deficiency $\longrightarrow$ type VIII

D Debranching enzyme; deficiency $\longrightarrow$ type III (Forbes)

E. Glucose-6-phosphatase; deficiency $\longrightarrow$ type I (von Gierke)

Types

All glycogen storage diseases can be separated into four categories:

1. Affects mostly liver with direct influence on blood glucose: types I, VI, VIII
2. Involves mostly muscle and affects anaerobic work: types V, VII
3. Affects both liver and muscle: type III
4. Affects various tissues yet *no* direct effect on blood glucose or anaerobic function: type II, IV

Neonatal diseases: von Gierke and Pompe

	Enzyme Deficiency	Organ	Clinical	Prognosis
Type I von Gierke	Glucose-6-phosphatase	Liver Kidney GI	Lactic acidosis (only this type), low glucose Hepatomegaly FTT, diarrhea Bleeding disorder	Poor prognosis Early death if no treatment Possible hematomas in late childhood
Type II Pompe	Lysosomal α-glucosidase	All organs (especially skeletal muscle and nerves)	Symmetric severe muscle weakness Cardiomegaly, CHF	Poor prognosis Usually death less than age 1 year
Type III Forbes	Debranching enzyme-amylo-1,6-glucosidase	Liver Muscle	Low glucose, ketonuria Hepatomegaly Muscle fatigue	No signs in neonatal period Good prognosis
Type IV Andersen	Branching enzyme	Liver Nerves	Cirrhosis beginning at several months of age Hypotonia Muscle weakness	No signs in neonatal period Very poor prognosis Death from liver failure less than 4 years of age
Type V McArdle	Muscle phosphorylase	Muscle	Muscle fatigue in adolescence	No signs in neonatal period Good prognosis
Type VI Hers	Liver phosphorylase	Liver	Mild hypoglycemia Hepatomegaly Ketonuria	No signs in neonatal period Usually good prognosis
Type VII Tarui	Muscle phosphofructokinase	Muscle	Similar to type V Muscle fatigue in adolescence	No signs in neonatal period Good prognosis
Type VIII	Phosphorylase kinase	Liver	Similar to type III yet without myopathy Low glucose Ketonuria Hepatomegaly	No signs in neonatal period Good prognosis

GI = gastrointestinal; FTT = failure to thrive; CHF = congestive heart failure. Modified from lecture by JF Nicholson, MD: Inborn errors of metabolism. Children's Hospital of New York-Presbyterian Medical Center, 1994.

Diagnosis

Administer glucagon and assess glucose and lactate levels (e.g., type I with increased lactate and normal glucose levels)

Assess enzyme levels [type III tested in white blood cells (WBCs), fibroblasts, liver, or muscle]

Examine glycogen structure in red blood cells (RBCs), muscle, and liver (ideal for type IV)

Electromyography (ideal for type II)

Muscle biopsy, liver biopsy (ideal to diagnosis type I and IV)

Check response of lactate to exercise (little change in type V)

Management

Maintain normal glucose levels so glycogen production not necessary (e.g., small frequent feeds, some disorders may require gastric feeds containing glucose during night)

Possible liver transplant (especially if type IV)

D. HEREDITARY FRUCTOSE INTOLERANCE

Pathway

$$\text{Fructose} \xrightarrow{\text{A}} \text{Fructose 1-phosphate} \xrightarrow{\text{B}}$$

A Fructokinase

B Fructose 1-phosphate aldolase, if absent or decreased leads to fructose intolerance with increased fructose-1-phosphate

Clinical

Autosomal recessive

Asymptomatic if breast feeding; symptoms begin after introduce cow's milk formula (contains sucrose) or when diet contains fruits and vegetables

Vomiting, lethargy, seizures; if prolonged symptoms → failure to thrive, liver disease (with hepatomegaly and bleeding disorder), proximal renal tubular dysfunction

May develop liver or kidney failure

Labs

Low glucose (due to blockage of glycogenolysis since fructose-1-phosphate inhibits phosphorylase activity and also due to inhibition of gluconeogenesis)

Absence of enzyme fructose 1-phosphate aldolase in liver, cortex of kidney, or intestinal mucosa, abnormal LFTs, urine reducing substances

Management

Eliminate fructose and sucrose from diet

III. Protein Abnormalities

A. UREA CYCLE DEFECTS (see also Section X)

Pathway

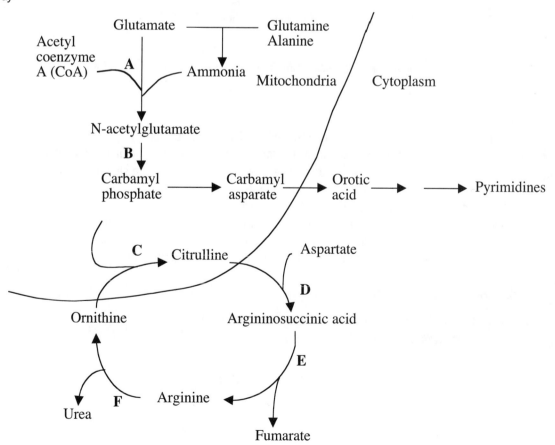

A N-acetylglutamate synthetase if deficiency → *normal or low orotic acid,* inconsistent amino acid profile

B Carbamyl phosphate synthetase

If deficiency → congenital hyperammonemia type I, autosomal recessive, hyperammonemia, *normal or low orotic acid,* increased glutamine and alanine, decreased citrulline, decreased arginine

C Ornithine carbamyl transferase

If deficiency → congenital hyperammonemia type II, *X-linked recessive* (yet many heterozygote females are also severely affected depending on type of mutation and result of random X inactivation of the abnormal gene)

Most common of all urea cycle abnormalities

Severe/lethal in males, partially defected females (with unaffected fathers)

Extremely *elevated urine orotic acid,* hyperammonemia, increased glutamine and alanine, decreased citrulline, decreased arginine

D Argininosuccinic acid synthetase if deficiency → *citrullinemia, brittle hair*

Hyperammonemia, *very high citrulline,* orotic aciduria, decreased arginine

E Argininosuccinic lyase if deficiency → argininosuccinic aciduria

Autosomal recessive, *brittle hair*

Orotic aciduria, some *increased citrulline,* decreased arginine

If severe deficiency, leads to hyperammonemia

F Arginase if deficiency → argininemia; autosomal recessive, typically presents with *spastic diplegia* that progresses, *orotic aciduria*

Clinical

Majority present after age 1 or 2 days (in contrast to transient hyperammonemia—see Section X), poor oral intake, vomiting, apnea, lethargy followed by hypotonia, seizures

Can present later with FTT, developmental delay, coma, mental deficiency

Labs

Severe hyperammonemia, primary *respiratory alkalosis* is common, normal glucose

Diagnosis

Serum amino acids, urine organic acids (orotic acid), fibroblast or hepatocyte enzyme activity

Management

Low protein diet

Supplement with arginine since produced by urea cycle (except if arginase deficiency)

Lactulose diet—intestinal bacteria will change lactulose to lactic acid and the low pH inhibits absorption of ammonia

Sodium benzoate (combines with glycine) and sodium phenylbutyrate (combines with glutamine), which leads to rapid excretion of these amino acids; thus, increased nitrogen excretion without requiring urea cycle pathway

If severe hyperammonemia: eliminate all protein from diet, provide intravenous glucose to meet energy requirements without requiring protein breakdown, administer sodium benzoate and phenylbutyrate, may require exchange transfusion or dialysis (hemodialysis more effective than peritoneal dialysis); currently, preferred method is hemodialysis in combination with extracorporeal membrane oxgyenation (ECMO) for hemofiltration

B. MAPLE SYRUP URINE DISEASE (MSUD)

Disorders of branched-chain amino acids (leucine, isoleucine, and valine)

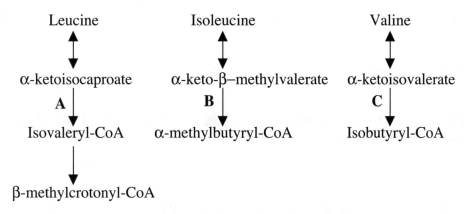

A, B, C All are ketoacid dehydrogenases that require thiamine; if deficiency → MSUD

Clinical
  Autosomal recessive
  Normal at birth
  Symptoms usually within first few days to weeks of life; death if untreated
  Poor feeding, vomiting, tachypnea, seizures, lethargy, can lead to coma
  Increased risk of mental deficiency (especially if late diagnosis)
  Often profound central nervous system (CNS) depression with alternating hypotonia and hypertonia
  Maple syrup odor in urine due to ketoacids in urine

Labs
  Metabolic acidosis typically later in course (can have anion gap), urine ketones, hypoglycemia

Diagnosis
  Newborn screen: increased leucine, isoleucine, and valine
  Urine dinitrophenylhydrazine test—if excess branched chain ketoacids will react with dinitrophenylhydrazine and form white precipitates
  Green-gray color with ferric chloride urine test, increased urine organic acids (elevated ketoacids of leucine, isoleucine, and valine)
  Definitive diagnosis: enzyme assay of skin fibroblasts or white blood cells (WBCs)

Management
  Emergent
  Restrict intake of branched-chain amino acids (need some, since all are essential)
  Possible thiamine supplementation
  If severe, may require dialysis or exchange transfusion to remove branched-chain ketoacids

C. PHENYLKETONURIA (PKU)

Pathway

Phenylalanine $\xrightarrow{\text{A}}$ Tyrosine $\xrightarrow{\text{C}}$ Dopamine
$\searrow$ B $\searrow$ Fumarate + acetoacetate

A Phenylalanine hydroxylase: produced in liver, requires tetrahydrobiopterin (BH_4)
B Fumarylacetoacetate hydrolase; if deficiency → tyrosinemia
C Tyrosine hydroxylase, requires BH_4

Types
　Classic: more common, secondary to phenylalanine hydroxylase deficiency, elevated phenylalanine with normal or low tyrosine
　Allelic variants of phenylalanine hydroxylase: may require dietary restriction
　Pterin defect: defect of tetrahydrobiopterin (important for phyenylalanine, tyrosine, and tryptophan hydroxylase reactions)
　　Leads to progressive lethal CNS disease
　Maternal PKU: effects fetus by leading to intrauterine growth restriction, microcephaly, and congenital heart disease; later in life, increased risk of FTT and mental deficiency

Clinical
　Autosomal recessive
　Musty or mousy urine odor (due to phyenylacetate), often normal at birth
　Primarily affects the brain and if untreated, evolves into severe mental deficiency; seizures may develop after several months
　Often with microcephaly, hypertonia; may have hypopigmentation

Diagnosis
　Newborn screen: measures whole blood phenylalanine (elevated by 12–24 hours of age)
　If screen demonstrates elevated phenylalanine, must then check tyrosine levels; if low or normal tyrosine levels → PKU; if high tyrosine → transient tyrosinemia since pathway develops late in gestation (thus, increased risk in premature infants)—this form has less permanent effects
　Classic: urine detection of phenylpyruvic acid (test by adding 10% *ferric chloride* to urine; positive if blue-green color)
　Pterin defect: measure dihydrobiopterin reductase in red blood cells; also measure biopterin metabolic products in urine

Management
　Classic: low phenylalanine diet (if initiated within 1st few weeks of life, may have normal intelligence); note: phenylalanine still required in diet since it cannot be synthesized (i.e., essential amino acid)
　　Best outcome if dietary control by 2 weeks of age
　Pterin defect: low phenylalanine diet and must replace tetrahydropterin (if decreased synthesis) or other agents (if tetrahydrobiopterin reductase deficiency); less successful therapy compared with classic form
　Note: time frame of low phenylalanine diet unclear

D. TYROSINEMIA

Pathway (see PKU section for pathway)
　Due to deficiency of fumarylacetoacetate hydrolase which leads to accumulation of metabolites that cause severe liver disease or can be due to severe liver disease

Clinical
　Autosomal recessive
　FTT, hepatomegaly, acute severe liver disease in first months of life or chronic liver disease in infancy or childhood
　Increased risk of hepatic malignancy later in life, may have hypopigmentation/albinism

Diagnosis
　Increased tyrosine levels, increased urinary levels of precursors of fumarylacetoacetate with normal blood phenylalanine levels
　Blood and urine succinylacetone elevation is pathognomonic
　Urine reducing substances, may have increased methionine levels

Management
Low phenylalanine and low tyrosine in diet
Liver transplant may prevent malignant transformation
New therapy —hydroxyphenylpyruvate dioxygenase inhibitor (e.g., NTBC) if no liver disease

E. HOMOCYSTINURIA

Pathway

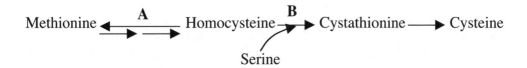

A Betaine-homocysteine methyltransferase and methyltetrahydrofolate-homocysteine methyltransferase (requires cobalamin/vitamin B12 as cofactor); required for converting homocysteine to methionine; thus, a defect in cobalamin metabolism will lead to impaired conversion to methionine and homocystinuria with *low methionine levels*
B Cystathionine synthetase, requires pyridoxine; if deficiency → excess homocysteine in blood and urine with *increased methionine levels* in blood due to increased reverse reaction, *most common etiology of homocystinuria*

Clinical (if cystathionine synthetase deficiency)
Autosomal recessive, asymptomatic in neonatal period
Involves eye, skeleton, central nervous system (CNS) and vascular system:
  Downward *dislocated lens* (note: if upward dislocation → Marfan syndrome), myopia, glaucoma
  Osteoporosis, scoliosis, increased risk of fractures, tall stature, arachnodactyly, decreased joint mobility (note: Marfan syndrome with joint laxity)
  Developmental delay, mental deficiency, seizure
  Increased risk of large thromboses and increased risk of bleeding

Diagnosis
Newborn screen: excess methionine in blood (won't detect abnormalities of A pathway); note: elevated methionine also found if tyrosinemia or liver disease
Excess homocysteine in blood and urine, positive nitroprusside test
Assess cystathionine synthetase levels in skin fibroblasts to confirm diagnosis

Management (if cystathionine synthetase deficiency)
Administer high amount pyridoxine to provide excess amounts of cofactor
Decrease methionine in diet and supplement with cysteine and folate
Consider betaine supplementation to increase synthesis of methionine from homocysteine
Overall good prognosis if obtain normal homocysteine levels

F. NON-KETOTIC HYPERGLYCINEMIA (NKH)

Pathway
Due to a defect in *glycine cleavage pathway:*

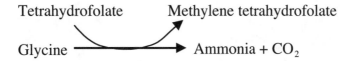

Clinical

Autosomal recessive

Does affect fetus—-associated with *agenesis of corpus callosum*

2/3 with symptoms by 48 hours of age, lethargy, profound CNS deterioration in early neonatal period with alternating hypertonia and hypotonia, seizures, coma

Respiratory depression, *hiccups*

Overall poor prognosis with high risk of death within first weeks of life

Labs

Elevated glycine [urine, plasma, cerebrospinal fluid (CSF)], no ketoacidosis

EEG: burst-suppression pattern during first few weeks of life; during 2nd month, may change to hypsarrhythmia

Diagnosis

Elevated glycine in CSF

Abnormal ratio of simultaneous glycine levels in CSF to plasma (>0.08)

Management

None

Can decrease incidence of seizures by treating with sodium benzoate (decreases plasma glycine) and diazepam (competes with glycine for CNS receptors)

Recent use of dextromethomorphan (an N-methyl-D-aspartate receptor antagonist) to prevent neuronal death and/or decrease seizure activity

G. HISTIDINEMIA

Pathway

Deficiency of histidase

Clinical

Autosomal recessive, rare

Impaired speech development, $+/-$ mental deficiency; other patients without symptoms

Labs

Increased blood histidine, excess urine imidazole pyruvic acid

Diagnosis

Add 10% aqueous *ferric chloride* to urine to detect imidazole pyruvic acid (turns blue-green)

H. CYSTINURIA

Pathway

Defect in amino acid transport across cell membranes leading to deficiency of cysteine

Clinical

Autosomal recessive

Urolithiasis (cysteine renal stones), hematuria, pyuria

Labs

Increased cysteine in urine with decreased cysteine levels in blood

Diagnosis
  Nitroprusside urine test

Management
  Hydration
  Alkalinization of urine (with sodium bicarbonate, potassium or sodium citrate)
  Restrict methionine in diet to decrease cysteine synthesis
  D-penicillamine

I. LYSINURIC PROTEIN INTOLERANCE

Pathway
  Abnormal amino acid transport across cell membrane leading to deficiency of lysine, arginine, and ornithine (last two are important in urea cycle)

Clinical
  If breast-fed, no symptoms until increase protein in diet
  Vomiting, coma, hepatosplenomegaly (HSM), FTT, osteoporosis, fractures

Labs
  Hyperammonemia, lysinuria with low plasma lysine levels

Management
  Citrulline supplementation; if hyperammonemia crisis⟶ eliminate all protein in diet, intravenous glucose to provide energy; sodium benzoate and sodium phyenylacetate

J. HARTNUP DISEASE

Pathway
  Defect in amino acid transport across cell membranes leading to decreased tryptophan availability

Clinical
  Autosomal recessive, presents in childhood or later in life
  Pellagra-like skin disease, ataxia, dystonia, may have mental deficiency or seizures
  Note: must differentiate from "blue diaper syndrome" in which there is an isolated abnormality of intestinal tryptophan transport (patients have indicanuria leading to blue-colored urine)

Labs
  Hyperaminoaciduria with normal or low levels in plasma

Management
  Oral nicotinamide, oral neomycin (to delay tryptophan degradation), avoid sunlight

IV. Organic Acidemias

A. ISOVALERIC ACIDEMIA

Pathway
  Due to abnormal leucine metabolism

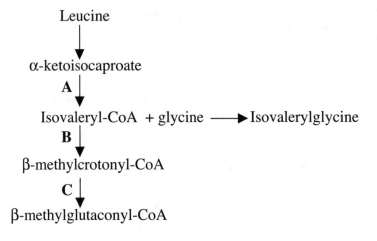

Leucine

↓

α-ketoisocaproate

A ↓

Isovaleryl-CoA + glycine ⟶ Isovalerylglycine

B ↓

β-methylcrotonyl-CoA

C ↓

β-methylglutaconyl-CoA

A If abnormal, leads to MSUD
B Isovaleryl-CoA dehydrogenase, if deficient → isovaleric acidemia
C Enzyme requires biotin, if deficient → β-methylcrotonyl glycinuria

Clinical
Autosomal recessive
Odor of sweaty feet (attributable to excess isovaleric acid)
Poor feeding, intermittent neurological signs (hypotonia, tremor, developmental delay), can lead to coma

Labs
Metabolic acidosis, urine ketones, hyperammonemia, majority with normal glucose, may have neutropenia and/or thrombocytopenia

Diagnosis
Increased urine isovalerylglycine and isovaleric acid

Management
Restrict protein intake
Glycine to increase non-toxic isovalerylglycine production
Carnitine to increase isovalerylglycine excretion
If severe, may require exchange transfusion or dialysis

B. β-METHYLCROTONYL GLYCINURIA—due to abnormal leucine metabolism

Pathway
See isovaleric acidemia, requires biotin

Clinical
Poor oral intake, vomiting, hypotonia, seizures

Labs
Metabolic acidosis, urine ketones, hyperammonemia, hypoglycemia, increased β-methylcrotonyl glycine in urine
Urine odor similar to *male cat urine*

Treatment
Biotin supplementation, restrict protein intake, oral glycine and carnitine may be beneficial

C. PROPIONATE PATHWAY ABNORMALITIES = *KETOTIC HYPERGLYCINEMIA*

Pathway

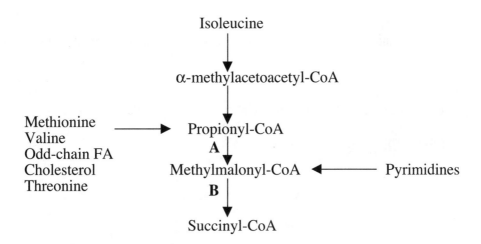

A Propionyl-CoA carboxylase, requires biotin
   If deficiency → *propionic acidemia*
B Methylmalonyl-CoA isomerase, requires cobalamin (vitamin B12)
   If deficiency → *methylmalonic acidemia*
Note: propionyl-CoA is a major metabolite of amino acids and lipids

Clinical
   Autosomal recessive, all with increased risk of bacterial infections, FTT, developmental delay, crises during catabolic
      stress, can lead to coma

Labs
   Ketoacidosis, hyperglycinemia, may have hypoglycemia, neutropenia, thrombocytopenia, *hyperammonemia*
   Increased blood and urine acylcarnitines

Management
   Vitamin B12 if methylmalonic acidemia
   In others—restrict protein intake or specific amino acid precursors of propionyl CoA (methionine, threonine, valine,
      isoleucine)
   Antibiotics to decrease intestinal bacteria that produce propionate
   Carnitine to decrease risk of carnitine deficiency since excrete excess organic acid esters with carnitine

D. MEVALONIC ACIDURIA

Pathway
   Defect of mevalonate kinase (a component of cholesterol synthesis pathway) with symptoms due to decreased end
      products

Clinical
   Autosomal recessive, rare
   Severe symptoms during infancy or early childhood
   FTT, developmental delay, dysmorphisms (large fontanel, high forehead, low-set ears, long philtrum), cataracts,
      malabsorption, recurrent episodes of fever, lymphadenopathy, HSM, arthralgia, hypotonia, ataxia

Labs
  No metabolic acidosis, normal glucose

Diagnosis
  Increased creatine kinase, increased LFTs, increased mevalonic acid, confirm with mevalonate kinase activity in WBCs or skin fibroblasts

Management
  Consider high cholesterol diet; consider ubiquinone; trial of corticosteroids during acute crisis

E. GLUTARIC ACIDURIA TYPE I

Pathway

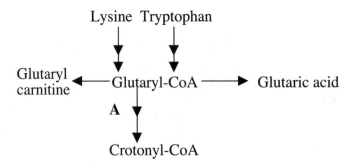

A Glutaryl-CoA dehydrogenase; if deficiency → type I glutaric aciduria

Clinical
  Autosomal recessive
  Typically diagnose after 1 year of age
  Macrocephaly, progressive neurologic symptoms (ataxia, myoclonus, stroke, choreoathetosis, dystonia), hepatic dysfunction, abnormal motor function, poor prognosis

Labs
  Low glucose, hyperammonemia, increased glutaric acid levels, secondary carnitine deficiency, some with acidosis

Diagnosis
  Neuroimaging often reveals *frontotemporal atrophy* and delayed myelination

Management
  Carnitine and riboflavin (B2) supplementation, low protein intake (specifically, decreased lysine and tryptophan)

F. HYDROXYMETHYLGLUTARYL-COA (HMG-COA) LYASE DEFICIENCY

This enzyme important in the last step of ketone synthesis from FA (also last step in leucine oxidation)
Seizures, hypotonia
Hypoketotic hypoglycemia (often leading to coma), acidosis
Treat with high carbohydrate diet, frequent feeds

V. Fatty Acid (FA) Abnormalities

Pathway

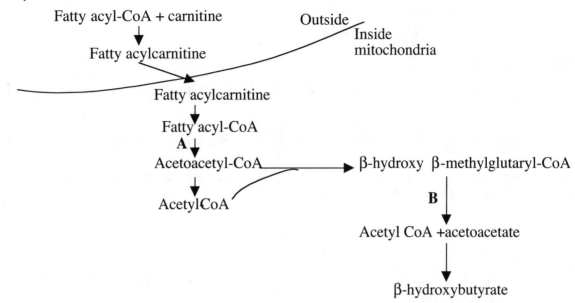

A Very long, medium, and short chain fatty acyl-CoA dehydrogenases and hydroxylase-CoA dehdydrogenases
B Hydroxymethylglutaryl-CoA lyase

A. MEDIUM CHAIN ACYL-COA DEHYDROGENASE DEFICIENCY (MCAD DEFICIENCY)

Most common and mildest FA oxidation disorder

Can't oxidize FA completely and thus
1. FA that are not oxidized will be excreted in urine as carnitine esters leading to carnitine deficiency
2. Inability to produce ketone bodies
3. If starvation, cannot produce glucose by fat breakdown and infant relies on carbohydrate breakdown for glucose production; hypoglycemia often results since carbohydrate reserves are insufficient; *hypoketotic hypoglycemia*
4. Encephalopathy due to hypoglycemia and hypoketonemia
5. Severe acidosis

Treat with high carbohydrate diet, frequent feeds, carnitine in diet

B. LONG CHAIN 3-HYDROXYACYL-COA DEFICIENCY (LCHAD)

Clinical
Autosomal recessive, cardiomyopathy, severe liver disease with cholestasis, FTT, feeding difficulty, hypotonia, high mortality (greater than MCAD deficiency)
Of note: heterozygous LCHAD-affected mother may have acute fatty liver disease, hypertension, elevated liver function tests, and low platelets during pregnancy

Labs
Hypoketotic hypoglycemia, increased serum creatinine kinase

Diagnosis
Increased 3-hydroxy-dicarboxylic acids, increased plasma 3-hydroxyacyl-carnitines

Measure LCHAD activity in lymphocytes, fibroblasts; muscle or liver biopsy

Management
Carbohydrate-rich, fat-restricted diet; avoid prolonged fasting
Supplement with medium-chain triglycerides to bypass defect

C. CARNITINE DEFICIENCY

Carnitine is made de novo by humans from lysine mostly in liver and kidney; it is also present in red meat and dairy products

Carnitine is an important cofactor to transport long-chain FA across mitochondrial inner membranes to be oxidized

Low levels common in premature infants and neonates receiving total parenteral nutrition without adequate carnitine supplementation (i.e., secondary carnitine deficiency)

Carnitine deficiency due to
· Failure to synthesize carnitine
· Defective carnitine transport
· Depletion of carnitine due to excretion of high amount of carnityl esters of organic acids (e.g., propionate pathway abnormalities, fatty acid disorders)

Clinical
Lethargy, muscle weakness, cardiomyopathy

Labs
Failure to produce ketones leading to *hypoketotic hypoglycemia*

Management
Carnitine supplementation

D. GLUTARIC ACIDURIA TYPE II

Pathway
Electron-transfer flavoprotein and electron-transfer flavoprotein dehydrogenase transfer electrons into the electron transport chain
If deficiency of these enzymes → glutaric aciduria II = multiple acyl-CoA dehydrogenase deficiency

Clinical
Hypotonia, coma, cardiomyopathy, dysmorphisms (high forehead, flat nasal bridge, short anteverted nose, ear anomalies), renal cysts, rocker bottom feet, hypospadias, macrocephaly, *sweaty feet*

Labs
Metabolic acidosis, low glucose, urine organic acid abnormalities

VI. Lysosomal Storage Diseases

Lysosome
Organelle that functions to degrade cellular products by hydrolysis so can reutilize these substances

If absence of one or more hydrolytic enzymes, leads to accumulation of non-degraded cellular material within the lysosome

Different tissues will have different manifestations since synthesis and degradation of compounds vary between tissues (if material turned over quickly, disease will manifest early in life)

Clinical

Over 100 types, majority with dysmorphisms

All progressive to varying degrees

Defects of bones and joints including dysostosis multiplex

Hepatosplenomegaly, gingival hyperplasia, degenerative CNS disease

Corneal clouding, retinal pigmentary changes

Rules

1. *Dysostosis multiplex* is pathognomonic of mucopolysaccharidoses
2. *Macular cherry red spots* is pathognomonic of lipid storage diseases affecting the brain
3. Rapid development of clinical symptoms over first few months will occur if there is more than one enzyme deficiency, often due to storage disorder of both lipids and mucopolysaccharides

A. MUCOPOLYSACCHARIDOSIS (MPS)

Majority with dysostosis multiplex + all with Alder-Reilly bodies (in white blood cells) + all with urine mucopolysaccharides

Type	Defect	Onset	Dys Mult	Ophtho Findings	Clinical Findings
MPS-I Hurler	α-iduronidase	1 yo	Yes	Cloudy cornea Normal retina	HSM Profound decrease in CNS function Short stature, coarse facial features, kyphosis, hirsutism, stiff joints
MPS-II Hunter	Iduronidase 2-sulfatase X-linked inheritance	1-2 yo	Yes	Clear cornea Retinitis papilledema *Only MPS with retinal abnormality	HSM Slow loss of CNS function Coarse facial features, short stature, stiff joints
MPS III Sanfilippo	Degrading heparin sulfates	3-4 yo	Mild	Clear cornea Normal retina	+/− hepatomegaly Rapid loss of CNS function
MPS IV Morquio	Galactosamine 6-sulfate-sulfatase	2 yo	No	Faint clouding of cornea Normal retina	Normal liver and spleen Normal CNS
MPS VI Maroteaux Lamy	N-acetylgalactosamine 4-sulfatase	2 yo	Yes	Cloudy cornea Normal retina	Normal liver and spleen Normal CNS
MPS VII Sly	β-glucuronidase	Varies	Yes	+/− cloudy cornea Normal retina	HSM +/− CNS abnormality

yo = year old; dys mult = dysostosis multiplex; ophtho = ophthalmologic; HSM = hepatosplenomegaly; CNS = central nervous system. Modified from lecture by JF Nicholson, MD: Inborn errors of metabolism. Children's Hospital of New York-Presbyterian Medical Center, 1994.

B. LIPIDOSES

Type	Defect	Onset	Ophtho Findings	CNS Liver Spleen	Bone Marrow and Other
Glucosylceramide = Lipidosis I = Gaucher I	Glucocerebrosidase	Any age	Normal	HSM Normal CNS	Gaucher cells in bone marrow Increased risk of fractures
Glucosylceramide Lipidosis II = Gaucher II	Glucocerebrosidase	Infant-2 yo	Normal	HSM Profound CNS loss	Gaucher cells in bone marrow
Sphingomyelin Lipidosis A Niemann-Pick A	Sphingomyelinase	First month	Clear cornea Cherry red spots in 1/2	HSM Profound CNS loss	Foam cells in bone marrow
Sphingomyelin Lipidosis B Niemann-Pick B	Sphingomyelinase	First month or later	Normal	HSM Normal CNS	Foam cells in bone marrow *(continued on following page)*

Type	Defect	Onset	Optho Findings	CNS Liver Spleen	Bone Marrow and Other
GM 2-ganglio-sidosis Tay-Sachs	Hexosaminidase A	3–6 months	Clear cornea Cherry red spots	No HSM Profound CNS loss	Normal bone marrow
Generalized gangliosidosis Infantile GM 1	β-galactosidase	Infant	Clear cornea Cherry red spots in 1/2	HSM Profound CNS loss	Inclusions in WBC
Metachromatic leukodystrophy	Arylsulfatase A	1–2 yo	Normal	No HSM Profound CNS loss	Normal bone marrow
Fabry disease	α-galactosidase	Early or late childhood	Cloudy cornea Normal retina	+/− hepatomegaly Normal CNS	Normal bone marrow X-linked
Galactosyl-ceramide lipidosis = Krabbe disease	β-galactosidase	First few months	Normal cornea Optic atrophy	No HSM Profound CNS loss	Normal bone marrow Storage is not lysosomal
Wolman disease	Acid lipase	Infant	Normal	Hepatomegaly Profound CNS loss Adrenal calcifications	Inclusions in WBC

ophtho = ophthalmologic; CNS = central nervous system; HSM = hepatosplenomegaly; WBC = white blood cells. Modified from lecture by JF Nicholson, MD: Inborn errors of metabolism. Children's Hospital of New York-Presbyterian Medical Center, 1994.

Disease	HSM	Cherry Red Spots	CNS Disease
Gaucher I	Yes	No	No
Niemann-Pick A	Yes	Yes (in 1/2)	Yes
Tay-Sachs	No	Yes	Yes

C. MUCOLIPIDOSES (ML)

Disease	Enzyme	Onset	Dys Mult	Clinical
ML I, sialidosis (type II)	Neuraminidase	Neonate	Yes	Cloudy cornea, cherry red spots HSM, profound CNS loss Oligosaccharides in urine Abnormal BM
ML I, sialidosis (type I)	Neuraminidase	> 8 yo	No	Clear cornea, cherry red spots No HSM, seizures Oligosaccharides in urine Sometimes abnormal BM
ML-II, I cell disease	Mannosyl phosphotransferase	Neonate	Yes	Late corneal clouding, normal retina HSM, profound CNS loss, cardiomyopathy Oligosaccharides in urine Cytoplasmic inclusions
ML-III, Pseudo-Hurler polydystrophy	Mannosyl phosphotransferase	4 yo	Yes	Late corneal clouding, normal retina No HSM, modest CNS abnormalities Oligosaccharides in urine
Multiple sulfatase deficiency	Sulfatase	1–2 yo	Yes	Normal eye findings HSM, profound CNS loss Acid mucopolysaccharides in urine Alder-Reilly bodies in WBCs
Aspartyl glycosaminuria	Aspartyl glucosaminidase	6 mo	Yes	Cataracts Early HSM, profound CNS loss Aspartyl glucosamine in urine Bone marrow with inclusion bodies
Mannosidosis	α-mannosidase	Neonate	Yes	Cloudy cornea, normal retina, cataracts HSM, profound CNS loss WBC inclusion bodies
Fucosidosis	α-fucosidase	Neonate	Yes	Clear cornea, retina can be pigmented HSM, profound CNS loss WBC inclusion bodies

Dys mult = dysostosis multiplex; HSM = hepatosplenomegaly; CNS = central nervous system; BM = bone marrow; WBCs = white blood cells. Modified from lecture by JF Nicholson, MD: Inborn errors of metabolism. Children's Hospital of New York-Presbyterian Medical Center, 1994.

VII. Mitochondrial Disorders

A. PYRUVATE DEHYDROGENASE COMPLEX DEFICIENCY

Pathway

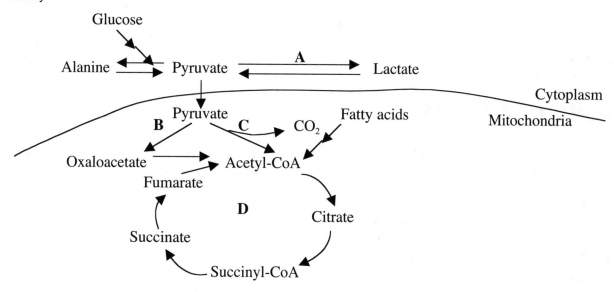

A Lactate dehydrogenase, ubiquitous
B Pyruvate carboxylase, requires biotin
C Pyruvate dehydrogenase complex, requires thiamine, oxidation pathway
D Krebs cycle, amino acids enter this cycle at several points

Clinical
May have *agenesis of corpus callosum*
Developmental delay, hypotonia, seizures, intermittent ataxia or choreoathetosis, cerebral and cerebellar atrophy
Dysmorphic features

Labs
Elevated pyruvate and lactate with normal lactate:pyruvate ratio (~20)
Metabolic acidosis

Diagnosis
Assay pyruvate dehydrogenase complex activity in WBCs and skin fibroblasts

Management
Ketogenic diet to increase acetyl-CoA levels
May give trial of biotin
Dichloroacetate treatment for lactic acidosis
Fatal despite therapy

B. PYRUVATE CARBOXYLASE DEFICIENCY

Clinical
Autosomal recessive
May present in neonatal period with neurological abnormalities (e.g., seizures, coma, hypotonia, hypertonia), hepatomegaly

More commonly presents at few months of age with developmental delay, FTT, lethargy, seizures, feeding difficulty, may develop proximal renal dysfunction

Labs

Metabolic acidosis, elevated pyruvate and lactate, ketonuria; if severe, often with hyperammonemia and citrullinemia since low oxaloacetate leads to decreased aspartate levels and decreased argininosuccinic acid

Management

No therapy (i.e., fatal); may give trial of biotin

C. RESPIRATORY CHAIN DISORDERS

Pathway

Respiratory chain leads to oxidative phosphorylation (i.e., ATP synthesis); during this process, electrons are transported to oxygen by multiple complexes

Clinical

Multiple modes of inheritance due to high number of genes in respiratory chain

Can present at any age (majority by 2 years of age)

Rapidly progressive, multi-organ involvement

Neonate: seizures, hypotonia, coma, hepatomegaly, sideroblastic anemia, cardiomyopathy, myopathy

1 month–2 years old: FTT, diarrhea, episodes of hypotonia, renal failure, coma, developmental delay

After 2 years of age: muscle weakness, ataxia, coma, seizures, developmental delay, MELAS syndrome (*m*yopathy, *e*ncephalopathy, *l*actic *a*cidosis, *s*troke-like episodes); ragged red fibers by muscle biopsy detected after adolescence

Labs

Lactic acidosis (lactate levels >> pyruvate levels; this is in contrast to pyruvate dehydrogenase complex deficiency with pyruvate levels approaching lactate levels)

Evidence of other organ involvement (e.g., increased LFTs)

Diagnosis

Measure respiratory enzyme activity for definitive diagnosis

Ragged red fibers consistent with muscle myopathy

Management

No therapy; treat symptoms and secondary effects; avoid valproate and barbiturates since may inhibit respiratory chain

VIII. Cofactor Abnormalities

Biotin	Biotinidase deficiency
	Propionic acidemia
	β-methylcrotonyl glycinemia
	Pyruvate carboxylase deficiency
Folic acid	Homocystinuria
	Non-ketotic hyperglycinemia
Riboflavin (B2)	Glutaric aciduria I
Pyridoxine (B6)	Homocystinuria
Thaimine (B1)	MSUD
	Pyruvate dehydrogenase complex deficiency
Tetrahydrobiopterin (BH₄)	PKU (pterin defects)
	Homocystinuria
Vitamin B12 = cobalamin	Methylmalonic acidemia
Vitamin C (ascorbic acid)	Transient tyrosinemia

A. BIOTINIDASE DEFICIENCY

Trait
Biotin is a ubiquitous vitamin, binds to carboxylases to enhance function
Biotinidase is an enzyme that allows release of biotin from the carboxylase so that it can be reutilized

Clinical
Autosomal recessive
Typically presents during infancy
Immune deficits, alopecia, rash, seizures, hypotonia, lethargy, ataxia, blindness or deafness if diagnosed later in life

Diagnosis
Newborn screen: low serum biotinidase
Organic aciduria, decreased plasma and urine biotin

Management
Oral biotin supplementation

IX. Other Metabolic Diseases

A. WILSON DISEASE

Trait
Abnormality of hepatic copper transport leading to copper deposition in liver, cornea, basal ganglia, and renal tubules
Decreased amount of copper into ceruloplasmin

Clinical
Autosomal recessive
Hepatic disease (majority present between 8 and 18 years of age)
Neurological disease with presentation between 20 and 40 years of age
Hemolysis, dysarthria, extrapyramidal movement disorder
Cornea with Kayser-Fleischer rings (golden-brown granular pigmentations) due to copper deposition

Diagnosis
Low ceruloplasmin levels with only slight decrease in copper; assay copper levels by liver biopsy

Management
D-penicillamine to chelate copper
A few patients may require liver transplant

B. MENKES DISEASE

Trait
Defect in a membrane copper transport channel leading to poor absorption and cellular distribution of copper

Clinical
X-linked recessive
Increased risk of premature rupture of membranes, increased risk hypothermia, unconjugated hyperbilirubinemia
Brittle, kinky, steely hair (may be evident at several months of age)
Developmental delay, seizures, unique facies (pudgy, sagging lips, abnormal eyebrow), skin and joint laxity, increased
  risk urinary tract infections, subdural hemorrhage, Wormian bones, osteoporosis, elongated tortuous arteries,
  progressive neurological deterioration

Diagnosis
Low ceruloplasmin and low copper levels

Management
Daily copper injections

C. DEFECTS OF BILE ACID SYNTHESIS

Pathway

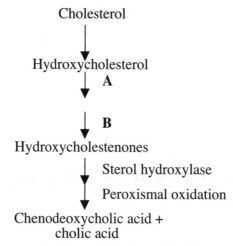

Cholesterol

↓

Hydroxycholesterol

↓ **A**

↓ **B**

Hydroxycholestenones

↓ Sterol hydroxylase

Peroxismal oxidation

Chenodeoxycholic acid +
cholic acid

A 3-β-dehydrogenase, if deficiency → prolonged neonatal hyperbilirubinemia, pale stools, rickets, fat-soluble vitamin malabsorption, giant cell hepatitis
Analyze bile acid levels in plasma or urine, assay enzyme in skin fibroblasts, treat with chenodeoxycholic acid

B 5-β-reductase, if deficiency → cholestatic jaundice, FTT, increased LFTs, giant cell hepatitis, assay plasma or urine bile acid levels, treat with chenodeoxycholic acid

D. ZELLWEGER SYNDROME

Pathway
Due to absence of peroxisomes leading to limited oxidation of long chain FA

Clinical
Presents at birth
Dysmorphic features (high forehead, flat orbital ridges, wide open fontanel, epicanthal folds, flat nasal bridge)
FTT, seizures, nystagmus, hypotonia, polycystic kidney disease, hepatomegaly, coma, deafness

Labs
Absent or decreased peroxisomes, increased very long chain FA, increased urine pipecolic acid, bile acid accumulation

Management
None, death usually by 1 year of age

X. Differential Diagnosis of Hyperammonemia

Clinical
Symptoms dependent on etiology, degree of elevated ammonia, rate of ammonia rise, degree of alkalosis (increased pH leads to increased distribution of ammonia to CNS), and age of patient
Hyperammonemia may present during neonatal period or later in life

Free ammonia has a direct neurotoxic effect

Severe neonatal hyperammonemia: complete block in urea cycle, presents during first few days of life with poor feeding, vomiting, seizures, coma; death in first week if untreated

Moderate neonatal hyperammonemia (ammonia levels = 200–400 mmoles/L): due to incomplete defects of urea cycle, often in organic acid disorders; poor feeding, vomiting, CNS depression, typically without seizures

Subclinical: chronic elevation of ammonia levels (100–200 mmoles/L); typically without symptoms

Transient neonatal hyperammonemia: self-limited, unknown etiology

Elevated ammonia levels shortly after birth (usually within first day of life) that may become so elevated that infant may require exchange transfusion or dialysis

Clinical symptoms may be severe but can survive without long-term effects

Usually in premature infants due to immature N-acetylglutamate synthetase activity

Flow chart for deciphering etiology of hyperammonemia

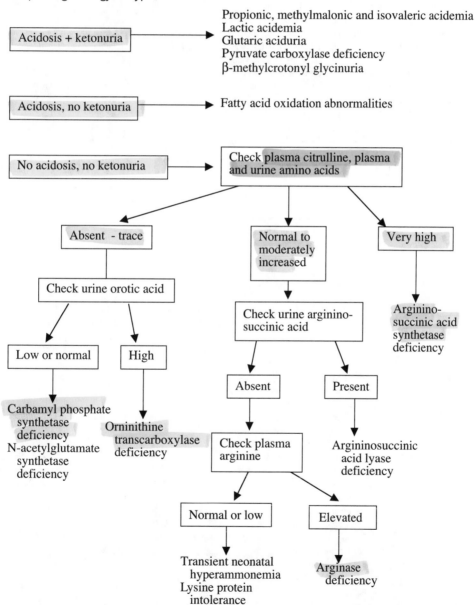

Modified from Ward JC. Inborn errors of metabolism of acute onset in infancy. *Pediatr Rev* 1990; 11(7):210 and "An Approach to Inborn Errors of Metabolism in the Neonate" Lecture by Mark Korson, MD. Boston, Children's Hospital, MA. August 1990.

XI. Clinical Traits Associated with Metabolic Diseases

Trait	Metabolic Disease
Alopecia	Biotinidase deficiency
Brittle hair	Argininosuccinic lyase deficiency, argininosuccinic acid synthetase deficiency, Menkes syndrome
Cardiomyopathy	Long-chain 3-hydroxyacyl-CoA dehydrogenase (LCHAD) deficiency, glutaric aciduria II, carnitine deficiency, Pompe disease, mitochondrial disorders of respiratory chain, mucolipidoses (I-cell disease)
Cataracts	Galactosemia, galactokinase deficiency, mevalonic aciduria
Coma/encephalopathy	Maple syrup urine disease, urea cycle defects, lysinuric protein intolerance, paroxysmal diseases, nonketotic hyperglycinemia, propionic, isovaleric, and methylmalonic acidemia, glutaric aciduria type II, HMG-CoA lyase deficiency, FA oxidation defects, pyruvate carboxylase deficiency, mitochondrial disorders of respiratory chain
Dysmorphisms	Zellweger: high forehead, flat orbital ridges, open wide fontanel, epicanthal folds, flat nasal bridge
	Homocystinuria
	Glutaric acidurias I: macrocephaly, II: rocker bottom feet, hypospadius, high forehead, flat nasal bridge, short anteverted nose, ear anomalies
	Lysosomal storage diseases (e.g., I-cell disease)
	Pyruvate dehydrogenase complex deficiency
	Mevalonic aciduria: large fontanel, high forehead, hypertelorism, epicanthal folds, low-set ears, long philtrum
Hepatomegaly	Galactosemia, glycogen storage disease, hereditary fructose intolerance, peroxismal diseases (e.g., Zellweger syndrome), tyrosinemia, LCHAD deficiency, Neimann-Pick disease, Gaucher disease, some mucopolysaccharidoses, some mucolipidoses, Wolman disease, pyruvate carboxylase deficiency, lysinuric protein intolerance
Hydrops (nonimmune)	Glucose-6-phosphate dehydrogenase deficiency, lysosomal storage disease, glycogen storage disease type IV
Sweaty feet odor	Isovaleric acidemia
	Glutaric aciduria type II
Thromboemboli	Homocystinuria

XII. Laboratory Blood Tests Associated with Metabolic Diseases

Laboratory Test	Metabolic Disease
Neutropenia, thrombocytopenia	Organic acidemias (propionic, isovaleric and methylmalonic acidemias)
Metabolic acidosis with elevated anion gap	Organic acidemias (propionic, isovaleric and methylmalonic acidemias)
	FA oxidation defects (short, medium, long and very long chain abnormalities), carnitine deficiency
	Congenital lactic acidosis (pyruvate dehydrogenase complex deficiency, pyruvate carboxylase deficiency, some mitochondrial disorders of respiratory chain)
	Secondary lactic acidosis: hereditary fructose intolerance, glycogen storage disease type I, FA oxidation defects, biotinidase deficiency, propionic, methylmalonic and isovaleric acidemias, HMG CoA lyase deficiency
	Other: prematurity (due to liver failure from total parenteral nutrition), hypoxic-ischemic encephalopathy, severe hepatitis, portal venous obstruction, abnormal mitochondrial oxidation from hypoxia
Normal anion gap	Diarrhea, renal tubular acidosis, galactosemia, tyrosinemia, some mitochondrial disorders of respiratory chain
Alkalosis	Urea cycle abnormalities (respiratory alkalosis)
Plasma amino acids, elevated	Maple syrup urine disease (increased leucine, isoleucine, valine)
	Organic acidemias (increased glycine)
	Tyrosinemia (increased methionine and tyrosine)
	Argininosuccinic acid synthetase deficiency and argininosuccinic acid lyase deficiency (increased citrulline)
	Hyperammonemia (increased glutamine)
	Lactic acidosis (increased alanine)
	Prolonged hyperalimentation in premature infants
Ketotic hyperglycinemia	Propionate pathway abnormalities
Ketotic hypoglycemia	Glycogen storage disease, organic acidemias (propionic, methylmalonic and isovaleric acidemia), short chain acyl-CoA dehydrogenase deficiency
Hypoketotic hypoglycemia	1. FA breakdown abnormalities: medium chain acyl-CoA dehydrogenase deficiency, LCHAD hydroxymethylglutaryl CoA lyase deficiency
	2. Carnitine deficiency
Newborn screen	Tests vary by state
	Often false-positive results in premature infants
	Due to recent advanced technology of tandem mass spectroscopy, will allow for expansion of metabolic testing

XIII. Urine Tests Associated with Metabolic Diseases

Urine organic acids, elevated	Methylmalonic acidemia
	MSUD
	FA oxidation defects
	Pyruvate abnormalities
	Mitochondrial disorders of respiratory chain
Urine, male cat odor (due to 3-hydroxyisovaleric acid)	β-methylcrotonyl glycinuria
	Multiple carboxylase deficiency
Urine, musty odor	PKU (due to phenylacetate)
Acetonuria	Organic acidemias
Clinitest = reducing substances	Nonenzyme assay for reducing substances
	Will detect galactose, fructose, and glucose
	Galactosemia (note: negative Clinistix), hereditary fructose intolerance, renal Fanconi syndrome, tyrosinemia, severe liver disease
Clinistix = glucose oxidase test	Only specific for *glucose*
Dinitrophenylhydrazine (DNPH) urine test —tests ketoacids	MSUD, PKU, tyrosinemia, histidinemia
Ferric chloride urine test—tests oxoacids	If blue-green → PKU (due to phenylpyruvic acid), histidinemia (due to imidazole pyruvic acid)
	If green-gray → MSUD (due to branch chain oxoacids, DNPH more common for MSUD diagnosis)
	If green → tyrosinemia (due to hydroxyphenylpyruvate)
p-nitroanilline urine test	Methylmalonic acidemia
Nitroprusside urine test—tests sulfur-containing acids	Homocystinuria
Urine ketones	Organic acidemias (e.g., MSUD)
	Glycogen storage disease (type I)

XIV. Neonatal Temperature Regulation

A. HEAT MAINTENANCE

Nonshivering thermogenesis
  Leads to heat production through oxidation of brown fat
  Mediated by catecholamines (e.g., norepinephrine)
  Leads to increased metabolic rate and increased oxygen consumption
  Impaired by hypoxemia and hypoglycemia

B. HEAT LOSS: NEONATE VS ADULT

Neonate more prone to heat loss due to:
  1. Decreased epidermal and dermal thickness → increased radiant and conductive heat loss
  2. Minimal subcutaneous fat → decreased response to cooling
  3. Immature nervous system → decreased response to cooling
  4. Increased surface area to body weight ratio (3× greater than adult ratio)

Neonatal heat loss ~4× greater than adult heat loss

Note: premature infant with even greater risk of heat loss compared with full-term infant

C. HEAT GAIN: NEONATE VS ADULT

Neonate with heat gain has more difficulty returning to normal body temperature due to:
  1. Additional thermal stresses (e.g., insulated clothing, phototherapy)
  2. Sweat glands not completely functional until several weeks of age

D. NEONATAL HYPOTHERMIA AND HYPERTHERMIA

	Hypothermia	Hyperthermia
Etiology	Heat loss is greater than heat prdouction (e.g., some cases of sepsis in which neonates have peripheral vasodilation and limited normal homeothermic response) Patients will have hypotension, bradycardia, slow and irregular respirations, decreased activity, decreased reflexes Laboratory results may demonstrate hypoglycemia and/or metabolic acidosis	Increased heat production (e.g., sepsis—typically infant with peripheral vasoconstriction leading to cool extremities and pale color) Decrease in heat loss and thus infant warm (e.g., overheated infant—infant with peripheral vasodilation leading to warm extremities and flushed skin) Can also be due to dehydration, medications, or abnormal nervous system responses
Management	Dry skin surface Place in thermally-controlled environment Increase incubator humidity Consider inner heat shield in incubator Evaluate for infection Monitor blood pressure and glucose	Evaluate for infection Maintain hydration, monitor electrolytes Remove excess heat source or extra clothing If severe, may require cooling techniques

E. TYPES OF NEONATAL HEAT LOSS

	Conductive	Convective	Evaporative	Radiant
Definition	Transfer of heat from neonate to a contacting solid object	Transfer of heat from neonate to surrounding gas The heated air expands and then travels upwards	Transfer of heat from skin and respiratory tract to a drier environment	Transfer of heat between neonate and surface that is *not* in contact with neonate Heat loss is in the form of electromagnetic waves
Examples	Cold blanket or mattress	Cool air Air currents will lead to more turbulence and displacement of heated gas ~40–50% of nonevaporative neonatal heat loss	Prematurity leading to immature stratum corneum and poor epidermal barrier function Younger postnatal age High velocity of surrounding air	Incubator walls, windows, chairs, light bulbs, other people
Prevention	Place infant on warm blanket or mattress	Maintain constant air temperature Limit air currents May require environmental temperature to be greater than skin temperature to maintain a normal core temperature	Plastic cover Increase incubator humidity	Protect incubator walls from excess cooling

F. INCUBATORS

Convective incubators
   Servocontrol of forced air by using skin or air temperature as a temperature control
   If infant placed inside, still has a large amount of radiant heat loss and some evaporative heat loss
   If *increase humidity* or swaddle infant, will *decrease evaporative* heat loss
   If *double-walled* incubator instead of single-walled incubator, will *decrease radiant* heat loss
   If add *plastic heat shields,* will *decrease radiant* heat loss
   If utilize *portholes* during care of neonate, will *decrease convective* heat loss
   If use *rubber foam mattress,* will *decrease conductive* heat loss

Radiant warmers
   Servocontrol of skin temperature by using infrared radiant warming
   Leads to a large difference in skin temperature between exposed and unexposed areas
   If infant placed inside, still has significant convective and evaporative heat losses
   Higher evaporative heat loss compared with convective incubators due to insensible water loss with greater skin-air temperature differences and a lower relative humidity compared with convective incubators
   If cover infant with *plastic film,* will decrease convective and evaporative heat losses

REFERENCES

Behrman RE, Kliegman R, and Jenson HB (eds): Nelson Textbook of Pediatrics (16th edition), Philadelphia, WB Saunders Company, 2000.

Cohen BA: Pediatric Dermatology (2nd edition). Philadelphia, Mosby, 1999.

den Boer ME, Wanders RJ, Morris AA, et al: Long chain 3-hydroxyacyl-CoA dehydrogenase deficiency: clinical presentation and follow-up of 50 patients. *Pediatrics* 2002; 109(1):99–104.

Dollberg S and Hoath SB: Temperature regualtion in preterm infants: role of the skin-environment interface." *NeoReviews* 2001; 2(12):e282–e291.

Erins GM and Packman S: Diagnosing inborn errors of metabolism in the newborn. *NeoReviews* 2001; 2(3):e183–e200.

Fanaroff AA and Martin RJ (eds): Neonatal-Perinatal Medicine (6th edition). St Louis, Mosby–Year Book Inc, 1997.

Fernandes J, Saudubray JM, Van den Berge G (eds): Inborn Metabolic Diseases: Diagnosis and Treatment (3rd edition) Berlin and New York, Springer-Verlag, 2000.

Lecture by JF Nicholson, MD: Inborn errors of metabolism. Children's Hospital of New York–Presbyterian Medical Center, 1994.

Ozand PT and Gascon GG: Organic acidurias: a review. *J Child Neurolog* 1991, 6:196–219 and 288–303.

Scriver CR (ed), Sly WS, Childs B, et al: The Metabolic and Molecular Bases of Inherited Disease (8th edition). McGraw-Hill, 2001

Ward JC. Inborn errors of metabolism of acute onset in infancy. *Pediatr Rev* 1990; 11(7):205–216.

CHAPTER 13

Dermatology

TOPICS COVERED IN THIS CHAPTER

I. Newborn vs Adult Skin

Component	Preterm Infant (~30 weeks)	Full-Term Infant	Adult	Neonatal Significance
Epidermis	~27 μm thickness	~50 μm thickness	~50 μm thickness	Premature skin with increased permeability and increased water loss
Dermis	Large decrease in collagen elastic fibers	Moderate decrease in collagen and elastic fibers	Normal	Neonates with decreased elasticity and greater tendency to blister
Melanosomes	1/3 # of full-term infant	Fewer # than adult	Normal	Increased photosensitivity
Eccrine glands (sweat glands)	Complete anhidrosis	Decreased activity for 1–7 days. Decreased neurologic control for up to 3 years	Normal	Decreased response to heat stress
Sebaceous glands	Large decrease in secretions	Moderate decrease in secretions	Normal	
Hair	Lanugo	Decreased terminal hair	Normal	Can assist in determining gestational age
Surface area-to-volume ratio	Significantly increased	Moderately increased	Normal	Increased surface area to volume ratio. Increased transcutaneous penetration of topical agents

Note: premature infants with greater risk of harlequin ichthyosis, collodion infant, lamellar ichthyosis and hemangiomas; Modified from Cohen BA: Pediatric Dermatology (2nd edition), Philadelphia, Mosby, 1999, p 13.

II. Benign Pustular Lesions

A. ERYTHEMA TOXICUM

Incidence
Most common pustular rash; occurs in 30–70% of full-term infants

Clinical
Benign, onset 2nd–3rd day of life (can occur up to 2–3 weeks of age)
1–3 mm erythematous macules and papules that may evolve into pustules on an erythematous base; palms and soles usually not involved
Isolated or clustered; fades over 5–7 days, may recur

B. NEONATAL PUSTULAR MELANOSIS

Incidence
Greater in dark-skinned infants; males = females

Three stages
1. Non-inflammatory pustules, no erythema
2. Ruptured pustules with *scale* surrounding hyperpigmented macule
3. Hyperpigmented macules (can last up to 3 months)

Clinical
Benign, usually present at birth (at any of the 3 stages)
Clusters under chin, forehead, neck or lower back; occasionally involving cheeks, trunks, extremities, and palms/soles
Pustules are fragile and can be wiped off easily
No treatment

C. MILIARIA

Due to obstruction of sweat glands leading to sweat retention

Intertriginous areas, face, scalp, and trunk

Worse in humid environment; improves when placed in a cooler environment

Types
Miliaria crystallina—superficial, thin-walled 1–2 mm vesicles, no inflammation
Miliaria rubra (obstruction within epidermis)—small red papules, = prickly heat
Miliaria profunda or pustular—rare, deeper blockage, nonerythematous pustules

D. MILIA

Pearly nonerythematous yellow papules over face, chin, and forehead
Cannot be removed easily
Due to small epidermal inclusion cysts
Resolve by 1–3 months of age
Pearls: large (usually single) milia located on genitalia, areola, mouth (= Epstein's pearls)

E. ACNE

20% neonates (males greater than females)
Closed or open comedones, papules, pustules, and/or cysts
Probably due to increased end-organ response to maternal or neonatal androgens
Majority resolve by 1 year of life

III. Vesiculobullous Lesions

A. BULLOUS IMPETIGO

Typically presents first few days of life with blisters that rupture easily leaving honey-colored crusts; located in genital
region, abdomen, inner thigh
Due to *Staphylococcus (Staph.) aureus*
Bullae are intraepidermal and contain polymorphonuclear cells
Treatment with antibiotics

B. STAPHYLOCOCCAL SCALDED SKIN SYNDROME

Etiology
Majority due to *Staph. aureus* (most common—group II phage) *exotoxin*

Clinical
Initially bright erythema on face, then severe bullous eruptions appear diffusely
Fever, irritability and tender skin; often with conjuctivitis and/or nasal congestion
Positive Nikolsky sign (epidermis can be detached by gentle traction)
Can shed in large sheets, crusting around mouth and eyes

Histology
Separation at granular layer, no inflammatory cells

Laboratory
Culture from bullae are NOT diagnostic since *fluid is sterile;* need to culture nasopharynx, conjuctivae, skin, blood

Management and outcome
Treat with antibiotics, fluid management; *no scarring,* rapid recovery

C. EPIDERMOLYSIS BULLOSA (EB)

Definition
Intraepidermal, junctional or subepidermal blisters following minor skin trauma

Characteristic	Junctional	Simplex = Epidermolytic	Dystrophic = Dermolytic
Scarring	No	Majority without scarring	Yes
Etiology and locale	Blisters at dermal and epidermal junction throughout body	Intra-epidermal blisters	Intra-dermal blisters
		Feet, hands, and scalp	Due to decrease in type VII collagen
	Nails (dystrophy), oral and anal mucosa involved		Increased collagenase
Genetics	Autosomal recessive	Many types	Both autosomal recessive and dominant types
		Autosomal dominant	
Clinical	Present at birth	Can be present at birth or soon after birth	Can be present at birth
	Most with short life span	Hemorrhagic bullae heal quickly	Autosomal recessive type more severe
	Electrolytes abnormal	Mild clinical course	Cycle of blistering, infection, and scarring
	May present with pyloric stenosis		Often hair loss, anemia, dysphagia, and poor growth

Modified from Cohen BA: Pediatric Dermatology (2nd edition), Philadelphia, Mosby, 1999, p 36.

D. INCONTINENTIA PIGMENTI

Genetics
X-linked dominant, majority female

Stages of skin lesions
1. *Linear inflammatory vesicles:* contain eosinophils; located along trunk and extremities during newborn period
2. Pigmented *warts* on red base
3. Macular hyperpigmented streaks and *whorls on trunk and extremities* during first year of life
4. Hypopigmented streaks that are atrophic later in childhood

Clinical
Seizures, mental deficiency, spastic paralysis
Abnormal dentition, alopecia, nail hypoplasia
Possible retinal vascular proliferation which can lead to retinal detachment and blindness
Mother of neonate often with subtle cutaneous findings

Management
Evaluate for associated defects (80%—typically central nervous system, eye, dentition)
No treatment

IV. Vascular Skin Lesions

A. HEMANGIOMAS = benign vascular endothelial cell tumors

Incidence
1–2% of all newborns; females greater than males; greater in premature infants (males similar to females)

Clinical
90% observed by second month of age

Face is most common location; initially appear as small telangiectasias or red macules that increase in size and color intensity

All increase during 6–8 months of age (due to rapid endothelial cell proliferation), 40–50% disappear by 5 years of age; 60–75% disappear by 7 years of age (growth slows, endothelial cells flatten, capillary lumina increase, and finally, involution of capillaries); this is in contrast to vascular malformations that grow proportionally with infant

Complications

Scarring may occur

Location may lead to complications (e.g., if around eye, may be associated with amblyopia and/or direct orbital damage; if involves buttocks, may ulcerate or become infected)

May have multiple hemangiomas that involve internal organs (lungs, liver, gastrointestinal tract, kidneys, central nervous system)

Kasabach-Merritt syndrome: may have multiple lesions that resemble hemangiomas or a single, large, rapidly growing hemangioma-like lesion (these hemangioma-like lesions have recently been noted to be Kaposi-like and consistent with hemangioendotheliomas); these lesions can lead to high-output heart failure, disseminated intravascular coagulation, and thrombocytopenia

Some hemangiomas may be associated with underlying abnormalities (e.g., if lumbosacral hemangioma, may have underlying vertebral or spinal abnormality; if upper face, may have thoracic anomaly; if scalp hemangioma, may have intracranial abnormality)

Management

If internal and/or systemic effects, treat with corticosteroids; interferon if life-threatening (less favorable due to association with spastic diplegia)

B. PORT-WINE STAIN

Etiology

Nevus flammeus; due to capillary malformation, permanent developmental defect

Clinical

Present at birth; remain the same size; may increase in color during adolescence

Majority located in head or neck

Sharp demarcation; flat in infancy and pebbly surface later in life

Observed in patients with:

Sturge-Weber syndrome: (see Neurology chapter) facial port-wine stain in first division of trigeminal nerve distribution, mental deficiency, seizures, hemiparesis contralateral to facial lesion, ipsilateral "tramline" intracortical calcifications, often with ipsilateral eye abnormalities such as glaucoma, optic atrophy, buphthalmos

Klippel-Trenaunay-Weber syndrome: superficial vascular abnormalities that are present at birth with underlying hypertrophy of bones or soft tissues, some with venous or lymphatic malformations

Beckwith-Weidemann syndrome and *Cobb syndrome* (cutaneomeningospinal angiomatosis)

Management

Treat with pulsed dye laser (often with very good outcome)

If involves periorbital or forehead regions, requires neurological and ophthalmologic evaluations

C. BLUE-RUBBER BLEB NEVUS SYNDROME

Rare, multiple venous malformations involving skin and intestines (can involve small intestine and large intestine; less commonly in liver, spleen and central nervous system)

Blue-purple rubbery, compressible blebs; can be present at birth; can be up to 3–4 cm in diameter with sparse or diffuse distribution

Often with anemia due to gastrointestinal bleeding

Don't regress spontaneously; need surgery if can resect

D. SALMON PATCHES

= vascular macules due to capillary malformation; also referred to as nevus flammeus simplex

60–70% neonates, usually on neck ("stork bite"), forehead ("angel's kiss"), upper eyelids

Pink color (may darken with physical exertion), irregular borders, blanches

Usually fade within first year of age (some may never fade)

E. TRANSIENT VASCULAR CHANGES

1. Cutis marmorata

Diffuse, reticulated, erythematous generalized pattern

Due to cold stress

Typically occurs < 1 month of age

If occurs beyond neonatal period, often associated with trisomy 18, trisomy 21, Cornelia de Lange syndrome or hypothyroidism

2. Harlequin color change

Occurs when infant horizontal and dependent half of body turns bright red in contrast to pale other half

Color may change when infant's position is altered; lasts from seconds to 1/2 hour

May recur up to 3–4 weeks of age

Not pathological

Etiology is most likely due to temperature imbalance of autonomic regulatory mechanism of cutaneous vessels

V. Hypopigmented Skin Lesions

A. PHENYLKETONURIA (PKU) AND CHEDIAK-HIGASHI SYNDROME

PKU (see Inborn Errors of Metabolism chapter)	Due to phenylalanine hydroxylase deficiency Neurological and cutaneous abnormalities Diffuse hypopigmentation Eczema, photosensitivity, seizures, mental deficiency
Chediak-Higashi syndrome	Neurological and cutaneous abnormalities Leukocytes and other cells with large granules Diffuse hypopigmentation Rare, autosomal recessive, fatal (due to infection or lymphoma-like process) Photophobia, hepatosplenomegaly, frequent infections, seizures

B. ALBINISM

1 in 17,000 in US, autosomal recessive

Pink pupils, yellow/white hair, decreased skin pigment, photophobia, nystagmus, cutaneous photosensitivity; decreased vision (central scotoma)

Due to deficiency of tyrosinase (tyrosine $\rightarrow$ dopamine pathway blocked and thus limited melanin production)

Partial albinism: = piebaldism, autosomal dominant, may be difficult to detect; normal pigmented areas adjacent to amelanotic regions; absent or deformed melanocytes

C. TUBEROUS SCLEROSIS (see Neurology chapter for nondermatologic manifestations)

Hypopigmented macule = ash-leaf spot in > 1/2 infants, present at birth or soon after, variable in number, greatest on trunk and buttocks

Wood's lamp assists in recognition of skin lesions
Often with café au lait spots

D. WAARDENBURG SYNDROME

Autosomal dominant
Lateral displacement of inner canthus, broad nasal root
Confluent eyebrows, variegation of pigment in iris (heterochromia iridis)
Congenital deafness, white forelock, cutaneous hypochromia

VI. Hyperpigmented Skin Lesions

A. CAFÉ AU LAIT SPOTS

Variable size, due to increased epidermal melanosis
Neurofibromatosis: increased risk if ≥ 6 spots and size greater than 0.5 cm (especially if axillary and inguinal location); also with Lisch nodules (small pigmented areas in iris); both lesions typically appear in first decade of life
May also be observed in patients with tuberous sclerosis

B. XERODERMA PIGMENTOSUM

Genetics
Autosomal recessive
DNA repair ability is decreased due to abnormally low endonuclease levels

Skin lesions
Skin initially normal but with increasing exposure to ultraviolet rays, skin alterations occur
Develop multiple hyperpigmented macules on sun-exposed areas
With time, skin becomes telangiectatic or atrophic
Increased risk of basal cell carcinomas, squamous cell carcinomas, and melanoma

Clinical
Cutaneous and ocular photosensitivity
May have progressive neurologic deterioration with decreased reflexes, mental deficiency, spasticity, peripheral neuropathy, cerebral and cerebellar dysfunction

Management
Light avoidance, protective clothing, sunscreen
Closely monitor skin exam for malignant changes

C. MASTOCYTOSIS

A spectrum of disorders with infiltration of mast cells in the skin or other tissues; majority are sporadic
Males = females; ~1/2 with clinical signs in first 2 years of life; overall good prognosis

Types
Mastocytoma: most common; typically in first 3 months of life
Presents with one or more skin-colored to light-brown oval or round macules (may be slightly elevated) along trunk, upper extremities, and neck

Urticaria pigmentosa: typically between 3 and 9 months of age
Presents with numerous reddish-brown macules, papules, and nodules that can coalesce
Majority located along trunk

Diffuse cutaneous mastocytosis: rare; most severe form; typically in first 3 years of life

Presents with generalized thick and edematous skin; patients often have Darier's sign (urticarial wheal and flare after firmly stroking lesion due to histamine release from mast cells)

May have pruritus and, less frequently, may have hepatosplenomegaly, lymphadenopathy, skeletal defects, diarrhea, abdominal pain, or hypotension

D. PEUTZ-JEGHER SYNDROME

Autosomal dominant with variable expression

Mucocutaneous pigmentation typically on lips and buccal mucosa (also involves face, fingers, elbows, palms); may be present at birth (rare)

During adolescence, increased risk of gastrointestinal polyps (can lead to rectal bleeding, intussuception, anemia)

VII. Hair and Nail Abnormalities

Hypertrichosis	Trisomy 18 (back and forehead)
	Cornelia de Lange syndrome (generalized)
	Turner syndrome (low occipital hairline)
	Mucopolysaccharidosis (generalized)
Hypotrichosis	Incontinentia pigmentosa
	Ectodermal dysplasia
Fine light-colored hair	Tyrosinemia
	Homocystinuria (fragile)
	Trisomy 21
	Phenylketonuria
Nail hypoplasia or dysplasia	Trisomy 13
	Trisomy 18
	Acrodermatitis enteropathica
	Epidermolysis bullosa
	Turner syndrome
Nail hypertrophy	Rubinstein-Taybi syndrome

VIII. Hairless Scalp Lesions

A. APLASIA CUTIS

Local or widespread congenital absence of skin

Clinical

Typically scalp erosion or ulceration (greatest in occiput, less commonly trunk and extremities) covered by crust or thin membrane followed by hairless, atrophic plaques

The benign form is autosomal dominant

Consider head imaging if large or unusual in appearance

Complications

May be associated with limb defects, epidermolysis bullosa, or chromosomal abnormalities (especially trisomy 13)

Symmetric truncal lesions can be associated with in utero fetal twin demise

B. NEVUS SEBACEOUS

1–4 cm yellowish, hairless, cobblestone-like plaque on scalp; a type of epidermal nevus

May involve head, neck (less commonly, trunk, extremities)

After neonatal period, becomes more verrucuous

10-15% associated with benign or malignant cutaneous tumors in adulthood and thus removal is often recommended in early childhood

IX. Nevi

A. EPIDERMAL NEVUS

Definition

Due to overgrowth of keratinocytes

Clinical

Verrucuous (wart-like) lesions that are linear and of variable size on limbs, trunk and scalp; often hyperpigmented with age

Can be associated with *skeletal defects* (shortened limbs, vertebral abnormalities, kyphoscoliosis)

Also can have *ocular complications* (eyelid/conjuctival nevi, coloboma, corneal opacity, nystagmus), *central nervous system disease* (mental deficiency, seizures, hemiparesis), tumors (neophroblastoma, Wilm's tumor, rhabdomyosarcoma), vitamin D–resistant rickets

B. MELANOCYTIC NEVI

Definition

Large cluster of melanocytes present at birth or in first few months of life

Types

Small: ≤ 1–1.5 cm during adulthood; most common of 3 types (1–2% of neonates)

Intermediate: 1–1.5 cm to 20 cm during adulthood; 0.6% of neonates

Large: >6–9 cm during adulthood; least common of 3 types (less than 0.02% of neonates)

Clinical

Tan, brown, or dark brown macules, papules, or plaques observed at brith

May be smooth or rough; may have hair

Large lesions are most commonly located on posterior trunk and have an increased risk of melanoma formation

Management

If small or intermediate, management is controversial due to uncertainty of risk of melanoma formation; during childhood, majority are observed and if there is a concerning change in appearance, excision is recommended

If large, typically manage by partial or complete excision

X. Scaly Disorders

A. ICHTHYOSIS

Abnormal keratinization

Patients have temperature instability, increased insensible water losses, increased risk infection

May improve with lubrication and some respond to oral retinoids (liver and skeletal toxicity)

Type	Transmission	Clinical	Pathology	Features
Congenital ichthyosiform erythroderma	Autosomal recessive 1 in 50–100,000	Onset: birth, can present as collodion infant Fine white scales (trunk, scalp, face)	Increased stratum corneum Increased granular layer	May have scarring, nail dystrophy, alopecia Increased risk heat intolerance *(continued on following page)*

Type	Transmission	Clinical	Pathology	Features
Epidermolytic hyper-keratosis = bullous ichthyosis	Autosomal dominant (sporadic) Rare	Large scale on extremities Onset: birth Widespread blisters and denuded skin at birth Blisters resolve and hyperkeratosis develops (increased in intertriginous and flexure areas)	Epidermolytic hyperkeratosis Vacuolization of epidermis Increased granular layer	Assess for neurological disorder Keratin mutations Increased scale with age Foul odor Bacterial overgrowth Often confused at birth with *Staph.* scalded-skin syndrome or epidermolysis bullosa Increased risk of infection, isolate
Ichthyosis vulgaris	Autosomal dominant with variable expression 1 in 250	Normal at birth Presents after 3 months of age with mild scales No flexure involvement	Decreased or absent granular layer Increased stratum corneum	Improves with age Defect in profilaggrin expression
Lamellar ichthyosis	Autosomal recessive 1 in 100,000	Onset: birth, can present as collodion infant Generalized, large, thick plate-like brown scales Ectropion, eclabion	Increased stratum corneum	Often premature Heat intolerance Assess for neurological disorder
X-linked ichthyosis	X-linked recessive 1 in 2,000–6,000 males	Onset: 0–3 mo Large, brown scales involving trunk and extremities (does not involve palms or soles) No flexure involvement	Secondary to steroid sulfatase deficiency Increased stratum corneum	Cryptorchidism in 1/4 males Increased incidence corneal opacities Female carriers with this deficiency often have low estradiol excretion and difficult labor

Modified from Cohen BA: Pediatric Dermatology (2nd edition), Philadelphia, Mosby, 1999, p 25.

Netherton's disease: abnormality of hair shaft circumflexa ("bamboo hair"), episodic skin changes after 2 years of age; typically without scalp hair

Generalized scaling erythroderma, failure to thrive with hypernatremic dehydration, diarrhea, increased risk infection

B. COLLODION INFANT

Clinical

Usually born premature with a brownish-yellow translucent shiny skin (cellophane-like membrane) that covers the body; desquamation (parchment-like) complete by 2–3 weeks of age; skin beneath is red

Defective cutaneous barrier function, increased insensible water loss, increased risk of hypothermia, infection (increased risk of pneumonia from aspiration of squamous cells)

Ectropion, eclabion, abnormal digits

Management

Lubrication of skin with bland emollients; high humidity environment

Prognosis

60–70% develop congenital ichthyosiform erythroderma (more uncommonly, may lead to lamellar ichthyosis or Netherton's disease); minority with normal skin

C. HARLEQUIN ICHTHYOSIS often fatal

Etiology

Rare, severe keratinization abnormality, majority autosomal recessive

Clinical

Thick, hardened, hyperkeratotic skin; inelastic skin

Ectropion due to rigidity of skin around eyes

Underdeveloped and distorted ears and nose; abnormal nails and hair

Majority infants are premature

Management

Often fatal due to dehydration, infection, or respiratory decompensation

Oral retinoids may improve survival

If survive, develop severe chronic ichthyosis

D. ECTODERMAL DYSPLASIA

Definition

A rare group of disorders due to abnormality of skin and its appendages

Clinical

Most common is X-linked recessive hypohidrotic ectodermal dysplasia:

Often presents with collodion membrane at birth

Facial findings include frontal bossing, depression of nasal bridge, periorbital wrinkling and hyperpigmentation, hypoplastic gum ridges, and everted lips

Decreased scalp and body hair, decreased ability to sweat, frequent fevers

Increased risk of asthma, allergies, eczema

XI. Other Skin Lesions

A. CUTIS LAXA

= generalized elastolysis

Can present in newborn period with skin changes and abdominal or inguinal hernias

Decreased skin resiliency, loose drooping skin leading to *bloodhound appearance*

Normal wound healing

Forms

Autosomal dominant—mildest, typically presents later in life, normal life span

Autosomal recessive—often presents at birth with flaccid skin; increased risk of congenital diaphragmatic hernia, emphysema early in life

X-linked recessive—bladder and gastrointestinal diverticulum, mild cognitive delay, bony protuberances of occiput with time, hip dysplasia

B. EHLERS-DANLOS SYNDROME

Multiple clinical forms

Hyperextensible skin, *joint hypermobility, soft tissue fragility,* and *easy bruisability*

Associations: intestinal or bladder diverticulum, umbilical or inguinal hernias, multiple dislocations, scoliosis, and aortic aneurysms

C. KERATOSIS PILARIS

Autosomal dominant, more common than acne

Increased incidence of eczema when older

No pustules or comedones

Keratotic papules surrounded by erythema on face, can spread to arms, lower body
"Plucked chicken skin"

D. LEINER SYNDROME

Clinical syndrome of generalized erythematous desquamative dermatitis with failure to thrive, diarrhea, and recurrent
   infections that presents within first few weeks of age; associated with functional complement 5 abnormality
Many are now recognized as Netherton's disease

E. SUBCUTANEOUS FAT NECROSIS

Incidence
   Often observed in infants with a history of difficult delivery, hypothermia, perinatal depression, maternal diabetes

Clinical
   Red nodules on cheeks, back, buttocks, arms, and legs at 1–6 weeks of age
   Usually firm and painless
   May be associated later with hypercalcemia

Histology
   Granulomatous reaction in fat with foreign body giant cells, fibroblasts, lymphocytes, and histiocytes

Prognosis
   Good prognosis, typically resolves spontaneously by 1–2 months with fibrosis formation
   If calcified, may lead to ulceration and drainage

XII. Dermatologic Infections

Etiology
   Bacterial, viral, fungal
   Localized or associated with systemic disease
   After birth, skin becomes colonized with organisms from maternal genital tract
   Subsequently, environmental or skin organisms predominate
   Staph. aureus, group A and B *Streptococcus, Listeria, Pseudomonas*, syphilis, herpes, *Candida*

Pathophysiology
   Break in skin and colonized organisms can now enter
   Increased risk of entry if abrasions (increased risk of abrasion if fetal scalp monitor, forcep usage, intravenous catheter
      usage, circumcision)

Clinical
   Pustules: Staph., Listeria, group B *Streptococcus* (GBS), multiple other organisms (including *Haemophilus,
      Pseudomonas, Klebsiella*)
   Vesicles: early stages of *Staph. aureus, Listeria*, GBS, *Pseudomonas*, herpes, varicella-zoster
   Bullae: typically *Staph.* can also be due to syphilis (palms and soles)
   Maculopapules: Staph. and *Streptoccocus* (Strep.), fungal, measles, enterovirus, rubella, syphilis (palms and soles,
      desquamating)
   Cellulitis: Strep.
   Impetigo: Strep., less likely—*Staph. aureus* and *E. coli*
   Abscesses: Staph. aureus, Strep., E. coli, Candida
   Pyoderma gangrenosum (necrotic, yellow-green pustules): *Pseudomonas*

Blueberry muffin spots (due to *dermal hematopoiesis*): rubella, cytomegalovirus, Coxsackie B2, parvovirus B19, twin-twin transfusion, hemolytic disease of the neonate, hereditary spherocytosis, neoplastic infiltrative diseases, congenital leukemia

XIII. Diagnosis of Dermatologic Diseases

Disease	Test	Finding
Bullous impetigo	Gram stain	Gram-positive cocci (most due to *Staph.*)
Candida	KOH	Pseudohyphae
	Gram stain	Yeast spore
Erythema toxicum	Wright's stain	Eosinophils, occasional neutrophils, negative Gram stain
Herpes	Tzanck smear	Multinucleated giant cells
Miliaria	Wright's stain	Some squamous cells or lymphocytes
		No organisms
Neonatal pustular melanosis	Wright's stain	Keratinosis debris
		Polymorphonuclear leukocytes
		Negative Gram stain
Scabies	Mineral oil preparation	Mites, ova, feces
Staph scalded-skin syndrome	Bullae	No inflammatory cells, sterile
Syphilis	Darkfield examination of skin lesions	*Treponema* visible

XIV. Nutrient Deficiencies Associated with Skin Manifestations

Deficiency	Skin Findings
Biotin	Alopecia, intertriginous and perioral dermatitis, scaling, seborrhea
Linoleic acid	Alopecia, coarse scaling, erosive intertriginous dermatitis
	Decreased wound healing
Niacin	Mucositis, symmetric hyperpigmented plaques at sun-exposed areas
Protein	Scaling, hypopigmentation
	Peripheral edema
Pyridoxine	Intertriginous and perioral dermatitis, mucositis
Riboflavin	Intertriginous and perioral dermatitis, mucositis
Vitamin A	Generalized scaling
Vitamin C	Poor wound healing, bleeding gums
Zinc	1. *Acrodermatitis enteropathica*
	Autosomal recessive; abnormality of zinc absorption or transport
	FTT, alopecia, diarrhea, diaper dermatitis (commonly perianal), ocular changes, rash (crusted, erythematous rash involving face, extremities, and anogenital region), nail hypoplasia or dysplasia
	During first few months of life and if breast-fed, symptoms will be delayed until after breast milk ceases
	Increased risk of secondary infections (*Candida, Staph*)
	Treat with zinc supplementation
	2. *Acquired*
	Premature infants receiving inadequate amounts of zinc
	Maternal zinc deficiency can lead to fetal growth deficiency, congenital anomalies
	Infants with malabsorption (e.g., cystic fibrosis)

Modified from Taeusch HW and Ballard RA (eds): Avery's Diseases of the Newborn (7th edition). Philadelphia, W.B. Saunders, 1998, p 1275.

References (please refer to these textbooks for pictorial review)

Cohen BA: Pediatric Dermatology (2nd edition), Philadelphia, Mosby, 1999.

Eichenfield LF, Frieden IJ and Esterly NB (eds): Textbook of Neonatal Dermatology. Philadelphia, WB Saunders, 2001.

Fanaroff AA and Martin RJ (eds): Neonatal-Perinatal Medicine (6th edition). St Louis, Mosby-Year Book Inc, 1997.

Fletcher MA: Physical Diagnosis in Neonatology. Philadelphia, Lippincott-Raven Publishers, 1998.

Vasiloudes P, Morelli JG and Weston WL. A guide to rashes in newborns. *Contemporary Pediatrics*, June 1997.

CHAPTER 14

Ophthalmology

TOPICS COVERED IN THIS CHAPTER

I. **Development of the Eye**

II. **Reflexes of the Eye**
   A. Pupillary light reaction
   B. Choroidal light reflex = red reflex

III. **Abnormalities of the Eye**
   A. Abnormal position of the eye
   B. Abnormalities of the eyelid
      1. Abnormal slanting of palpebral fissures
      2. Ptosis
   C. Associations with specific abnormalities of the eye

IV. **Disorders of the Eye**
   A. Retinopathy of prematurity (ROP)
      1. Incidence

2. Pathogenesis
3. Classification
4. Screening and monitoring
5. Management
6. Prognosis
   B. Cataracts
   C. Congenital glaucoma
   D. Retinoblastoma

V. **Associations with Eye Abnormalities**
   A. Syndromes associated with the eye
   B. Infectious diseases associated with the eye
      1. Conjunctivitis
      2. Chorioretinitis

I. Development of the Eye

Embryology of the eye
  Development of the eye begins in the fifth week of gestation
  The retina is derived from the neuroectoderm of the forebrain
  The vascular and sclerocorneal layers of the eye are derived from the mesoderm
  The lens is derived from surface ectoderm

Functional development of the eye
  30 weeks gestation: eyelid closes in response to light; pupils reactive to light (may not respond until 32 weeks gestation; well-developed at age 1 month)
  Full-term infants: conjugate horizontal gaze, visual fixation (well-developed at age 2 months)
  Age 2 months: conjugate vertical gaze
  Age 3 months: visual following is well-developed
  Age 6 months: visual evoked potential reaches adult level
  By 2 age years: optic nerve myelination is complete

II. Reflexes of the Eye

A. PUPILLARY LIGHT REACTION

Application
  Evaluates pupillary response to light (need to compare response of each eye and assess the degree of pupillary constriction)
  The pupillary response to light tests for intact afferent and efferent pathways of cranial nerve III; suggests visual function of subcortex (note: may be present despite cortical blindness)

Developmental changes
  In premature infants, the ability of the pupil to respond to light increases with advancing gestational age (GA), and the pupillary diameter decreases with GA until ~30 weeks
  The reactivity of pupil to light may be observed at 30 weeks gestation but can appear at 32 weeks gestation; it is well developed at age 1 month

Abnormalities
  Unreactive bilateral pupils with increased size can be observed in infants with late signs of hypoxic-ischemic encephalopathy (may also have decreased pupillary size and sometimes can be reactive), intraventricular hemorrhage, infantile botulism
  Unreactive unilateral pupil with increased size in infants with subdural hematoma or other unilateral mass

B. CHOROIDAL LIGHT REFLEX = RED REFLEX

Application
  Detects retinal blood vessels that appear as a red glow when viewed through an ophthalmoscope
  Demonstrates lack of obstruction between external corneal surface and retina

Developmental changes
  Premature infants < 28 weeks gestation may not demonstrate choroidal reflex because of unclear corneas and vitreous

Abnormalities
  Leukocoria (*white reflex*): most commonly caused by cataracts

May also be attributed to retinoblastoma, coloboma, retinopathy of prematurity, persistent hyperplastic primary vitreous, retinal detachment or dysplasia, vitreous hemorrhage, intraocular inflammation, medulloepithelioma, myelinated nerve fibers

III. Abnormalities of the Eye

A. ABNORMAL POSITION OF THE EYE

Hypotelorism	Hypertelorism
Decreased intraorbital distance	Widely spaced eyes (increased intraorbital distance)
	Note: a low nasal bridge may give false impression of hypertelorism, so confirm by measuring
High association with holoprosencephaly	May be associated with syndromes, including Apert syndrome, cat-eye syndrome, CHARGE association, cri du chat syndrome, Crouzon syndrome, deletion 13q,
May also be associated with syndromes such as Meckel-Gruber syndrome, trisomy 13, Williams syndrome	DiGeorge sequence, Holt-Oram syndrome, Noonan syndrome, trisomy 8
	Teratogenic effect of hydantoin, isotretinoin

B. ABNORMALITIES OF THE EYELID

1. Abnormal slanting of palpebral fissures

Down-slanting	Upslanting
Abnormal if intersection of the two lines through the medial and lateral canthus of each eye is *above* the line connecting the medial canthus of both eyes	Abnormal if intersection of the two lines through the medial and lateral canthus of each eye is *below* the line connecting the medial canthus of both eyes
Probably caused by the *greater* growth rate of the brain above the eye compared with the facial area below the eye (e.g., maxillary hypoplasia)	Probably caused by the *smaller* growth rate of the brain above the eye compared with the facial area below the eye (e.g., microcephaly)
Associated with Apert syndrome, Noonan syndrome, cri du chat syndrome, Rubenstein-Taybi syndrome, Treacher Collins syndrome	Associated with trisomy 21
May also be associated with other syndromes, including cat-eye syndrome, DiGeorge sequence	May occasionally be associated with hydantoin teratogenic effect, Prader-Willi syndrome, trisomy 13, and trisomy 18
Teratogenic effect of isotretinoin	Note: mild degrees of upslanting have been observed in ~4% of nonsyndromic children

2. Ptosis

Definition: the upper eyelid cannot rise to normal level, leading to decreased vertical space between the upper and lower eyelids; unilateral or bilateral

Pathogenesis: usually caused by dysfunction of the levator palpebral muscle (cranial nerve III)

Etiology:

Isolated autosomal dominant disorder with variable penetrance

Cranial nerve palsy: Horner's syndrome (can be observed with Klumpke's palsy)

Associated with specific syndromes, including deletion 13q, Fanconi pancytopenia syndrome, fetal alcohol syndrome, Mobius sequence, Noonan syndrome, Smith-Lemli-Opitz syndrome, WAGR syndrome

Also observed with chronic eyelid inflammation and trauma

Diagnosis: when eye is in the neutral position, the upper eyelid should move above the middle of the pupil

Often difficult to diagnose in neonate unless it is unilateral

C. ASSOCIATIONS WITH SPECIFIC ABNORMALITIES OF THE EYE

Eye abnormality	Specific associations
Cherry red spot (macular spot of epithelium that is of normal color but visible because of thinning of the cell layer in the center of the macula)	Lipidoses (e.g., Niemann-Pick A disease and Tay-Sachs disease), mucolipidoses (e.g., sialidosis)
Coloboma (tissue or gap)	Cat-eye syndrome (iris), CHARGE association (80%; usually retina), deletion 13q, Treacher Collins syndrome (eyelid), trisomy 8 (iris)

(continued on following page)

Eye abnormality	Specific associations
Epicanthal folds (represent redundant skin folds usually caused by a low nasal bridge)	Cri du chat syndrome, deletion 13q, fragile X syndrome, Noonan syndrome, Smith-Lemli-Opitz syndrome, Stickler syndrome, trisomy 21, Williams syndrome
	Fetal alcohol syndrome, *in utero* methotrexate exposure, teratogenic effect of valproic acid
Lens, dislocation	Homocystinuria, Marfan syndrome
Sclera, blue	Type I and II osteogenesis imperfecta (type III with blue sclera during infancy that later normalizes and type IV with normal sclera)
	May also be seen in Russell-Silver syndrome, Ehlers-Danlos syndrome, incontinentia pigmentosa, Marfan syndrome, Turner syndrome
	Because premature infants have thin scleras, may appear blue
Telecanthus (inner canthi are laterally displaced, leads to false impression of hypertelorism and strabismus)	Waardenburg syndrome

IV. Disorders of the Eye

A. RETINOPATHY OF PREMATURITY (ROP)

1. Incidence
Risk and severity of ROP increases with decreasing GA and birth weight

Almost all infants $<$ 27 weeks gestation develop some form of ROP

Increasing incidence of ROP caused by increased survival of very low-birth-weight premature infants

2. Pathogenesis
Retinal vascularization progresses from the inner retina and proceeds outward

Infants who are born prematurely do not have complete retinal vascularization, and the growing retinal blood vessels are extremely sensitive to stress (e.g., prolonged hyperoxia, intraventricular hemorrhage, pneumothorax, shock, sepsis)

During the time of illness, the retinal blood vessels may become injured, resulting in a period of no growth

Afterwards, the avascularized retinal region usually becomes extremely hypoxic, inciting excess amount of vascular growth factors (e.g., vascular endothelial growth factor [VEGF])

When retinal vascularization begins again (i.e., neovascularization) at ~30 to 34 weeks gestational age, the vascular growth factors induce erratic and excessive blood vessel growth (i.e., ROP)

3. Classification
Zone = location where abnormal retinal vessels end

    I: most posterior part of retina with vessels closest to optic disc, most immature zone with greatest risk for progession to stage 5 (particularly if evidence of "plus disease")

    II: area between zone I and II (defined more distinctly by region from edge of zone I to a point tangential to nasal ora serrata to the temporal anatomic equator)

    III: most anterior part of retina, most mature zone, most common area involved in ROP

Stage = severity of transition site of the vascularized and avascular retina

    1: distinct demarcation line (usually white or yellow) separating transition of vascularized posterior retina and avascular anterior retina

        flat, mildest form

    2: demarcation line is thickened and elevated; forms a ridge; abnormally growing immature vessels are still within the retina

    3: ridge with extraretinal neovascularization and retinal vessels enter the vitreous space

    4: partial retinal detachment

        a. extrafoveal

        b. includes fovea

    5: complete retinal detachment; severest form

Clock hours = extent

Describes the number of clock hours within the retina that shows evidence of ROP

Other descriptive terms of ROP disease

"*Plus disease*": findings of dilated, tortuous vessels that demonstrate advanced vascular disease; always evident before retinal detachment; may also have iris vascular engorgement, pupillary rigidity, vitreous haze or hemorrhage

"*Threshold disease*": ROP in zone I or II with at least five contiguous clock hours or eight total clock hours; must be accompanied by plus disease

50% progress to stage 5

"*Prethreshold disease*":

= any ROP in zone I that is not threshold

= ROP in zone II, stage 2 with plus disease

= ROP in zone II, stage 3 without plus disease

= ROP in zone II, stage 3 and plus disease but inadequate clock hours to meet threshold disease

4. Screening and monitoring

Current screening recommendations in the United States:

Examine infants ≤ 28 weeks gestation

Examine infants ≤ 1500 g birth weight

Examine older premature infants if they are unstable (independent of birth weight)

Perform examination on above infants at 4 to 6 weeks after birth or at 31 to 33 weeks postconceptional age

Continue examinations until the retina is completely vascularized

Monitoring:

Prethreshold disease requires follow-up exam within 1 week

Milder ROP requires monitoring every 2 weeks unless there is progression to zone III (low risk; can monitor less frequently)

5. Management

Threshold disease requires laser or cryotherapy (less common) within 2 to 3 days; this technique ablates the retina and decreases production of vascular growth factors

After laser or cryotherapy (immediate postoperatively): often increased risk for apnea and local swelling; majority with good outcome; however, retinal detachments can occur

If partial retinal detachment: in some cases, scleral buckling (to move sclera closer to retina) may allow the retina to reattach

If retinal detachment: difficult to reattach retina; vitrectomy may rescue light/dark perception or provide ambulatory vision yet typically, there is no change in visual acuity

Referral to early intervention program if there is an increased risk of blindness

6. Prognosis

All premature infants with increased risk for amblyopia and refractive errors with increasing severity depending on degree of ROP

If ROP as neonate, increased risk of retinal detachment during adulthood (especially if stage 3 because residual scars may predispose to retinal thinning and holes, thus increasing risk for detachment)

Infants who had received laser or cryotherapy have unknown long-term outcome because the oldest group consists of teenagers

B. CATARACTS

Definition

Nonspecific reaction to a change in lens metabolism leading to lens opacification

Pathogenesis
Caused by any process that alters the glycolytic pathway or epithelial cell mitosis of the avascular lens

Etiology
Isolated autosomal dominant (25%)
May be associated with other eye abnormalities
Congenital infections: herpes simplex virus, varicella syndrome, rubella syndrome (50%), toxoplasmosis (5%)
Metabolic: galactosemia, galactokinase deficiency, mevalonic aciduria, some mucolipidoses, hypocalcemia, vitamin A or D deficiency
Associated with specific syndromes, including Smith-Lemli-Opitz syndrome, Stickler syndrome, trisomy 21, WAGR syndrome
In utero radiation exposure
Trauma

Diagnosis
White pupillary reflex = leukocoria

Management
Surgery
Attempt to identify an underlying etiology

Prognosis
If untreated, may lead to visual loss, poor fixation, nystagmus, ambylopia, or strabismus

C. CONGENITAL GLAUCOMA

Definition
Increased intraocular pressure in the aqueous humor (anterior fluid of eye)

Pathogenesis
Majority caused by obstruction of aqueous humor outflow

Etiology
Primary (caused by structural abnormality): 1/10,000 births
Typically autosomal recessive
Males > females
Presents at birth
Secondary: presents after neonatal period; can be caused by homocystinuria, congenital rubella syndrome, retinopathy of prematurity, and numerous syndromes (e.g., Sturge-Weber syndrome [30%], Stickler syndrome)
Symptoms similar to those of primary glaucoma

Clinical
Bilateral involvement with corneal cloudiness (caused by corneal edema), photophobia, lacrimation, buphthalmos (i.e., enlargement of globe), eye rubbing

Diagnosis
Measure intraocular pressure (precision is difficult in neonates)

Management
Periodic observation; consultation with an ophthalmologist

Consider medical therapy, but patients usually require surgery to increase drainage
Monitor vision

Prognosis
The sooner the treatment, the better the outcome
Increased risk for blindness if untreated

D. RETINOBLASTOMA (see Hematology and Oncology chapter)

V. Associations with Eye Abnormalities

A. SYNDROMES ASSOCIATED WITH THE EYE

Syndrome	Eye manifestations
Trisomy 13	Hypotelorism Microophthalmia Colobomas (iris) Retinal dysplasia Less common: slanting palpebral fissures, hypertelorism, cyclopia, hypotelorism, anopththalmos
Trisomy 18	Short palpebral fissures May also have hypoplasia of orbital ridges, inner epicanthal folds, ptosis, corneal opacity Less frequently ($< 10\%$) with slanted palpebral fissures, hypertelorism, colobomas (iris), cataracts, microphthalmos
Trisomy 21	Brushfield spots Lens opacities Myopia Nystagmus Strabismus Blocked tear duct Cataracts (adults)
Deletion 13q	Colobomas Small eyes Hypertelorism Increased risk of retinoblastoma (usually bilateral) Ptosis Epicanthal folds

B. INFECTIOUS DISEASES ASSOCIATED WITH THE EYE

1. Conjunctivitis (ophthalmia)
Incidence: 1% to 12% of neonates
Etiology and clinical manifestations:

Type	Onset	Characteristics
Chemical	Within 24 hours after exposure	After prophylaxis Decreased incidence because there is less usage of 1% silver nitrate for prophylaxis Negative culture findings Spontaneously resolves within 48 hours
Acute purulent	Age 24–48 hours (can be later in life)	Infections caused by *Staphylococcus aureus* (most frequent organism; golden crust around eyelids), group B *Streptococcus, Haemophilus influenzae* (dacrocystitis), *Streptococcus pneumoniae* (dacrocystitis), *Pseudomonas aeruginosa*

(continued on following page)

Type	Onset	Characteristics
Gonorrheal	Age 2–5 days	Abrupt onset of extremely copious, prurulent bilateral discharge
		Medical emergency because it can progress to involve cornea and ulceration or perforation if untreated
		Treat with third generation cephalosporin
		Can prevent with prophylaxis (0.5% erythromycin most common; ideal if applied < age 1 hour, decreases incidence of gonorrheal conjunctivitis from 10% to 0.5%)
Chlamydia	Age 5–14 days (can be earlier if premature rupture of membranes)	~ 8/1000 births
		Most common cause of conjunctivitis in first month of life
		In ~1/2 of infants with colonized mothers
		Typically bilateral
		Initially watery discharge that becomes prurulent
		Often associated with chlamydia pneumonia
		Diagnose by Giemsa stain of conjunctival scrapings
		Treat with oral erythromycin for 14 days (20% require second course)
Herpes simplex	Broad range (age 4 days–3 weeks)	Most frequent viral etiology
		May also have keratitis, chorioretinitis, retinal dysplasia
		Assess for systemic herpes and herpes encephalitis

Differential diagnosis: trauma, foreign body, glaucoma, obstructed nasal lacrimal duct
Possible complications: infiltrates, corneal epithelial erosions, visual loss

2. Chorioretinitis

Etiology:

Early congenital *syphilis*: may be bilateral; "*salt and pepper*" appearance to fundus

Perinatal or congenital *herpes* simplex virus: typically severe, yellow-white exudates and retinal necrosis

Congenital *rubella* syndrome: occurs in ~5% of affected infants; unilateral or bilateral diffuse granular pigmented areas; "*salt and pepper*" appearance; no alteration in vision

Congenital *cytomegalovirus*: occurs in ~20% of affected patients; bilateral involvement evident by numerous yellow-white fluffy retinal lesions; hemorrhage present; treat with ganciclovir

Congenital *toxoplasmosis*: occurs in large number of affected patients (80% to 90%), usually bilateral, necrotizing retinitis resulting in large, atrophic, retinal scars that often involve the macula

Candidiasis: appearance of fluffy white balls

References

Fletcher MA. Physical Diagnosis in Neonatology. Philadelphia, Lippincott-Raven Publishers, 1998.

Jones KL: Smith's Recognizable Patterns of Human Malformations (5th edition). Philadelphia, WB Saunders, 1997.

Phelps DL. Retinopathy of prematurity: history, classification and pathophysiology. *NeoReviews.* 2(7), 2001: c153–c166.

Phelps DL. Retinopahty of premtaurity: clinical trials. *NeoReviews.* 2(7), 2001:c167–c173.

Phelps DL. Retinopathy of prematurity: a practical clinical approach. *NeoReviews.* 2(7), 2001:c174–c179.

Pickering LK (ed): 2000 Red Book: Report of the Committee on Infectious Diseases (25th edition). Elk Grove Village, IL, American Academy of Pediatrics, 2000.

Zitelli BJ, Davis HW (eds): Atlas of Pediatric Physical Diagnosis (4th edition). Philadelphia, Mosby, 2002.

CHAPTER 15

Pharmacology

TOPICS COVERED IN THIS CHAPTER

I. Drug Disposition
 A. Absorption
 B. Distribution
 C. Metabolism
 D. Excretion

II. Pharmacokinetics
 A. Zero-order kinetics
 B. First-order kinetics
 C. Compartment models
  1. One-compartment model
  2. Two-compartment model

D. Loading dose
E. Clearance
F. Steady-state
G. Half-life (t $\frac{1}{2}$)
H. Drug monitoring

III. Clinical pharmacology
 A. Human teratogens
 B. Drugs and lactation
 C. Drugs that interfere with fetal and neonatal oxidation of vitamin K
 D. Drug effects on bilirubin levels

I. Drug Disposition

A. ABSORPTION

Definition
Process by which drug moves from administration site to circulation

Influences
1. Biochemical factors of drug: molecular weight, lipid solubility, degree of ionization
2. Neonatal factors: gastric acidity, gastric emptying time, intestinal surface area, amount of bile available, bacterial colonization of gastrointestinal (GI) tract, presence of underlying disease
3. Drug bioavailability
4. Other factors: drug formulation and route of administration

Modes of transport across cell membranes
1. Simple (passive) diffusion: transport directly related to concentration gradient with compound moving from area of high concentration to area of low concentration
   Dependent on lipid solubility of the drug, ionization of the drug, and molecular weight of the compound (i.e., drug will diffuse more rapidly if it is lipid soluble, not ionized, and smaller in size)
   Transport method used by most compounds
2. Facilitated passive diffusion: transport mediated by a carrier that moves compound *along* the concentration gradient; no energy required
   Dependent on carrier availability and carrier specificity
   Transport method for glucose
3. Active transport: transport mediated by a carrier that moves compound *against* the concentration gradient; requires energy
   Dependent on carrier availability, carrier specificity, and energy availability
   Transport method for drugs that are similar to endogenous compounds
4. Pinocytosis: compounds are engulfed and packaged by cell; requires energy; transport method for minority of drugs

B. DISTRIBUTION

Definition
Process by which drugs moves from intravascular space to extravascular tissues

Influences
Dependent on rate of blood flow to tissues, drug ability to bind to tissues, permeability of cell membranes, pH, protein-binding ability of drug, drug composition, and body compartments

Volume of distribution (V_d) (L/kg)
Volume of fluid in which drug distributes
Large V_d suggests distribution into many tissues and usually drug with long half-life
Small V_d occurs with highly protein-bound drugs

$$V_d = \frac{\text{total amount of drug in body (mg)}}{\text{plasma concentration of drug (mg/L)} \times \text{weight (kg)}}$$

Premature neonates have a greater V_d compared with full-term infants

Protein-binding
Drugs within plasma that are bound to proteins (e.g., phenytoin and diazepam)
Only free (unbound) drug is active

While acidic drugs typically bind to albumin, basic drugs bind to α-glycoproteins and lipoproteins

High protein-binding leads to decreased V_d

Neonates have decreased protein-binding ability because of decreased total protein, albumin, and glycoprotein levels

Blood–brain barrier (BBB)

Bloodstream barrier restricts drug distribution to brain

Drugs bound tightly to proteins and ionized forms enter brain very slowly

Clindamycin is an example of a drug that minimally crosses the BBB

C. METABOLISM

Definition

Process by which drugs are altered

Majority of changes occurs in liver with contributions from kidney, lungs, intestines, and skin

Most drugs are lipophilic, and biotransformation is required to make them more water-soluble so they can be excreted

Types

Phase I reactions: modification(s) of drug via oxidation, reduction, hydrolysis, or demethylation

75% of drugs are modified this way

Cytochrome P_{450} metabolism: most important enzyme system in phase I reactions; microsomal enzymes that transfer electrons from NADPH to cytochrome P_{450}

Enzymes lack substrate specificity (i.e., few enzymes metabolize many drugs)

Important for metabolism of phenobarbital, theophylline, caffeine, and phenytoin

Some drugs can induce the cytochrome system (e.g., rifampin), and others can inhibit the system (e.g., ranitidine)

Drugs can displace each other, leading to decreased metabolism

Phase II reactions: conjugation(s) of drug with endogenous components (glycine, glucuronic acid, sulfate, glutathione, or hippurate)

Glucuronidation: the most common phase II reaction

Important for metabolism of morphine and acetaminophen

Neonates have undeveloped liver enzymes and slower rates of glucuronidation

D. EXCRETION

Definition

Elimination of drug or metabolite from body (majority by the kidneys)

Some contribution from the biliary system (when enterohepatic cycling is incomplete)

II. Pharmacokinetics

A. ZERO-ORDER KINETICS

Characteristics

Excrete a *constant* amount of drug per unit time regardless of the serum drug concentration

There is a linear decrease of serum concentration over time

The half-life is dependent on drug dosage (larger doses are cleared more slowly, so they have longer half-lives)

The fraction of drug that is eliminated (i.e., elimination rate constant) is not constant

Drugs that demonstrate zero-order kinetics include aspirin, chloramphenicol, ethanol, and diazepam

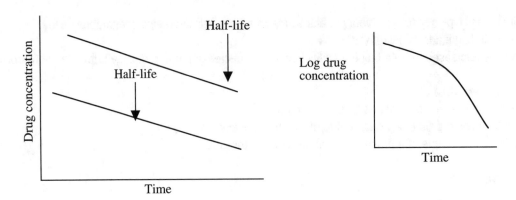

B. FIRST-ORDER KINETICS

Characteristics

Excrete a certain *percentage* of drug per unit time, so the rate of drug elimination is directly proportional to the serum drug concentration

There is an exponential decrease of serum concentration over time

The half-life is independent of drug dosage

The *fraction* of drug that is eliminated (i.e., elimination rate constant) is constant

Most drugs have this type of kinetics, including phenobarbital and theophylline

$$\frac{\text{dose}_1}{[\text{SS}]_1} = \frac{\text{dose}_2}{[\text{SS}]_2}$$

Dose_1 = First dose of drug
Dose_2 = Second dose of drug; usually solving for this
$[\text{SS}]_1$ = Steady-state concentration achieved with first dose
$[\text{SS}]_2$ = Desired steady-state concentration

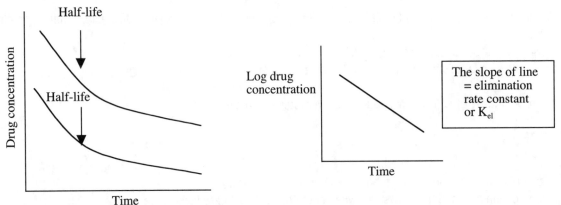

C. COMPARTMENT MODELS

1. One-compartment model

Assumes that a drug distributes equally to all areas of the body

Assumes that a drug *rapidly* equilibrates with peripheral tissues

Assumes first-order kinetics (linear if log drug concentration plotted vs time)

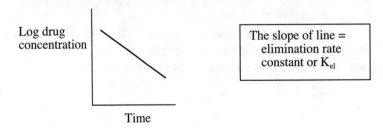

Aminoglycosides rapidly equilibrate with tissues, so the one-compartment model can be used

2. Two-compartment model

Assumes that a drug initially rapidly equilibrates with central compartment and then more *slowly* equilibrates with peripheral compartment

Vancomycin slowly equilibrates with tissues, so the two-compartment model can be used

Biphasic line if log drug concentration is plotted over time with the initial phase = distribution phase (half-life = t 1/2) and the second phase = elimination phase (half-life = β t 1/2)

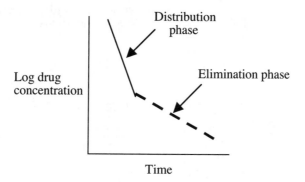

D. LOADING DOSE

$$\text{Loading dose} = \frac{\text{Volume of distribution (L/kg)} \times C_p \text{ (mg/L)}}{S \times F}$$

Loading dose in mg/kg; C_p = plasma concentration in mg/L (or C_p desired − C_p current); S = fraction of drug which is active; F = fraction of drug which is bioavailable; multiply by weight for total dose in mg only; if S and F not specifically given, assume it to be 1.

For drugs with small volume of distribution, smaller loading dose required

E. CLEARANCE

= degree of efficiency a drug is removed from body over time

Because it is a first-order process, the amount of drug removed depends on the drug concentration

Clearance also depends on the infant's body weight, surface area, cardiac output, and renal and liver function as well as the protein binding of drug

Elimination rate constant (K_{el}) is the *fraction* of the drug eliminated over time and is represented by the slope of the log serum concentration decay curve

$$\text{Clearance} = \text{elimination rate constant} \times \text{volume of distribution}$$

$$\text{Thus, elimination rate constant } (K_{el}) = \frac{\text{Clearance of drug}}{\text{Volume of distribution}}$$

$$\text{Clearance also} = \frac{\text{Dose/interval}}{\text{Average steady-state concentration}}$$

F. STEADY-STATE

Defined as the equilibrium point at which the amount of drug administered equals the amount of drug that is excreted

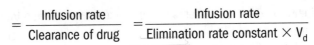

$$= \frac{\text{Infusion rate}}{\text{Clearance of drug}} = \frac{\text{Infusion rate}}{\text{Elimination rate constant} \times V_d}$$

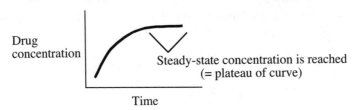

Drug concentration / Time

Steady-state concentration is reached (= plateau of curve)

G. HALF-LIFE (t 1/2)

Defined as the time required for the serum drug concentration to decrease by 1/2

$$\text{Elimination half-life } (t_{1/2}) = \frac{0.693}{K_{el}} = \frac{0.693}{\text{Clearance of drug}/V_d} = \frac{0.693 \times V_d}{\text{Clearance of drug}}$$

~Five half-lives needed to reach steady state

t 1/2	Amount of drug (%)
1	50.000
2	75.000
3	87.500
4	93.750
5	96.875

H. DRUG MONITORING

Serum level
Drug monitoring of serum levels is important for drugs with narrow therapeutic range, drugs with unpredictable dose/response relationship, drugs with severe toxic effects, and neonates with liver or renal disease
Should be drawn during the elimination phase (after distribution is completed) and when steady-state is reached (five half-lives)

Peak level
Dependent on the infusion rate (the longer the infusion rate, the lower the peak level)
Dependent on dosage of drug (if high peak level, decrease dose of drug)
Clinical peak of aminoglycosides is measured 30 minutes after the end of the infusion
Peak levels are not as useful for antibiotics that display time-dependent killing (e.g., vancomycin)

Trough level
Dependent on interval of drug (if high trough level, extend interval of drug)
Trough levels are most valuable in assessing toxicity risk
Clinical trough of aminoglycosides is measured 30 minutes before the administration of the next dose
For antibiotics with time-dependent killing (e.g., vancomycin), need to keep trough level at least 2 two times the minimum inhibitor concentration (MIC) for specific organism

Dosing interval
To minimize plasma fluctuations in drug levels, maintain dosing interval $\leq$ half-life

Therapeutic window
The range of plasma drug concentration with good therapeutic success and minimal toxicity
Warfarin and digoxin have narrow therapeutic indexes
Penicillin has a wide therapeutic index

III. Clinical Pharmacology

A. HUMAN TERATOGENS (see Maternal-Fetal Medicine chapter)

B. DRUGS AND LACTATION

Excretion of drugs into breast milk depends on the total amount of the drug, transport and metabolism of the drug, biochemical properties of the drug, size of the drug's rate of milk production, and composition of the milk

Drugs excreted into breast milk typically have low molecular weight, high lipid solubility, low protein binding, and decreased ionization

Examples of drugs contraindicated in nursing mothers are cyclosporine, lithium, methotrexate, phencyclidine, and radioactive agents

C. DRUGS THAT INTERFERE WITH FETAL AND NEONATAL OXIDATION OF VITAMIN K

Anticonvulsants (e.g., phenytoin and phenobarbital)

Antituberculosis medications (e.g., isoniazid and rifampin)

Other: warfarin and cephalosporins

D. DRUG EFFECTS ON BILIRUBIN LEVELS

Increase bilirubin levels by binding albumin and displacing unconjugated bilirubin from albumin:
Ceftriaxone
Sulfonamides
Indomethacin

Decrease bilirubin levels by increasing P_{450} metabolism and increasing the conjugation of bilirubin:
Phenobarbital
Rifampin

References

Beers MH, Berkow R, Burs M (eds): The Merck Manual of Diagnosis and Therapy (17th edition). Whitehouse Station, NJ, Merck Research Laboratories, 1999.

Benitz WE, Tatro DS. The Pediatric Drug Handbook. St. Louis, Mosby, 1995.

Bhat R. Neonatology Pharmacology I. Specialty Review in Neonatology/Perinatology. National Center for Advanced Medical Education, Chicago, IL, 1995.

Boroujerdi M. Pharmacokinetics: Principles and Applications. New York, McGraw-Hill, 2001.

Hatzopoulos FK. Neonatology Pharmacology II. Specialty Review in Neonatology/Perinatology. National Center for Advanced Medical Education, Chicago, 1995.

CHAPTER 16

Statistics

TOPICS COVERED IN THIS CHAPTER

I. Study Designs
- A. Cohort study
- B. Case-control study
- C. Interventional trial
- D. Cross-sectional survey

II. Data Types
- A. Nominal or categorical
- B. Ordinal
- C. Ranked
- D. Discrete
- E. Continuous

III. Measures of Central Tendency
- A. Mean
- B. Median
- C. Mode

IV. Measures of Dispersion
- A. Range
- B. Interquartile range
- C. Standard deviation
- D. Standard error of the mean

V. Measures of Disease Frequency
- A. Incidence
  1. Cumulative incidence
  2. Incidence rate
  3. Approximation of cumulative incidence with incidence rate
- B. Prevalence

VI. Measures of Association
- A. Risk ratio or relative risk (RR)
- B. Risk difference (RD) or attributable risk (AR)
- C. Odds ratio (OR)
- D. Attributable risk percent (AR%)
- E. Population attributable risk percent (PAR%)

- F. Number needed to treat (NNT)

VII. Screening
- A. Sensitivity
- B. Specificity
- C. Positive predictive value (PPV)
- D. Negative predictive value (NPV)
- E. False-negative
- F. False-positive

VIII. Hypothesis Testing
- A. Null hypothesis
- B. One-tail vs two-tail hypothesis
- C. P-value
- D. Confidence interval

IX. Parametric vs Non-parametric
- A. Parametric
- B. Non-parametric

X. Precision and Accuracy
- A. Precision
- B. Accuracy

XI. Types of Errors
- A. Type I or α error
- B. Type II or β error

XII. Power

XIII. Stratification vs Matching

XIV. Rates
- A. Prematurity rate
- B. Fetal mortality rate
- C. Perinatal mortality rate
- D. Neonatal mortality rate
- E. Postneonatal mortality rate
- F. Infant mortality rate
- G. Birth weight specific mortality rate

I. Study Designs

A. COHORT STUDY

Study groups characterized by exposure status to a specific risk factor (present [R+] or absent [R−]), and followed for the development of the outcome or disease of interest (present [D+] or absent [D−])

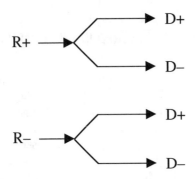

Can be prospective or retrospective
Prospective
    At initiation of study, all individuals in study group are free of the disease of interest
    Study group followed for a *period of time* and assessed for disease outcome
Retrospective
    Events, exposure, and outcome have already occurred when study is initiated
    However, still evaluate by identifying cohort based on risk status and then determine disease outcome (R → D)

Types
  1. Closed-cohort
    Fixed follow-up for all subjects
    Can calculate cumulative incidence, not incidence rate
  2. Open-cohort
    Can change exposure status
    Each individual contributes *person-time years* (the total time period each person contributed to the cohort; does not have to be contiguous as a person can enter and leave the cohort at different times)
    Can calculate incidence rate, not cumulative incidence

Strengths
  Ideal when exposure is rare
  Able to examine multiple effects of a single exposure
  Able to examine temporal relationships between exposure and disease
  If prospective:
    Minimizes bias in exposure ascertainment
    Decreases selection and information bias
  Allows calculation of *incidence* of disease in exposed versus non-exposed

Weaknesses
  Inefficient for studying rare diseases
  If prospective: expensive and time-consuming
  If retrospective: requires availability of medical records
  Potential for bias if follow-up is incomplete

B. CASE-CONTROL STUDY

Study groups defined by disease status

Comparison of risks between individuals with disease of interest (cases [D+]) and individuals without disease (controls [D−])

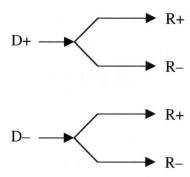

Controls should be free of disease but at *risk* for disease with the same exposure status

Strengths
  Inexpensive, quick
  Good for diseases with long latency periods
  Good for rare diseases
  Able to examine multiple etiologic factors for a single disease

Weaknesses
  Bias—recall, reporting, selection
  Inefficient for rare exposures
  Unable to calculate incidence rates
  Temporal relationships difficult to establish

C. INTERVENTIONAL TRIAL

"Gold-standard" of research studies

Ideally, the exposure should be randomly allocated
  Randomization—if properly done will equally allocate all variables (potential confounders) to the exposed and unexposed groups making them comparable; this is true for *known and unknown variables*

To ethically conduct a randomized trial, *equipoise* (*equal and sufficient arguments*) must exist between offering the exposure (treatment) and withholding the exposure (treatment)

Strengths—provides strong direct evidence between exposure or treatment and outcome of interest

Weaknesses—interventional trials are time-consuming and costly

D. CROSS-SECTIONAL SURVEY

Descriptive

Exposure and disease status are measured together at one point in time

Requires a large sample size

Provides information about disease *prevalence*

Often used as a first step for a cohort study

Unable to explore temporal relationships between exposure and outcome (will not be able to determine if exposure of interest preceded or followed outcome)

II. Data Types

A. NOMINAL OR CATEGORICAL

Arbitrarily assign numbers, code, or labels

Order and magnitude of the number not important

Dichotomous/binary (0,1) or categorical (≥ 2 categories)

e.g., 0 = male, 1 = female, race categories

B. ORDINAL

Order among categories important

Magnitude not important (difference between two ordered groups is not the same for another two)

e.g., grading of severity, Apgar scoring, intraventricular hemorrhage grading, neonatal intensive care unit level of care, retinopathy of prematurity staging

C. RANKED

Ordered by magnitude, then assigned number rank

Once assigned number rank, magnitude disregarded between items

e.g., ranked list of leading causes of death

D. DISCRETE

Integer or counts (no fractional or intermediate values)

Ordering and magnitude important

e.g., actual counts—number of accidents, number of kids

E. CONTINUOUS

Data represent measurable quantities

Fractional values possible

e.g., lab results such as aminophylline level; weight

III. Measures of Central Tendency

A. MEAN

$$= \frac{\text{sum of observations}}{\text{number of observations}}$$

Most frequent measure of central tendency

Extremely sensitive to outlying values

B. MEDIAN

Middle value of a set of measurements when sequentially ordered (lowest to highest or highest to lowest)

Robust, less sensitive to outlying data points

When data not symmetric, median best measure of central tendency

C. MODE

Observation that occurs most frequently

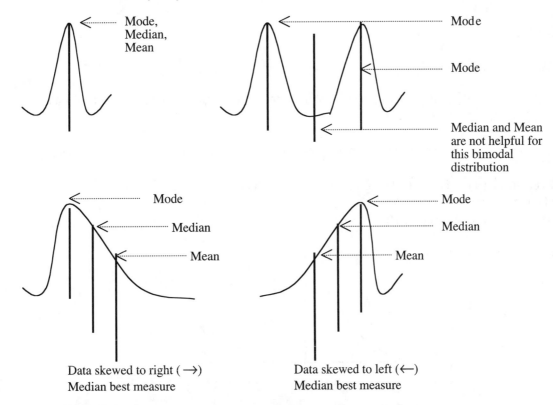

IV. Measures of Dispersion

A. RANGE

Largest number to the smallest number

Can be misrepresentative when extremes in the ends of the distribution exist (similar to mean)

B. INTERQUARTILE RANGE

Distance between the 25th and the 75th percentiles of the data

More representative of the data and less influenced by extreme values

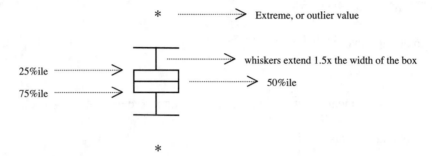

C. STANDARD DEVIATION (SD)

Amount of variability or spread about the mean of a sample

Standard deviation is also sensitive to large and small values

$$SD = \sqrt{var}$$

$$var = variance = \sum_{i=1}^{n} (X_i - \bar{X})^2 / n\text{-}1$$

If there is a large spread about the mean, the SD will be large, reflecting greater amount of variability among subjects (may be a result of small sample size)

Likewise, if there is a small spread about the mean, the SD will be small, reflecting more homogenous population

One SD from mean (μ) = 68.2% of the total sample or population (34.1% $\times$ 2)
Two SD from mean = 95.4% [(34.1% + 13.6%) $\times$ 2]
Three SD from mean = 99.8% [(34.1% + 13.6% + 2.2%) $\times$ 2]

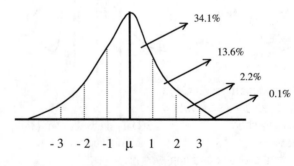

Standard Deviation

D. STANDARD ERROR OF THE MEAN (SEM)

Measure denoting the certainty with which the mean computed from a random sample estimates the true mean of the total population

There is less variability among the sample means than among the individual observations

As n increases, sampling variation decreases

If n is large enough, it will approximate the normal distribution = *"central limit theorem"*

$$\text{SEM} = \frac{\text{SD}}{\sqrt{n}}$$

V. Measures of Disease Frequency

A. INCIDENCE

= number of *new* cases of disease that develop in a population over a specified time interval

1. Cumulative incidence

$$= \frac{\text{number of new cases in a given time period}}{\text{total population at risk}}$$

=%, or a proportion
Provides an estimate of the probability (or risk) that an individual will develop a disease during a specified period of time
Value starts at 0 and increases with time
Does not account for varying time periods of exposure
Survival probability = 1−cumulative incidence

2. Incidence rate

$$= \frac{\text{number of new cases of disease in a given time period}}{\text{person-time years of observation}}$$

Denominator is the sum of each individual's time at risk, or sum of time that each person remained under observation and free from disease
Accounts for varying time periods of risk exposure
Value may go up or down with time
Rate, not a proportion

3. Approximation of cumulative incidence with incidence rate
Cumulative incidence will approximate incidence rate when:
    Period of observation is extremely short
    Prevalence of disease is low
    Duration of disease same among exposed and non-exposed

B. PREVALENCE

Proportion of individuals in a population with disease at a specific point in time

$$= \frac{\text{number of cases at a point of time}}{\text{total population at risk}} \times 100\%$$

= true-positives (TP) plus false-negatives (FN) divided by the sum of true positives (TP), false negatives (FN), false positives (FP) and true negatives (TN)

$$= \frac{TP + FN}{TP + FN + FP + TN} \quad (see\ section\ VII)$$

Also referred to as "point prevalence"
Proportion, not a rate

VI. Measures of Association

		Disease	
		+	−
Exposure +		a	b
−		c	d

A. RISK RATIO OR RELATIVE RISK (RR)

Estimates the magnitude of an association between exposure and disease and indicates the likelihood of developing the disease in the exposed group relative to the non-exposed group

$$RR = \frac{risk\ in\ exposed}{risk\ in\ non\text{-}exposed} = \frac{[a\ /\ (a+b)]}{[c\ /\ (c+d)]}$$

If RR 1.0, then no association between exposure and disease

If RR $>$ 1.0, then positive association, or increased risk of disease given exposure

If RR $<$ 1.0, then negative association, or decreased risk of disease given exposure

e.g., RR $=$1.4 indicates a 40% increased risk of disease if exposed

B. RISK DIFFERENCE (RD) OR ATTRIBUTABLE RISK (AR)

Measure of association that provides information about the absolute effect of the exposure or the excess risk of disease in those exposed compared with those non-exposed

$$= [a\ /\ (a+b)] - [c\ /\ (c+d)]$$

Value indicates the number of cases of the disease among the exposed that can be attributed to the exposure itself

Common public health impact measure

C. ODDS RATIO (OR)

Gives odds of disease in exposed over odds of disease in non-exposed (a ratio)
   e.g., OR of 1.3 indicates a 1.3 fold increase in odds of developing disease if exposed compared to those non-exposed

Measures strength of association

$$= \text{"cross product ratio"} = \frac{a \times d}{b \times c}$$

If rare disease, then OR is very close or approximates RR

OR is symmetric, RR is not

Often used with case-control studies

D. ATTRIBUTABLE RISK PERCENT (AR%)

The % of disease in the *exposed* population that is attributable to the exposure or can be eliminated if the exposure were eliminated

Defines the excess risk of disease in those *exposed* compared with those not exposed

$$= \frac{AR}{[a / (a+b)]} \times 100$$

E. POPULATION ATTRIBUTABLE RISK PERCENT (PAR%)

The % of disease in the total population that is attributable to the exposure, or can be eliminated if the exposure were eliminated

$$= AR\% \times Pe \text{ (proportion of exposed cases)}$$

$$= AR\% \times [a / (a+c)]$$

Meaningful measure only when the true ratio of exposed and unexposed individuals in source population is reflected in the study population

F. NUMBER NEEDED TO TREAT (NNT)

A way to measure the benefit of an intervention (a medical therapy)

$$= 1 / \text{(events in the control/non-exposed group} - \text{events in the treated/exposed group)}$$

If A = events in the control/non-exposed group = c/(c+d)

B = events in the treated/exposed group = a/(a+b)

Then, NNT = $\dfrac{1}{A - B}$

A value of 10 suggests that 10 patients need to be treated to avoid 1 death (or any other outcome studied)

VII. Screening

	Disease +	Disease −
Test +	a	b
Test −	c	d

a = true positives (TP)
b = false positives (FP)
c = false negatives (FN)
d = true negatives (TN)

A. SENSITIVITY

= % of true disease correctly identified by screening test

= probability of test being positive when true disease is present

$$= \frac{a}{a + c} = \frac{TP}{TP + FN}$$

B. SPECIFICITY

= % of population free of disease correctly identified as not having the disease by screening test

= probability of test negative when true disease is absent

$$= \frac{d}{b + d} = \frac{TN}{FP + TN}$$

C. POSITIVE PREDICTIVE VALUE (PPV)

= % of individuals who tested positive that do have true disease

= probability of having true disease when test is positive

$$= \frac{a}{a + b} = \frac{TP}{TP + FP}$$

Increased PPV with:
1. Increased prevalence
2. Increased specificity
3. To a lesser degree, increased sensitivity

D. NEGATIVE PREDICTIVE VALUE (NPV)

= % of individuals who tested negative that do *not* have true disease

= probability of not having true disease when test is negative

$$= \frac{d}{c + d} = \frac{TN}{FN + TN}$$

E. FALSE-NEGATIVE

= 1 − sensitivity

To decrease false-negative rate, increase sensitivity

F. FALSE-POSITIVE

= 1 − specificity

To decrease false-positive rate, increase specificity

VIII. Hypothesis Testing

A. NULL HYPOTHESIS

Hypothesis of no association between two variables

B. ONE-TAIL VS TWO-TAIL HYPOTHESIS

One-tail hypothesis: assess change in only one direction

Two-tail hypothesis: hypothesis can be utilized in either direction

C. P-VALUE

Probability of obtaining by chance a value as extreme as or more extreme than the observed value given that the null hypothesis is true

So, if p-value set at 0.05 → 5% probability that finding is due to chance alone

D. CONFIDENCE INTERVAL

A range of values that is intended to contain the parameter of interest with a certain degree of confidence (95% confidence, 99% confidence)

The larger the level of confidence, the larger the interval

As sample size increases, the width of the confidence interval decreases

When being applied for RR or OR estimates, if the interval crosses 1 (= no association), the association being tested is not considered statistically significant and the null hypothesis cannot be rejected

IX. Parametric and Non-Parametric Testing

A. PARAMETRIC

Assumes an underlying distribution to the data, a *normal distribution* or approximately so

Normal distribution:
When data points are plotted, the graph has an appearance of a "bell-shaped" curve (also known as a *Gaussian* distribution)

The mean and variance are not dependent on one another

Example parametric tests:
   Pearson's R (measure of correlation), t-test (comparison of means), chi-square (comparison of proportions)
   Data types: nominal, categorical, continuous

B. NON-PARAMETRIC

Makes no assumption about the underlying distribution of the data

Example non-parametric tests:
   Spearman's Rho (measure of correlation from ranked data), Mann-Whitney (non-parametric alternative to the independent t-test using ranked data), Wilcoxon test (non-parametric matched t-test alternative from ranked data)
   Data types: ordinal, continuous

Appropriate statistical test depending on data type and population sample					
	Unmatched		Matched		Correlation
Data Type	2 Groups of Different Individual	3+ Groups of Different Individuals	Before/After, Same Individuals	Multiple Treatments, Same Individuals	Association Between 2 Variables
Continuous, normal	Unpaired t-test	ANOVA	Paired t-test	Repeated ANOVA	Pearson's R (>2 variables, linear regression)
Categorical, or Nominal	Chi-square	Chi-square	McNemar's	Cochrane	Relative risk odds ratio (>2 variables, logistic)
(Small #)	(Fischer exact)	(Fischer exact)	(Sign test)		

Modified from Glanz, SA: Primer of Biostatistics (4th ed). New York, McGraw-Hill, 1997, inside cover.

X. Precision and Accuracy

A. PRECISION

Measurement that has nearly the same value each time it is assessed:
   Reproducible
   Consistent
   Reliable

Affected by:
   Random error
   Measuring technique of variables
   Observer bias
   Subject bias
   Instrument bias

Enhanced by:
   Increasing the size of the study
   Increasing efficiency with which the information is collected
   Standardization of measurement methods
   Trained observers
   Repetition
   Calibration

B. ACCURACY

Degree that a variable actually represents what it is supposed to represent:
Valid

Affected by:
Sensitivity
Specificity
Positive predictive value
Negative predictive value
Observer bias
Subject bias
Instrument bias

Enhanced by:
Calibration
Blinding

XI. Types of Errors

A. TYPE 1 OR α ERROR

Reject null hypothesis when the null hypothesis is true
i.e. a study shows a difference in outcome between two treatments when there is truly no difference

$=$ false-positive

Probability of committing this error is determined by the significance level of the test
If significance level is 0.05, then one will reject the null hypothesis even though it is true 5% of the time

B. TYPE 2 OR β ERROR

Do not reject the null hypothesis when the null hypothesis is false
i.e. study shows no difference in outcome between two treatments when there really is a difference

$=$ false-negative

Usually due to inadequate sample size
Also dependent on magnitude of difference between the two populations

XII. Power

Probability of rejecting the null hypothesis when the null hypothesis is false

$= 1 - $ type 2 error

To increase power:
1. Increase α value
2. Increase sample size
3. Increase the magnitude of difference between the two populations

XIII. Stratification vs. Matching

Stratification
  Separation of data by levels of a specific variable (e.g., age, marital status, race)
  One method to adjust for confounding
  Advantages: easily understood, flexible, can do after study is completed
  Disadvantages: limited number of variables that can be controlled simultaneously

Matching
  Pair subjects by variables which may represent potential confounders (pair by gestational age, weight)
  Advantages: eliminates confounding variables
  Disadvantages:
    Must do at beginning of study and thus requires early decisions
    Time-consuming
    Data always need to stay together, cannot evaluate matched variable as an independent factor

XIV. Rates

A. PREMATURITY RATE

$$\frac{\text{number of births} < 37 \text{ weeks gestational age}}{\text{total number of births}} \times 1000$$

B. FETAL MORTALITY RATE

$$\frac{\text{fetal deaths of} \geq 28 \text{ weeks gestation}}{\text{number of live births and fetal deaths of} \geq 28 \text{ weeks}} \times 1000$$

C. PERINATAL MORTALITY RATE

$$\frac{\text{fetal deaths of} \geq 28 \text{ weeks and infant deaths} < 7 \text{ days}}{\text{number of live births and number of fetal deaths of} \geq 28 \text{ weeks}} \times 1000$$

D. NEONATAL MORTALITY RATE

$$\frac{\text{number of neonatal deaths less than 28 days}}{\text{number of live births}} \times 1000$$

E. POSTNEONATAL MORTALITY RATE

$$\frac{\text{number of postneonatal deaths, 28 days to 1 year of age}}{\text{number of live births}} \times 1000$$

F. INFANT MORTALITY RATE

$$\frac{\text{number of infant deaths during the first year of life}}{\text{number of live births}} \times 1000$$

G. BIRTH WEIGHT SPECIFIC MORTALITY RATE

$$\frac{\text{number of deaths in a specific birth weight category}}{\text{number of births in same birth weight category}} \times 1000$$

1. Normal birth weight $= \geq 2500$ grams
2. Low birth weight (LBW) $= < 2500$ grams
3. Very low birth weight (VLBW) $= < 1500$ grams
4. Extremely low birth weight (ELBW) $= < 1000$ grams

References

Hennekens CH. and Buring, JE: Mayrent, SL(ed). Epidemiology in Medicine. Boston, Little, Brown and Company, 1987.

Hermansen, M: Biostatistics: Some Basic Concepts. Patterson, NJ, Caduceus Medical Publishers, Inc., 1990.

Norman, GR and Streiner DL: Biostatistics: The Bare Essentials (2nd ed). St.Louis, Mosby, 2000.

Pagano M and Gauvreau K: Principles of Biostatistics (2nd ed). Belmont, Duxbury Press, 2000.

Rothman KJ and Greenland S: Modern Epidemiology (2nd ed). Philadelphia, Lippincott-Raven Publishers, 1998.

Formulas

Airway resistance	$= \dfrac{\text{length} \times \text{viscosity}}{(\text{radius})^4}$
Altitude effect on paO_2 (arterial oxygen)	$= (p_{B\#1} - p_{H20}) \times FiO_{2\#1} = (p_{B\#2} - p_{H20}) \times FiO_{2\#2}$ $p_{B\#1}$ and $p_{B\#2}$ = barometric pressure in location 1 and 2 $FiO_{2\#1}$ and $FiO_{2\#2}$ = oxygen requirement in location 1 and 2 p_B at sea level = 760 mm Hg pH_2O = atmospheric pressure of water = 47 mm Hg
Alveolar–arterial gradient of oxygen	$= [FiO_2(p_B - p_{H20})] - (paCO_2/RQ) - (paO_2)$ p_B = barometric pressure p_{H20} = 47 $paCO_2$ = arterial content of CO_2 paO_2 = arterial content of O_2 RQ = respiratory quotient, usually 0.8 FiO_2 is in decimal form
Alveolar gas equation	$= [FiO_2(p_B - p_{H20})] - (paCO_2/RQ)$
Alveolar minute ventilation	$= (\text{tidal volume} - \text{dead space}) \times \text{respiratory rate}$
Anion gap	$= (Na) - (Cl + HCO_3)$
Cardiac output	$= \text{heart rate} \times \text{stroke volume}$ $= \dfrac{\text{systemic blood pressure}}{\text{total peripheral vascular resistance}}$
Cerebral blood flow	$= \dfrac{\text{cerebral perfusion pressure}}{\text{cerebral vascular resistance}}$
Cerebral perfusion pressure	$= \text{mean arterial pressure} - \text{intracranial pressure}$
Clearance of drug	$= \text{elimination rate constant} \times \text{volume of distribution}$
Compliance	$= \dfrac{\text{change in volume (cc)}}{\text{change in pressure (cm } H_2O)}$
Dead space, anatomic (Bohr equation)	$= \dfrac{(\text{end tidal } CO_2 - \text{expired } CO_2) \times (\text{tidal volume})}{\text{end tidal } CO_2}$
Elastance (inverse of compliance)	$= \dfrac{\text{change in pressure (cm } H_2O)}{\text{change in volume (cc)}}$
Elimination half-life ($t_{1/2}$)	$= \dfrac{0.693}{K_{el}} = \dfrac{0.693}{\text{clearance of drug}/V_d} = \dfrac{0.693 \times V_d}{\text{clearance of drug}}$ K_{el} = elimination rate constant V_d = volume of distribution
Elimination rate constant (K_{el})	$= \dfrac{\text{clearance of drug}}{\text{volume of distribution}}$
FENA or urinary fractional excretion of Na (%)	$= \dfrac{\text{urine Na concentration} \times \text{plasma creatinine concentration}}{\text{urine creatinine concentration} \times \text{plasma Na concentration}} \times 100$
Henderson-Hasselbalch equation	Hydrogen concentration $= \dfrac{(24 \times pCO_2)}{\text{bicarbonate concentration}}$
Laplace's law	Distending pressure $= \dfrac{2 \times \text{surface tension}}{\text{radius}}$
Loading dose (mg/kg)	$= \dfrac{\text{volume of distribution (L/kg)} \times C_p \text{ (mg/L)}}{S \times F}$

C_p = plasma concentration in mg/L (or C_p desired $-$ C_p current)
S = fraction of drug that is active
F = fraction of drug that is bioavailable
Multiply by weight for total dose in mg only
If S and F not specifically given, assume it to be 1

Mean airway pressure (MAP)	= K(PIP-PEEP) $\times$ I time (I time + E time) + PEEP K = constant PIP = peak inspiratory pressure PEEP = positive end expiratory pressure I time = inspiratory time and E time = expiratory time
Minute ventilation	= tidal volume $\times$ respiratory rate
Osmolality of serum	$2\,(Na) + \dfrac{\text{glucose (mg/dL)}}{18} + \dfrac{\text{BUN (mg/dL)}}{2.8}$
Oxygen carrying capacity = O_2 content of blood	= O_2 bound to Hb + dissolved O_2 O_2 bound to Hb = [(1.34 cc O_2/g Hb) $\times$ Hb (g/dL) $\times$ O_2 sat (decimal)] Dissolved O_2 = [(0.003 cc O_2/ dL torr) $\times$ paO_2 (torr)]
Oxygen consumption = Fick principle	= CO (dL/min) $\times$ (CaO2 $-$ CvO2) = CO $\times$ (1.34 cc/g Hb) (Hb concentration) (arterial sat–venous sat) CO = cardiac output CaO2 = oxygen content of arterial blood CvO2 = oxygen content of mixed venous blood Use decimal for sat (saturation)
Oxygen delivery (cc/kg/min)	To alveoli: (alveolar minute ventilation) $\times$ (FiO$_2$) To tissues: (O_2 carrying capacity)(cardiac output)(10)
Oxygen index (OI)	$= \dfrac{(\text{MAP} \times \text{FiO}_2)}{\text{postductal pa}O_2} \times 100$ MAP = mean airway pressure FiO$_2$ is in decimal form
Poiseuille's law for laminar flow	Flow = $\dfrac{\text{change in pressure} \times \pi \times (\text{radius})^4}{8\,(\text{length} \times \text{viscosity})}$
Power	= work (kg cm) $\times$ frequency (per minute)
Renal clearance (ml/min)	$= \dfrac{U \times V}{P}$ U = urinary concentration of solute (mg/dL) V = urinary volume divided by length of time collected (ml/min) P = plasma concentration of solute (mg/dL)
Resistance	$= \dfrac{\text{change in pressure (cm } H_2O)}{\text{change in flow (L/sec)}}$
Saturation level for cyanosis	= % oxygen saturation $= \dfrac{HbO_2}{\text{total Hb = reduced Hb + Hb } O_2}$
Shunt equation	$= \dfrac{\text{content pulmonary cap } O_2 - \text{content pulm art } O_2}{\text{content pulm cap } O_2 - \text{content pulm mixed venous } O_2}$ cap = capillary; pulm=pulmonary
Steady state concentration	$= \dfrac{\text{infusion rate}}{\text{clearance of drug}} = \dfrac{\text{infusion rate}}{V_d \times \text{elimination rate constant}}$ V_d = volume of distribution
Stroke work	Mean arterial pressure $\times$ stroke volume
Time constant	Resistance (cm H_2O/cc/sec) $\times$ compliance (cc/cm H_2O)
Volume of distribution (L/kg)	$= \dfrac{\text{total amount of drug in body (mg)}}{\text{plasma concentration of drug (mg/L)} \times \text{weight (kg)}}$
Work of breathing	= Pressure (or force) $\times$ volume (or displacement)

INDEX

Page numbers in **boldface type** indicate complete chapters.

Intelligence quotient (IQ), in mental deficiency, 154
Interferon-alpha, 213
Interleukin-1, 213
Interquartile range, 390
Interventional trials, 387
Intracranial pressure, increased, 134
Intrauterine growth restriction, 23–25
  lupus-related, 9
  symmetric *vs.* asymmetric, 24
Introns, 158
Inversions, chromosomal, 162
Iodide-containing contrast media, 280
Iron, 251
  breast milk, cow's milk, and colostrum content of, 253
Iron deficiency anemia, 251, 287
Ischemia, cerebral, 139–140
Isochromosomes, 162
Isoimmunization, 289–290
Isoleucine, 247
Isoleucine disorders, 332–333
Isomil, 253, 254
Isoniazid, 190, 191
Isoproterenol, 117
Isotretinoin, teratogenicity of, 38, 39
Isovolumic contraction, 90
Isovolumic relaxation, 90

J
Jatene (arterial switch) procedure, 119
Jaundice
  breast feeding, 302
  nonphysiologic or pathologic, 302
  physiologic, 301–302
Jejunum, atresia of, 267
Jeune syndrome, 239
Job's syndrome, 213
Junctional ectopic tachycardia, 111

K
Keratinization, abnormal, 364
Keratinocytes, overgrowth of, 363
Keratosis pilaris, 366
Ketones, urinary, 351
Kidney. *See also* Renal disease
  agenesis of, 234, 235
  blood flow in, 229
  congenital anomalies of, 234–238
    ultrasound detection of, 16
  ectopic, 238
  function of, 229
    evaluation of, 231–234
    glomerular and tubular, 230–231

Kidney (*Cont.*)
  hormonal control of, 231
  renal acid-base regulation, 224
  horseshoe, 234, 238
  morphogenesis of, 228–229
    abnormalities of, 234–239
  pelvic, 234
Klebsiella infections, 192
  antibiotic therapy for, 210
Kleihauer-Betke test, 286
Klinefelter syndrome, 176, 315
  advanced maternal age as risk factor for, 165
Klippel-Feil syndrome, 178
  cardiac defects associated with, 119
Klippel-Trenaunay Weber syndrome, 178
Klumpke's palsy, 144
Krabbe disease, 344

L
Labor, 29–30
Lactalbumin, breast milk and cow's milk content of, 253
Lactase, intestinal, 262
  absorption of, 260
Lactation, physiology of, 251
Lactobacilli, breast milk-enhanced growth of, 251
Lactoferrin, 209
Lactoperidoxalase, 209
Lactose, 248–249
  breast milk content of, 252
Laminar flow, 56
Laplace's law, 50, 401
Large intestine
  digestion and absorption function of, 262
  ultrasound visualization of, 279
Laryngomalacia, 77
Learning disability, 155
Lecithin/sphingomyelin ratio, 49
Left bundle branch block, 112
Left ventricular hypertrophy, EKG findings in, 110
Leiner syndrome, 367
Lens, dislocation of, 372
Leptomeningeal inflammation, 136
Leucine, 247
Leucine disorders, 332–333, 338
Leukemia, congenital, 299
Leukocoria, 370–371
Leukocytosis, pregnancy-related, 3
Leukodytrophy, metachromatic, 344
Leukomalacia, periventricular, 140–141

Leukotrienes, 212
Limb anomalies
  hypertrophic, 180
  ultrasound detection of, 15
Linkage studies, 160
Linoleic acid, 248
  deficiency of, cutaneous manifestations of, 368
  parenteral nutrition content of, 255
Linolenic acid, 248
Lipases
  breast milk content of, 252
  gastric, 261
  intestinal, 262
  lingual, 261
Lipidoses, 343–344
Lipids, parenteral nutrition content of, 254
Lipogenesis, 248
Lipoma, 124
Lissencephalopathy, 124, 136
Listeria infections, 186
  antibiotic therapy for, 210
Lithium
  as congenital heart disease cause, 120
  as contraindication to breast feeding, 253, 383
  teratogenicity of, 39
Liver
  digestion and absorption function of, 261
  hematopoiesis in, 282
Loading dose, 381, 401
Lockjaw, 208
Locus, of genes, 159
Long chain 3-hydroxyacyl-CoA deficiency, 341–342
Lower motor neuron disorders, 145–148
Lowe syndrome, 236
Lung
  congenital malformations of, 78–81
  morphologic development of, 45–46
  perfusion of, 53–55
  ventilation of, 53
  volume-pressure curves of, 58–59
Lung capacity, in hyaline membrane disease, 57
Lung disease, chronic, 73–74
  water balance in, 220
Lung fluid, fetal, 46–47
Lung maturity testing, fetal, 49
Lung tissue resistance, 56
Lung volume, in hyaline membrane disease, 57

Myasthenia gravis (*Cont.*)
congenital neonatal, 145, 147
maternal, fetal effects of, 9–10
Mycobacterium tuberculosis, 190–191
Mycoplasma hominis, 206
Mycoplasma infections, antibiotic therapy for, 210
Myelination, 124
disorders of, 124
Myelocystocele, 124
Myelomeningocele, 124, 125–126
Myelopathy, hypoxic-ischemic, 145
Myeloschisis, 124
Myoglobinuria, 234
Myopathy, congenital or myotubular, 146
Myotonic dystrophy, congenital, 146, 147–148
prenatal diagnosis of, 160
Myxoma, cardiac, 105

N
Nails, abnormalities of, 362–363
Natriuretic agents, 221
Necrosis
cortical, 240
medullary, 240
selective neuronal, 139
subcutaneous fat, 367
Necrotizing enterocolitis, 275–276
radiographic features of, 279
Negative predictive value (NPV), 394
Neisseria gonorrhoeae infections, 189, 209
Neocate, 254
Neonatal mortality rate, 398
Neosure, 253, 254
Nephrocalcinosis, 241
Nephrogenesis, 228–229
Nephropathy, sodium ion-losing, 220
Nephrotic syndrome, congenital, 234–235
Nerve injuries, at birth, 144–145
Nervous system, development of, 124
Netherton's disease, 365
Neural proliferation, 124
Neural tube defects
in utero surgical treatment of, 41
as mental deficiency cause, 153
recurrence risk of, 165
Neuroblastoma, 299
Neurocutaneous syndromes, 151–152
Neurofibromatosis, 129, 151, 361
Neurological anomalies, ultrasound detection of, 15–16
Neurological studies, 133–135
Neuromuscular disorders, 145–148

Neuromuscular disorders (*Cont.*)
with hypotonia and weakness, 148
of lower motor neurons, 145–148
Neuronal migration, 124
Neuropathy
chronic renal failure-related, 243
congenital hypomyelinating, 145
congenital motor and sensory, 145
Neurulation, 124
Neutropenia, 214
Escherichia coli-related, 192
Neutrophilia, 214
Neutrophils, 212
Nevi
epidermal, 363
melanocytic 364
Nevus sebaceus, 363
Niacin deficiency, cutaneous manifestations of, 368
Niemann-Pick disease, 343
Nikolsky sign, in staphylococcal skin syndrome, 358
Nitric oxide (NO), 70–71
p-Nitroaniline urine test, 351
Nitroprusside, 117
Nitroprusside urine test, 351
Nominal data, 388
Non-parametric testing, 396
Nonstress test (NST), 18
Noonan syndrome, 171–172, 179, 298
cardiac defects associated with, 120
Norepinephrine, 117
Northern blot analysis, 159
Norwood procedure, 119
Nosocomial infections, parenteral nutrition-related, 256
Null hypothesis, 395
false, 397–398
Number needed to treat (NNT), 383
Nutramigen, 254
Nutrient deficiencies, cutaneous manifestations of, 368
Nutrition, **245–257**
Nystatin, 205

O
Oculocerebrorenal syndrome, 236
Odds ratio, 393
Oleic acid, 248
Oligohydramnios, 22, 239
Omega-3 fatty acids, 248
Omega-6 fatty acids, 248
Omphacele, 273–275
differentiated from gastroschisis, 275

Omphalitis, 183–184
Oncology, 299–300. *See also* specific types of cancer
One-tail *vs.* two-tail hypothesis, 395
Ophthalmia, 375–376
Ophthalmology, **369–376**
abnormalities of the eye, 371–372
conditions associated with eye abnormalities, 375–376
development of the eye, 370
disorders of the eye, 372–375
reflexes of the eye, 370–371
Ordinal data, 388
Ornithine carbamyl transferase deficiency, 332
Osmolality, of serum, 402
Osteodystrophy, renal, 243
Osteogenesis imperfecta, 172
advanced paternal age as risk factor for, 165
Osteomyelitis, 183
Osteopenia, of prematurity, 324–325
Otitis media, respiratory syncytial virus-related, 194
Oxygen carrying capacity, 63, 402
Oxygen consumption, 63
Oxygen delivery, 62, 402
Oxygen index, 67, 402
Oxygen physiology, 61–64
Oxygen transfer, 64
Oxyhemoglobin dissociation curve, 62
Oxytocin, 251

P
Pachygyria, 124
Pacing reflex, 133
Palmar grasp, 132
Palmitic acid, 248
breast milk content of, 252
Palpebral fissures, abnormal slanting of, 371
Pancreas, digestion and absorption function of, 261
Pancreatic insufficiency, 272
Panhypopituitarism, 320
PaO$_2$ (partial pressure of oxygen in arterial blood), effect of altitude on, 61, 401
Parametric testing, 395–396
Parasagittal cerebral injury, 139
Parathyroid hormone, pregnancy-related increase in, 4
Parenteral nutrition, 254–256
complications of, 255–256